D1596775

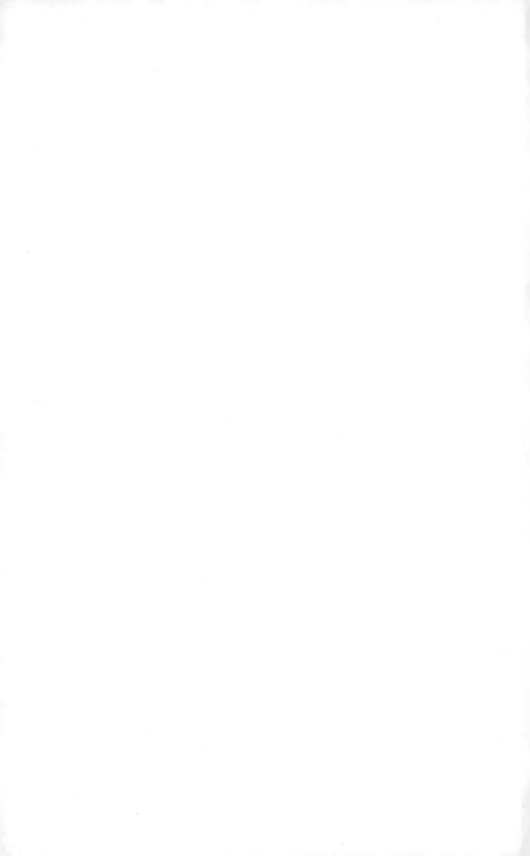

Coronary Thrombolysis in Perspective

FUNDAMENTAL AND CLINICAL CARDIOLOGY

Editor-in-Chief
Samuel Z. Goldhaber, M.D.
*Harvard Medical School
and Brigham and Women's Hospital
Boston, Massachusetts*

Associate Editor, Europe
Henri Bounameaux, M.D.
*University Hospital of Geneva
Geneva, Switzerland*

Additional Volumes in Preparation

Coronary Thrombolysis in Perspective

Principles Underlying Conjunctive and Adjunctive Therapy

Edited by

Burton E. Sobel

*Washington University School of Medicine and
Barnes Hospital
St. Louis, Missouri*

Désiré Collen

*University of Leuven
Leuven, Belgium*

Marcel Dekker, Inc.   New York • Basel • Hong Kong

Library of Congress Cataloging-in-Publication Data

Coronary thrombolysis in perspective : principles underlying
  conjunctive and adjunctive therapy / edited by Burton E. Sobel,
  Désiré Collen.
        p.   cm -- (Fundamental and clinical cardiology ; 16)
     Includes bibliographical references and index.
     ISBN 0-8247-9154-1 (alk. paper)
     1. Thrombolytic therapy. 2. Myocardial infarction--Chemotherapy.
  3. Myocardial infarction--Adjuvant treatment.   I. Sobel, Burton E.
  II. Collen, D. (Désiré) III. Series.
     [DNLM: 1. Thrombolytic Therapy. 2. Coronary Disease--drug
  therapy. 3. Fibrinolytic Agents--therapeutic use.   W1 FU538TD v.16
  1993 . WG 300 C825655 1993]
  RC685.I6C696 1993
  616.1'23061--dc20
  DNLM/DLC
  for Library of Congress   93-23997
                                                                       CIP

The publisher offers discounts on this book when ordered in bulk quantities.
For more information, write to Special Sales/Professional Marketing at the
address below.

This book is printed on acid-free paper.

MARCEL DEKKER, INC.
270 Madison Avenue, New York, New York 10016

Current printing (làst digit):
10 9 8 7 6 5 4 3 2 1

PRINTED IN THE UNITED STATES OF AMERICA

Series Introduction

Marcel Dekker, Inc., has focused on the development of various series of beautifully produced books in different branches of medicine. These series have facilitated the integration of rapidly advancing information for both the clinical specialist and the researcher.

My goal as editor of the Fundamental and Clinical Cardiology series is to assemble the talents of world-renowned authorities to dicuss virtually every area of cardiovascular medicine. In the current monograph, Burton E. Sobel and Désiré Collen have edited a much needed and timely book. Future contributions to this series will include books on molecular biology, interventional cardiology, and clinical management of such problems as coronary artery disease and ventricular arrhythmias.

Samuel Z. Goldhaber

Preface

Coronary thrombolysis has rapidly become the initial treatment of acute myocardial infarction caused by thrombotic occlusion of culprit coronary arteries. Its emergence has been propelled by DeWood's pivotal angiographic studies demonstrating the frequent presence of intracoronary thrombi very early after the apparent onset of infarction, by advances in coronary arteriography that have made feasible the acquisition of definitive end points of therapeutic efficacy, and by the development of diverse fibrinolytic agents, some of which exhibit considerable fibrin selectivity. Recently, the extent to which initially rapid recanalization and maintenance of patency require interdiction of competing processes such as coagulation has become a focus of research. Because of the seminal importance of anticoagulation and inhibition of activation of platelets for optimal thrombolysis, such measures, which we consider conjunctive therapy, have changed the face of coronary thrombolysis. What has previously been conceptualized as monotherapy is now recognized to require conjunctive treatment as well.

Progress in the care of patients with acute myocardial infarction has reflected the importance of another therapeutic principle as well—namely, the retardation or inhibition of myocardial injury associated with ischemia, reperfusion, or both. Measures to protect jeopardized ischemic and reperfused myocardium constitute adjunctive therapy, which is designed to attenuate and limit the extent of irreversible myocardial injury.

The importance of conjunctive therapy is evident from several considerations. In more than 90% of instances, coronary thrombosis occurs in the immediate vicinity of a complex atherosclerotic plaque undergoing rupture, fissuring, and intramural hemorrhage. These processes are most often accelerated in lipid-laden plaques rather than in mature lesions with fibrous caps, regardless of the extent to which the lipid-laden lesions themselves limit flow in an epicardial coronary artery. All of the activators of the fibrinolytic system used clinically induce conversion of plasminogen to plasmin and consequent lysis of fibrin within clots. It has been recognized, however, that all the agents available and used intravenously in clinically effective doses paradoxically induce sufficient plasminemia to activate the coagulation system. Thus, plasmin-mediated conversion of prothrombin to thrombin, activation of other procoagulants including factor V and factor X, and consequent augmentation of thrombin activity can retard clot lysis, predispose to reocclusion, or both.

Interest in adjunctive therapy is intense as well. Although the mechanisms underlying myocardial stunning have not yet been elucidated definitively, it appears that early reperfusion can compromise the integrity of jeopardized ischemic myocardium, despite producing overall benefit. Diverse agents, including calcium channel blockers, scavengers of oxygen-centered free radicals and inhibitors of their generation, β-adrenergic blocking agents, inhibitors of inflammation, and agents designed to sustain microcirculatory function, are being explored in the search for improved myocardial protection.

Conjunctive and adjunctive therapy are the focus of this monograph. Contributors are internationally respected authorities who have acquired pivotal information in each of their areas of expertise and who have provided information for investigators and clinicians who seek to maximize the efficacy of coronary thrombolysis. Several chapters address the history of coronary thrombolysis, the evolution of the use of specific activators of plasminogen, the nature of atherosclerotic lesions underlying acute coronary thrombosis, and the objectives of therapy with respect to early and late induction of coronary patency. The clinical importance of time to treatment and the paradoxical procoagulant effects of fibrinolytic agents are the focus of subsequent chapters. Other chapters consider the interactions between fibrinolytic agents and platelets and the importance of activation of coagulation pathways with respect to early, thrombotic reocclusion. Several chapters address specific strengths and limitations of specific anticoagulation regimens; interpretation of results with end points such as ventricular function, coronary patency, and mortality; and the relative value of diverse conjunctive measures in defined clinical settings. The importance of adjunctive therapy is considered in chapters focusing on reperfusion injury, therapeutic regimens designed to protect ischemic myocardium, and interpretation of results of mechanistic and large-scale multicenter clinical trials.

Our objectives in developing this monograph are (1) to provide critical review of the major advances in coronary thrombolysis that have done so much to enhance its efficacy, (2) to provide practical information needed to minimize untoward effects and maximize prompt and sustained induction of patency in thrombotically occluded coronary arteries, (3) to highlight areas of rapidly evolving investigation elucidating fundamental mechanisms that can compromise coronary thrombolysis, and (4) to provide the information needed for prompt and effective implementation of conjunctive and adjunctive measures so necessary when coronary thrombolysis is employed clinically.

Burton E. Sobel
Désiré Collen

Contents

Contributors

Dana R. Abendschein, Ph.D. Research Associate Professor of Medicine, Cell Biology, and Physiology, Cardiovascular Division, Department of Internal Medicine, Washington University School of Medicine, St. Louis, Missouri

Steven R. Bergmann, M.D., Ph.D. Associate Professor of Medicine, Cardiovascular Division, Department of Internal Medicine, Washington University School of Medicine, St. Louis, Missouri

Stanley D. Bleich, M.D. Assistant Clinical Professor of Medicine, Cardiovascular Specialists Research Group, Tulane University School of Medicine, Metairie, Louisiana

Désiré Collen, M.D., Ph.D. Professor of Medicine, Center for Molecular and Vascular Biology, University of Leuven, Leuven, Belgium

David de Bono, M.D., F.R.C.P. Professor, Department of Cardiology, University of Leicester and Glenfield General Hospital, Leicester, United Kingdom

Paul R. Eisenberg, M.D., M.P.H. Associate Professor of Medicine, and Director, Cardiac Care Unit, Cardiovascular Division, Department of Internal Medicine, Washington University School of Medicine, St. Louis, Missouri

Erling Falk, M.D., Ph.D. Visiting Associate Professor of Medicine, Harvard Medical School and Massachusetts General Hospital, Boston, Massachusetts

Jack Hirsh, M.D. Director, Hamilton Civic Hospitals Research Centre, and Professor, Department of Medicine, McMaster University, Hamilton, Ontario, Canada

Ik-Kyung Jang, M.D., Ph.D. Assistant Professor of Medicine, Harvard Medical School and Massachusetts General Hospital, Boston, Massachusetts

Karl-Ludwig Neuhaus, M.D. Professor of Medicine and Chief of Medical Clinic II, Kassel, Germany

Edward F. Plow, Ph.D. Head of Research, Center for Thrombosis and Vascular Biology, The Cleveland Clinic Foundation, Cleveland, Ohio

Burton E. Sobel, M.D. Lewin Professor of Medicine and Head, Cardiovascular Division and Center for Cardiovascular Research, Washington University School of Medicine, and Cardiologist-in-Chief, Barnes Hospital, St. Louis, Missouri

Alan J. Tiefenbrunn, M.D., F.A.C.C. Associate Professor of Medicine, Cardiovascular Division, Washington University School of Medicine, St. Louis, Missouri

Frans Van de Werf, M.D. Professor of Medicine and Head of Clinic, Division of Cardiology, University of Leuven and University Hospital Gasthuisberg, Leuven, Belgium

Jean-Louis J. Vanoverschelde, M.D. Research Fellow, Cardiovascular Division, Washington University School of Medicine, St. Louis, Missouri

Marc Verstraete, M.D., Ph.D., F.R.C.P. (Edin), F.A.C.P. (Hon) Professor of Medicine, Center for Molecular and Vascular Biology, University of Leuven, Leuven, Belgium

Uwe Zeymer, M.D. Medical Clinic II, Kassel, Germany

1

Coronary Thrombolysis
Background and Factors Underlying Its Emergence

Burton E. Sobel
Washington University School of Medicine and Barnes Hospital
St. Louis, Missouri

I. INTRODUCTION

In 1789 when Morgagni recognized that cadaver blood remained fluid (i.e., uncoagulated), the conceptual framework for fibrinolysis was initiated. A century later, in 1889, Denys and Zimmerman recognized that human blood contained fibrinolytic activity that could result in lysis of fibrin over intervals of 12–24 hours. In fact, because it was believed historically that blood was rich in the fibrinolytic moiety, some had thought that it might be suitable for transfusion.

Denys and coworkers identified a thermolabile proteolytic substance in serum that was extractable with chloroform and exhibited fibrinolytic properties. Their observations led ultimately to the recognition by Tillet and Garner in 1933 that extracts from hemolytic streptococci could induce fibrinolysis of human plasma clots as well. The active substance, eventually named streptokinase, was activating what we now know is a zymogen in blood, plasminogen, by forming proteolytic complexes (SK–plasminogen complexes and their derivatives) with fibrinolytic activity. Ironically from today's perspective, strep-tokinase is a misnomer. In contrast to other activators of plas-minogen, the protein is not an enzyme, let alone a kinase (i.e., a phosphorylating enzyme).

In 1941, Millstone and coworkers showed that streptoki-nase required a cofactor found in euglobulin fractions of hu-man blood for fibrinolytic activity, an observation that led to the demonstration a few years later by Christensen and Kaplan that the zymogen, plasminogen, was converted to plasmin by the streptokinase–plasminogen proteolytic complex. The "ac-tivated" plasminogen, which was in fact plasmin, was soon shown to be an enzyme with properties similar to those of trypsin and recognized to be the active proteolytic enzyme re-sponsible for degradation of fibrin and the lysis of clots.

II. ORIGINS OF THE MODERN CONSTRUCT

Over time, inhibitors of plasmin such as α_2-antiplasmin were identified. Of particular importance, a theoretical construct was developed, largely by Sherry and coworkers, that attrib-uted fibrinolytic activity in human blood to the conversion of clot-associated plasminogen to plasmin by endogenous or exogenous plasminogen activators (e.g., streptokinase, uroki-nase, or tissue-type plasminogen activator [t-PA]) with conse-quent dissolution of fibrin and clots.

In the late 1940s, these workers demonstrated that intra-pleural administration of streptokinase could liquify loculated empyema. Soon thereafter, in 1958, they sought to determine whether treatment of patients with acute myocardial infarction was feasible by lysis of putative coronary thrombi.

At this point in the evolution of the field, fibrinolysis of intravascular thrombi was known to depend upon activation of plasminogen. Sherry and coworkers were among the first to appreciate the importance of clot selectivity, namely, the tar-geting of fibrinolysis to the plasminogen associated with fibrin in the domain of thrombi as opposed to free plasminogen cir-culating in the blood stream.

However, at this time the paradigm according to which clinicians conceptualized acute myocardial infarction was very different from the one appreciated today. Despite Herrick's pivotal observations in 1912, it was not yet generally accepted that myocardial infarction was frequently a manifestation of acute thrombotic coronary arterial occlusion. In fact, many believed that coronary thrombosis was an epiphenomenon reflecting and resulting from rather than underlying impaired coronary flow. Accordingly, initial attempts to treat myocardial infarction with fibrinolytic agents were largely disregarded despite some favorable reports from subsequent large-scale multicenter trials demonstrating apparent benefit.

During the next 10 years, much of the research in ischemic heart disease was dominated by the concept that preservation of jeopardized, ischemic myocardium could be best accomplished through reduction of myocardial oxygen demands. Several studies had demonstrated that increased oxygen requirements exacerbated the severity of infarction in hearts of experimental animals and patients and that reduction of myocardial oxygen requirements could exert salutary effects. It soon became clear that the most effective means of ameliorating the imbalance between myocardial oxygen requirements and oxygen delivery was potentiation of perfusion. Furthermore, DeWood and coworkers soon showed that acute transmural myocardial infarction in patients was virtually invariably associated with complete thrombotic coronary occlusion as judged from angiograms acquired early in its course.

The therapeutic potential of coronary thrombolysis was soon appreciated. Salient features underlying its enthusiastic acceptance included the availability of definitive end points of efficacy including angiography performed in critically ill patients spurred by pioneering investigators such as Maseri and colleagues, who were studying coronary vasospasm as a cause of acute coronary syndromes. The dissolution of clots occluding coronary arteries was readily demonstrable angiographically, and the causative role of such thrombi in the initiation of acute myocardial infarction soon appeared to be unequivocal.

When angiographically documented restoration of patency of infarct-related thrombotically occluded coronary arteries was accompanied by prompt resolution of the chest pain associated with infarction and hemodynamic stability in pioneering studies by Chazov and by Rentrop, it was difficult to deny that coronary thrombolysis was a potentially powerful therapeutic intervention.

Simultaneously, much progress was being made in the elucidation of the nature of acute myocardial infarction itself. Recognition that the phenomenon was a dynamic one in which the ultimate outcome was determined by the overall mass of myocardium undergoing irreversible injury grew based on results of studies in laboratory animals and in patients. The protective effects of diverse interventions, each of which improved the balance between myocardial oxygen requirements and myocardial oxygen supply, lent credence to the notion that the extent of injury sustained was modifiable and that its magnitude was the prime determinant of the ultimate extent of ventricular dysfunction and mortality. Unfortunately, however, interventions that proved to be promising in studies of laboratory animals in which myocardial oxygen requirements could be reduced immediately before or after the onset of experimentally induced myocardial infarction were not fulfilled in clinical studies, perhaps because myocardial oxygen requirements could not be reduced as completely or promptly after the onset of ischemic injury in patients as in animals or at a time when myocytes would still be amenable to salvage.

III. EVOLUTION OF CORONARY THROMBOLYSIS

The convergence of these diverse threads of investigation demonstrating that thrombosis was the proximate cause of acute myocardial infarction, that the balance between myocardial oxygen demand and oxygen supply determined the extent of myocardial injury and the ultimate fate of the heart and the organism, and that restitution of coronary artery patency early after the onset of thrombotic occlusion could confer salutary effects set the stage for acceptance of coronary thrombolysis as primary therapy. Availability of angiographic end points in critically ill patients made it possible to determine the extent to which induction of fibrinolysis restored coronary artery patency and the extent to which recanalization was accompanied by clinical benefit including improved survival. Surprisingly, however, the importance of prompt and sustained recanalization was often rejected by skeptics despite its being the only credible means by which coronary thrombolysis confers benefit.

In the past 10 years, one other factor has contributed dramatically to the evolution of coronary thrombolysis as primary treatment for acute myocardial infarction, namely, the development of so-called fibrin-selective activators of the fibrinolytic system (see Chapter 2). It had been known for many years that the fibrinolytic system functioned endogenously in a highly targeted fashion. The presence of an intravascular thrombus elicits the elaboration from adjacent endothelium of proteins capable of activating (converting) fibrin-bound plasminogen to fibrin-bound plasmin. Such proteins, generally called tissue-type plasminogen activators (t-PAs), can induce fibrinolysis without inducing plasminemia. Accordingly, the proteolytic phenomena unleashed physiologically are highly specific and focused on the offending thrombi.

In the early 1980s, we and others sought to determine whether proteins of this type (t-PAs) would have favorable therapeutic properties for use in lysing occlusive coronary thrombi. We found that human t-PA harvested from supernatant fractions of conditioned media of melanoma cell cultures could elicit clot lysis in coronary arteries of laboratory animals promptly and without perturbation of hemostasis or induction of plasminemia comparable to that seen with nonselective agents. We found subsequently that similar effects were inducible in patients with evolving myocardial infarction with consequent restoration of patency of infarct-related coronary arteries in the absence of hemostatic breakdown. In six of the first seven patients with total thrombotic coronary occlusions in whom parenterally administered human t-PA was administered, reperfusion was elicited within 19–57 minutes without appreciable fibrinogenolysis.

Soon thereafter many studies were performed with t-PA produced by recombinant DNA technology. The results were remarkably similar, with frequent and prompt induction of coronary patency within 60–90 minutes (approximately 75–80% of infarct-related arteries being rendered patent) without depletion of fibrinogen or manifestations of the systemic lytic state seen with first-generation, non–fibrin-selective agents.

In concert, observations in laboratory animals in which thrombotic coronary occlusion was relieved with fibrinolytic agents, in patients with acute myocardial infarction associated with thrombotic occlusion of infarct-related arteries, and ultimately in large-scale clinical studies in which acute myocardial infarction was treated by administration of clot-selective fibrinolytic agents validated the hypothesis that prompt recanalization of thrombotically occluded coronary arteries with prompt intravenous administration of fibrinolytic agents was a practical means for salvaging jeopardized ischemic myocardium and improving outcome early after the onset of infarction. The net result of treatment predicated on this hypothesis has been a substantial reduction in mortality associated with acute myocardial infarction, from an overall early mortality of approximately 10% in patients hospitalized in coronary care units in the prethrombolytic era to as low as 5% presently in patients 75 years of age or less treated with clot-selective fibrinolytic agents such as t-PA.

The efficacy of this approach in reducing mortality, preserving jeopardized ischemic myocardium and consequently left ventricular pump function, avoiding late ventricular arrhythmia, and improving the quality of life by preventing congestive heart failure and other derangements depends, however, not only on the rapidity and frequency with which infarct-related thrombotically occluded arteries can be recanalized but also on the extent to which recanalization can be sustained. Unfortunately, many studies of thrombolytic agents have failed to evaluate or assess the efficacy of the intervention with respect to the induction of sustained rather than simply transitory recanalization. Accordingly, results and conclusions may have been unnecessarily ambiguous. It is clear that early recanalization can salvage jeopardized ischemic myocardium. It is clear also that salvage of jeopardized ischemic myocardium can preserve ventricular function and reduce mortality after acute myocardial infarction. The linkage between restoration of perfusion and clinical benefit has sometimes been obfuscated in studies in which early reperfusion is likely to have been compromised because of omission of measures necessary to consolidate the gains of initial recanalization. One objective of this monograph is to provide information pertinent to interpretation of the results of diverse studies in which thrombolytic agents have been assessed under circumstances in which sustained reperfusion was either vigorously pursued or neglected.

Fibrinolysis is not monotherapy. Its ultimate benefits depend, at least in part, on the extent to which recanalization is sustained by concomitant measures including vigorous anticoagulation, amelioration of the thrombogenicity of the underlying atheromatous plaque giving rise to the thrombus initiating the index infarct, sufficient recanalization of still compromised vessels by subsequent angioplasty, atherectomy, or surgery, and regression of atherosclerosis. Coronary thrombolysis clearly can "buy time," salvage jeopardized ischemic myocardium, and provide a substrate for improved prognosis. Coupled with appropriate conjunctive measures designed to accelerate and sustain recanalization, it is a powerful therapeutic advance.

PERTINENT REFERENCES

Bergmann S R, Fox K A A, Ter-Pogossian M M, Sobel B E, Collen D: Clot-selective coronary thrombolysis with tissue-type plasminogen activator. *Science* 1983;220:1181–1183.

Bergmann S R, Sobel B E: The impact of coronary thrombolysis and tissue-type plasminogen activator (t-PA) on acute myocardial infarction, in

Collen D, Verstraete M (eds): *Thrombolysis*. Edinburgh, Churchill Livingstone, 1985, pp. 61–84.

Chazov E I, Matveeva L S, Mazaev A V, Sargin K E, Sadovskaia G V, Ruda M I: Intracoronary administration of fibrinolysis in acute myocardial infarction. *Ter-Arkh* 1976;48:8–19.

Christensen L R: The activation of plasminogen by chloroform. *J Gen Physiol* 1946;30:149–157.

Christensen L R, MacLeod C M: A proteolytic enzyme of serum: characterization, activation, and reaction with inhibitors. *J Gen Physiol* 1945;28:559–583.

Collen D, Lijnen H R, Verstraete M: *Thrombolysis: biological and therapeutic properties of new thrombolytic agents*. Edinburgh, Churchill Livingstone, 1985.

Collen D, Stassen J M, Verstraete M: Thrombolysis with human extrinsic (tissue-type) plasminogen activator in rabbits with experimental jugular vein thrombosis. Effect of molecular form and dose of activator, age of the thrombus, and route of administration. *J Clin Invest* 1983;71:368–376.

Collen D, Topol E J, Tiefenbrunn A J, Gold H K, Weisfeldt M L, Sobel B E, Leinbach R C, Brinker J A, Ludbrook P A, Yasuda T, Bulkley B H, Robison A K, Hutter A M, Jr., Bell W R, Spadaro J J, Jr., Khaw B A, Grossbard E B: Coronary thrombolysis with recombinant human tissue-type plasminogen activator: a prospective, randomized, placebo-controlled trial. *Circulation* 1984;70:1012–1017.

Denys J, De Marbaix H: Les peptonisations provoquees par le chloroforme. *Cellule* 1889;5:197.

DeWood M A, Spores J, Notske R N, Mouser L T, Burroughs R, Golden M S, Lang H T: Prevalence of total coronary occlusion during the early hours of transmural myocardial infarction. *N Engl J Med* 1980;303:897–902.

European Cooperative Study Group: Streptokinase in acute myocardial infarction. *N Engl J Med* 1979;301:797–802.

Fletcher A P, Sherry S, Alkjaersig N, Smyrniotis F E, Jick S: The maintenance of a sustained thrombolytic state in man. II. Clinical observations on patients with myocardial infarction and other thromboembolic disorders. *J Clin Invest* 1959;38:1111–1119.

Geltman E M, Ehsani A A, Campbell M K, Schechtman K, Roberts R, Sobel B E: The influence of location and extent of myocardial infarction on long-term ventricular dysrhythmia and mortality. *Circulation* 1979;60:805–814.

Ginks W R, Sybers H D, Maroko P R, Covell J W, Sobel B E, Ross J, Jr.: Coronary artery reperfusion. II. Reduction of myocardial infarct size at one week after the coronary occlusion. *J Clin Invest* 1972;51:2717–2723.

Herrick J B: Clinical features of sudden obstruction of the coronary arteries. *JAMA* 1912;59:2015.

Kaplan M H: Nature and role of lytic factor in hemolytic streptococcal fibrinolysis. *Proc Soc Exp Biol Med* 1944;57:40–43.

Maroko P R, Kjekshus J K, Sobel B E, Watanabe T, Covell J W, Ross J, Jr., Braunwald E: Factors influencing infarct size following experimental coronary artery occlusions. *Circulation* 1971;43:67–82.

Maseri A, L'Abbate A, Baroldi G, Chierchia S, Marzilli M, Ballestra AM, Severi S, Parodi O, Biagini A, Distante A, Pesola A: Coronary vasospasm as a possible cause of myocardial infarction. A conclusion derived from the study of "preinfarction" angina. *N Engl J Med* 1978;299:1271–1277.

Milstone H: A factor in normal human blood which participates in streptococcal fibrinolysis. *J Immunol* 1941;42:109–116.

Morgagni J B: *The seats and causes of diseases investigated by anatomy*, Vol. 3. London, 1769, pp. 185–190.

Rentrop K P, Blanke H, Karsch K R, Wiegand V, Kostering H, Oster H, Leitz K: Acute myocardial infarction: intracoronary application of nitroglycerin and streptokinase. *Clin Cardiol* 1979;2:354–363.

Roberts R, Croft C, Gold H K, Hartwell T D, Jaffe A S, Muller J E, Mullin S M, Parker C, Passamani E R, Poole W K, Raabe D S, Jr., Rude R E, Stone P H, Turi Z G, Sobel B E, Willerson J T, Braunwald E, for the MILIS Study Group: Effect of propranolol on myocardial-infarct size in a randomized, blinded, multicenter trial. *N Engl J Med* 1984;311:218–225.

Sherry S: The fibrinolytic system and its pharmacologic activation for thrombolysis. *Cardiol Clin* 1987;5:1–11.

Sobel B E: Safety and efficacy of tissue-type plasminogen activator produced by recombinant DNA technology (rt-PA). *J Am Coll Cardiol* 1987;10 (suppl. B): 40B–44B.

Sobel B E: Thrombolysis in the treatment of acute myocardial infarction, in Fuster V, Verstraete M (eds): *Thrombosis in cardiovascular disorders*. Philadelphia, W.B. Saunders, 1992, pp. 289–326.

Sobel B E, Bresnahan G F, Shell W E, Yoder R D: Estimation of infarct size in man and its relation to prognosis. *Circulation* 1972;46:640–648.

Sobel B E, Collen D: Questions unresolved by the Third International Study of Infarct Survival. *Am J Cardiol* 1992;70:385–389.

Sobel B E, Geltman E M, Tiefenbrunn A J, Jaffe A S, Spadaro J J, Jr., Ter-Pogossian M M, Collen D, Ludbrook P A: Improvement of regional myocardial metabolism after coronary thrombolysis induced with tissue-type plasminogen activator or streptokinase. *Circulation* 1984;69:983–990.

Sobel B E (guest ed): Thrombolysis and the heart. *Cardiol Clin* 1987;5:1–145.

Tiefenbrunn A J, Sobel B E: Factors contributing to the emergence of coronary thrombolysis. *Cardiol Clin* 1987;5:49–53.

Tillett W S, Garner R L: The fibrinolytic activity of hemolytic streptococci. *J Exp Med* 1933;58:488–502.

Van de Werf F, Bergmann S R, Fox K A A, de Geest H, Hoyng C F, Sobel B E, Collen D: Coronary thrombolysis with intravenously administered human tissue-type plasminogen activator produced by recombinant DNA technology. *Circulation* 1984;69:605–610.

Van de Werf F, Ludbrook P A, Bergmann S R, Tiefenbrunn A J, Fox K A A, de Geest H, Verstraete M, Collen D, Sobel B E: Coronary thrombolysis with tissue-type plasminogen activator in patients with evolving myocardial infarction. *N Engl J Med* 1984;310:609–613.

Verstraete M, van de Loo J, Jesdinsky H L (eds): Streptokinase in acute myocardial infarction. *Acta Med Scand* 1991;suppl 648:1–117.

2

Thrombolytic Agents

Désiré Collen and Marc Verstraete
University of Leuven
Leuven, Belgium

Thrombolytic agents are compounds that induce conversion of plasminogen, the inactive proenzyme of the fibrinolytic system in blood, to the proteolytic enzyme plasmin. Plasmin dissolves the fibrin of a thrombus but may also degrade normal components of the hemostatic system and other blood proteins. Five thrombolytic agents are presently in or approaching clinical use. The oldest is streptokinase, which activates plasminogen indirectly, and of which more recently an anisoylated complex with plasminogen (APSAC, anistreplase) has been developed. The other three are human proteins that directly activate plasminogen: single-chain urokinase-type plasminogen activator (scu-PA, pro-urokinase), two-chain urokinase-type plasminogen activator (tcu-PA, urokinase), and tissue-type plasminogen activator (t-PA, alteplase).

I. STREPTOKINASE

A. Physiochemical Properties

Streptokinase is a bacterial protein secreted by several strains of hemolytic streptococci. Streptokinase used for therapeutic thrombolysis is derived from a nonpathogenic, group C (Lance-field) strain of the organism and was originally called strepto-coccal fibrinolysin. It is a single-chain polypeptide with a molecular weight of 43,000 and contains 415 amino acids with very little carbohydrate and no disulfide bonds. The region comprising amino acids 1–230 shows some homology with trypsinlike serine proteinases, but lacks the active site serine residue. Streptokinase has neither peptidase nor amidase activity. Early preparations of streptokinase were relatively impure, with some containing only about 10% active drug; current preparations have a purity of greater than 95%.

B.   Mechanism of Plasminogen Activation

Streptokinase activates plasminogen to plasmin indirectly, following a three-step mechanism. In the first step, it reacts rapidly and stoichiometrically with plasminogen to form a streptokinase–plasminogen complex, whereby plasminogen undergoes a conformational change resulting in the exposure of an active site. In the second step, this active site catalyzes the activation of plasminogen to plasmin. In a third step, plas-minogen–streptokinase molecules are converted to plasmin-streptokinase complex with preservation of activator activity. The activation of Glu-plasminogen by the plasminogen–strep-tokinase complex is enhanced 6.5-fold in the presence of fibrin and 2-fold in the presence of fibrinogen, although fibrin does not contain specific binding sites for streptokinase. The plas-minogen–streptokinase complex is not inhibited by plasma protease inhibitors and hydrolyzes the chromogenic plasmin substrate D-Val-Leu-Lys-p-nitroanilide. These phenomena form the basis for the spectrophotometric determination of plasmi-nogen activity in plasma after addition of excess streptokinase.

Conversion of the equimolar plasminogen–streptokinase complex to the plasmin–streptokinase complex occurs rapidly by proteolytic cleavage of both the plasminogen and the strep-tokinase moieties. In plasminogen, the Arg^{560}-Val^{561} and the Lys^{77}-Lys^{78} peptide bonds are cleaved. Four modified forms of streptokinase differing in molecular weight by 4000–5000 have been observed with canine plasminogen and a major proteolytic derivative with molecular weight of 36,000 with human plasminogen. Plasmin and streptokinase react rapidly, with a rate constant of $3–5 \times 10^{-7}$ $M^{-1}s^{-1}$, to form a noncovalent complex with a dissociation constant of 5×10^{-11} M. The active site residues in the plasmin-streptokinase complex are the same as those in plasmin, but their interaction with plasminogen and with α_2-antiplasmin is very different. Plasmin, in contrast to its complex with streptokinase, is unable to activate plasminogen, while the plasmin(ogen)–streptokinase complex, unlike plasmin, is insensitive to α_2-antiplasmin.

Streptokinase induces a "systemic fibrinolytic state" in blood, characterized by plasminogen activation in plasma (hyperplasminemia), depletion of α_2-antiplasmin, and breakdown of fibrinogen, factor V, and factor VIII. The breakdown products of fibrinogen (FDPs) that are formed also impede blood coagulation. These effects significantly prolong the activated partial thromboplastin time (APTT), the thrombin clotting time, and the prothrombin time (PT), assays frequently used in laboratory monitoring. In addition, plasmin also degrades components of the extracellular matrix, including fibronectin and laminin; it activates latent tissue collagenases capable of degrading interstitial collagens of types I, II, and III or basement membrane collagen type IV.

C. Pharmacokinetic Properties

In vivo, the fibrinolytic activity of streptokinase is cleared via the reticuloendothelial system with a half-life of 18–25 minutes. The level of antistreptokinase antibodies, which may result from previous infections with β-hemolytic streptococci, varies widely among individuals. Approximately 350,000 units of streptokinase are required to neutralize the circulating antibodies in 95% of a healthy population, with individual requirements ranging between 25,000 and 3,000,000 units. A few days after streptokinase administration, the antistreptokinase titer rises rapidly to 50–100 times the preinfusion value and remains high for at least 4–6 months, during which period renewed thrombolytic treatment with streptokinase or compounds containing streptokinase is impracticable.

D. Dosage

The dosage of streptokinase at which systemic fibrinolysis occurs is dependent mainly on the plasma levels of antistreptococcal antibodies. The initial dose for an individual patient can be either determined by the streptokinase resistance test (if laboratory facilities are available and time permits), or a standard initial intravenous dose of 500,000 units can be given over a period of 10–30 minutes, followed by a continuous intravenous maintenance dose of 100,000 units hourly for 1 or more days. Such a fixed dosage regimen produces a satisfactory thrombolytic effect in the vast majority of patients without requiring laboratory monitoring.

During the last decade, high-dose (1,500,000 units), short-term (3–60 minutes infusion) streptokinase treatment has routinely been used in patients with acute myocardial infarction. Local infusion of 2000–4000 units streptokinase/minute over 60–120 minutes is used in occlusions of pulmonary and limb arteries. Intracoronary infusion of streptokinase with a loading dose of 10,000–20,000 units followed by 5000 units/min (range 2000–6000) for 60 minutes was used in the early 1980s.

E. Adverse Effects

Transient hypotension and bradycardia occur frequently during streptokinase therapy and may be related to histamine or/ and bradykinin release. Incidences of transient hypotension as high as 40% have been reported, but clinically relevant hypotension is noted in only a few percent of treated patients. Hypotension is usually halted by cessation of the infusion and is more likely to occur when streptokinase is rapidly infused. The incidence of hypotension does not seem to be affected by premedication with steroids. With the conventional dose of 1.5 million units streptokinase over 1 hour, in patients treated for acute myocardial infarction, the mean blood pressure decreases by an average of about 10 mm after about 20 minutes. The most common adverse reaction is mild to moderate (but occasionally severe) fever. This complication occurs in some 5–30% of patients, usually with a delay in onset of several hours.

Streptokinase is antigenic in humans and may provoke serious allergic reactions (urticaria, bronchospasm, angioneurotic or periorbital edema). In the large ISIS-3 trial, the incidence of some allergic reactions with streptokinase was only 3.6%. Major anaphylactoid reactions to streptokinase are rare (0.3%). In detailed reports shivering, chills, rashes, flushing, nausea, or musculoskeletal pain appear in 10% of patients during or shortly after streptokinase infusion. Serum sickness symptoms have occasionally been reported. Agonizing interscapular low thoracic back pain as well as severe lower abdominal pain have been repeatedly described during or after infusion of streptokinase; hemorrhage into the iliopsoas muscles has been documented.

Streptokinase infusion, if repeated between 5 days and 6 months following the initial infusion, may be clinically ineffective as a result of a high titer of circulating antibodies. In a recent study, it was found that 3 months after streptokinase treatment, antibody titers were still sufficiently high to fully neutralize 1.5 million units of streptokinase. Repeated administration of streptokinase is therefore best avoided between about 5 days and 1–2 years after the first use. If repeated thrombolysis is required during this time window, nonantigenic drugs such as urokinase and alteplase are recommended.

Hemorrhage is the most common complication of streptokinase administration. Minor bleeding (not requiring transfusion) occurs in 3–4% of patients. These occurrences are usually related to puncture or injection sites, but microscopic hematuria and blood-streaked sputum or vomit are frequently noted. Significant or major bleeding (potentially life threatening or requiring transfusion) occurs in 2% (range 0.4–10%); in the ISIS-3 trial the incidence among 13,780 patients was 1%. Anticoagulant and/or aspirin treatment may also enhance the frequency of bleeding, as do invasive catheter approaches.

The most serious complication is cerebral bleeding, which occurs with an incidence of 0.1–0.5%, while ischemic stroke during streptokinase treatment of myocardial infarction occurs in 0.8–1.5% of patients. In the large trials there is an excess of "early" hemorrhagic or other strokes on the day of streptokinase treatment. However, there are fewer strokes thereafter, rendering the overall risk of stroke similar in streptokinase and placebo-treated patients. The risk of intracranial bleeding appears to be greater with advanced age and hypertension; this devastating event is not to be underrated when deciding to start thrombolytic treatment with any of the currently available agents, as they cause most often permanent disability and may be fatal in up to half of the cases.

II.   ANISOYLATED PLASMINOGEN STREPTOKINASE ACTIVATOR COMPLEX

Anisoylated plasminogen streptokinase activator complex (APSAC, anistreplase, Eminase[R]) is an equimolar noncovalent complex between human Lys-plasminogen and streptokinase in which the active site in the plasminogen moiety is reversibly blocked by acylation. This compound was designed to prolong the half-life of streptokinase and to make treatment more convenient by allowing intravenous bolus injection of the drug.

A.   Physicochemical Properties

Human plasminogen with NH_2-terminal lysine (Lys-plasminogen) rather than glutamic acid (native or Glu-plasminogen) is used to produce the anistreplase complex because it has a higher affinity for fibrin than Glu-plasminogen. Specific acylation of the catalytic center is achieved by the use of a reversible acylating agent, p-amidinophenyl-p'-anisate-hydrochloride (APAN). The cationic amidino group is positioned to interact with the anionic carboxyl group of Asp^{735} within the catalytic center of plasminogen. The anisoyl head is located at a position near the Ser^{741} residue of the active center, so that the required acyl transfer can take place. Following bolus injection, the complex deacylates slowly to regenerate active complex.

B.   Pharmacokinetic Properties

In the circulation, streptokinase dissociates very slowly from the plasminogen–streptokinase complex with a rate constant of less than 2×10^{-5} per second. The deacylation rate constant on the other hand, is much greater, which means that the activity of the complex will be controlled by the deacylation rate rather than by dissociation. In healthy volunteers, an apparent clearance half-life of 70 minutes was found for anistreplase, as compared to 25 minutes for the plasminogen–streptokinase complex formed upon administration of streptokinase alone. With the recommended dose of 30 units (mg) of anistreplase in patients with acute myocardial infarction, the plasma fibrinogen level decreases to 14% of the baseline value and almost all of the α_2-antiplasmin is consumed. These findings are similar to those reported following the intravenous administration of 1.5 million units of streptokinase.

C.   Dosage

The recommended standard dose in acute myocardial infarction is 30 U of anistreplase to be given as a bolus injection, which contains approximately 1,250,000 units of streptokinase. In aggregate, comparative studies indicate that the efficacy for coronary thrombolysis (angiographic patency at 90 minutes) with anistreplase is comparable or somewhat higher than that of intravenous streptokinase.

D.   Adverse Effects

The overall incidence of "allergic reactions" to APSAC is around 5%. Serious allergic reactions such as anaphylaxis and bronchoconstriction are rare (0.2–0.4%); more commonly, fever, flushing, or chills have been observed (5–10%).

   As anticipated, in comparative trials of anistreplase (30 U bolus) versus streptokinase (1.5×10^6 units over 60 minutes), the same fall in fibrinogen concentrations and a comparable incidence of adverse events were noted. When compared with alteplase, anistreplase administration resulted in greater and more prolonged reduction of both circulating fibrinogen (to 28% vs. to 65% of baseline) and plasminogen (to 23% vs. to 58% of baseline).

Cerebrovascular accidents related to anistreplase treatment have been reported in 10 (0.6%) of 1598 patients, which is comparable to the rate observed with other thrombolytic agents. The stroke rate in the ISIS-3 trial was 0.9, 1.1, and 1.2% in patients treated with streptokinase, anistreplase, or t-PA (duteplase), respectively.

Anistreplase causes immunization, and the antibody titer increases up to 60-fold after 2–3 weeks, to remain very high after 3 months.

III. SINGLE-CHAIN UROKINASE-TYPE PLASMINOGEN ACTIVATOR

Single-chain urokinase-type plasminogen activator (scu-PA, pro-urokinase) is a human protein first identified in cell culture fluid and later produced by recombinant DNA technology. The human gene responsible for its synthesis is located on chromosome 10; it is about 6.4 kb long, organized in 11 exons, and gives rise to a 2.5-kb-long messenger RNA, which transcribes a single-chain glycosylated polypeptide. The single-chain protein is synthesized principally by renal epithelial endothelial cells but also by a variety of cultured normal, transformed, and malignant cell types.

A. Physiochemical Properties

scu-PA is a single-chain glycoprotein with a molecular weight of 54,000 containing 411 amino acids. The molecule comprises an NH_2-terminal domain, which is homologous with the growth factor domain of several other proteins, a kringle domain, homologous to the kringles in plasminogen, tissue-type plasminogen activator, and several other proteins and a serine protease domain. However, the kringle domain of scu-PA does not confer fibrin-binding properties to the enzyme. The single glycosylation site of the protein is located at asparagine 302. The molecule expressed by *Escherichia coli* lacks the carbohydrate, which reduces the molecular weight to 47,000 daltons (specific activity 175,000 IU/mg).

scu-PA is a precursor of urokinase. Limited hydrolysis by plasmin or kallikrein of the Lys^{158}-Ile^{159} peptide bond converts the molecule to two-chain urokinase-type plasminogen activator (tcu-PA) which is held together by one disulfide bond. A fully active tcu-PA derivative is obtained after additional proteolysis at position Lys^{135}-Lys^{136}. Specific hydrolysis of the Glu^{143}-Leu^{144} peptide bond in scu-PA yields a low molecular weight scu-PA of 32,000 daltons (scu-PA-32k). Thrombin, on the other hand, cleaves the Arg^{156}-Phe^{157} peptide bond in scu-PA, resulting in an inactive double-chain molecule.

B. Mechanism of Plasminogen Activation

In purified systems, scu-PA has some intrinsic plasminogen-activating potential, which is, however, ≤0.5% that of tcu-PA. Conversion of scu-PA to tcu-PA in the vicinity of a fibrin clot apparently constitutes a significant positive feedback mechanism for clot lysis in human plasma in vitro. This conversion may, however, play a less important role in in vivo thrombolysis, due to preferential fibrin-associated activation of plasminogen by scu-PA.

Several cell types, such as human peripheral monocytes and fibroblasts, express specific high-affinity binding sites for scu-PA and tcu-PA on their surface. Cell-bound scu-PA and tcu-PA are thought to be involved in the generation of pericellular proteolysis during cell migration and tissue remodeling.

C. Pharmacokinetic Properties

scu-PA is rapidly cleared from the blood following a biphasic pattern, which can be described by two exponential terms with half-lives of 7.9 ± 1.2 and 48 ± 8 minutes, respectively. The

NH$_2$-terminal region and carbohydrate moieties appear not to be critical for clearance because the pharmacokinetics of natural glycosylated scu-PA, of recombinant nonglycosylated scu-PA, and of the truncated low molecular weight variant, scu-PA-32k, are very similar. These findings suggest the need for continuous intravenous infusion in order to achieve and maintain steady-state plasma levels required for thrombolytic efficacy. Postinfusion clearance of scu-PA occurs with similar rapidity, suggesting nonsaturability of the clearance mechanism.

D. Dosage

There is still limited clinical experience with recombinant scu-PA. The generic name for full-length unglycosylated human recombinant scu-PA obtained from *E. coli* is saruplase. The dose used successfully in patients with acute myocardial infarction was 20 mg given as a bolus and 60 mg in the next 60 minutes, immediately followed by an intravenous heparin infusion (20 U/kg/h) for 72 hours. This dosage regimen was found to cause extensive systemic activation of the fibrinolytic system and fibrinogen degradation, which was due, at least in part, to conversion of scu-PA to tcu-PA in the circulation.

E. Adverse Effects

In a direct double-blind comparison between intravenous saruplase (80 mg over 60 minutes) and streptokinase (1.5 million units over 60 minutes) in 401 patients with acute myocardial infarction, a somewhat smaller reduction in circulating fibrinogen levels was observed in patients treated with saruplase. There were significantly fewer bleeding episodes in the saruplase group than in the streptokinase group (14 vs. 25%), and less need for transfusion (4 vs. 11%).

IV. UROKINASE

The fibrinolytic activity in human urine, originally described by Williams and Astrup et al. and presently identified as urokinase, is isolated for therapeutic use from tissue cultures of human embryonic kidney cells.

A. Physicochemical Properties

Urokinase is a trypsinlike serine proteinase composed of two polypeptide chains (molecular weight 20,000 and 34,000). It may occur in two molecular forms designated S_1 (molecular weight 31,600, 276 amino acids: low molecular weight urokinase) and S_2 (molecular weight 54,000, 411 amino acids: high molecular weight urokinase), the former being a proteolytic degradation product of the latter. The high molecular weight form is predominant in preparations obtained from urine, whereas the low molecular form is obtained from long-term cultures of human fetal kidney cells collected at 26–32 weeks of gestation. Both molecular forms of urokinase have comparable pharmacological properties in vivo and do not differ in terms of clinical results.

The complete primary structure of high molecular weight urokinase has been elucidated: the light chain contains 158 amino acids and the heavy chain 253. The catalytic center is located in the COOH-terminal chain and is composed of Asp^{255}, His^{204}, and Ser^{356}. The NH_2-terminal chain contains a growth factor domain and one kringle domain. A low molecular weight tcu-PA (molecular weight 33,000) can be generated with plasmin by hydrolysis of the Lys^{135}-Lys^{136} peptide bond following previous cleavage of the Lys^{158}-Ile^{159} peptide bond.

B. Mechanism of Plasminogen Activation

Urokinase activates plasminogen directly following Michaelis-Menten kinetics. It has no specific affinity for fibrin and activates fibrin-bound and circulating plasminogen relatively indiscriminately. Extensive plasminogen activation and depletion of α_2-antiplasmin may occur following treatment with urokinase, leading to degradation of several plasma proteins including fibrinogen, factor V, and factor VIII.

Several inhibitors of plasminogen activators (PAI) have been described. Plasminogen activator inhibitor 1 (PAI-1) is released by endothelial cells and different neoplastic cell lines and is also found in platelets and plasma. Plasminogen activator inhibitor 2 (PAI-2) was first detected in placental extracts and is also released from cell lines and macrophages. These PAIs are proteins with a molecular weight of about 50–60 kd and differ in immunological reactivity and several other physiological characteristics; both belong to the serpin (serine protease inhibitor) superfamily.

C. Pharmacokinetic Properties

The half-life of urokinase is approximately 15 minutes. Urokinase is cleared mainly by the liver, with about 3–5% being cleared by the kidneys.

D. Dosage

For more than a decade, an initial intravenous dose of 4000 units/kg body weight over 10 minutes followed by the same maintenance dose per kg hourly was recommended for the treatment of acute major pulmonary embolism. Intravenous infusion of 3,000,000 units of urokinase (1,000,000 units over 10 minutes and 2,000,000 units over the next 110 minutes) is presently being tested.

In the early trials in acute myocardial infarction, intracoronary urokinase (6,000 U/min) has been given for 90–120 minutes. At present, the systemic dose of urokinase is 2,000,000 units given as an intravenous bolus or 3,000,000 units administered over 60–90 minutes.

E. Adverse Effects

Purified urokinase preparations are nonantigenic, nonpyrogenic, and their proper use is most often associated with a milder coagulation defect than that with streptokinase, but with a similar incidence of bleeding. As the level of inhibitors in plasma is relatively constant, a fixed dosage regimen can readily be used.

V. TISSUE-TYPE PLASMINOGEN ACTIVATOR

The plasminogen activator, which is synthesized by endothelial cells and secreted into the blood, has been identified as tissue-type plasminogen activator (t-PA). Antigen levels of t-PA in normal plasma are about 5 ng/ml. Tissue-type plasminogen activator has been purified from the tissue culture fluid of stable human melanoma cell lines in sufficient amounts to study its biochemical and biological properties; it is presently produced for clinical use by recombinant DNA technology. The human t-PA gene, located on chromosome 8 (bands 8.p.12→9.11.2), is divided into 14 exons that code for specific domains of the protein.

A. Physicochemical Properties

Tissue-type plasminogen activator is a serine proteinase with a molecular weight of about 70,000, composed of a single polypeptide chain of 527 amino acids with Ser as the NH_2-terminal amino acid. The complete 2530-base-pair cDNA sequence has been elucidated. It was subsequently shown that native t-PA contains an NH_2-terminal extension of three amino acids (Gly-Ala-Arg-).

The mature, secreted molecule contains five domains: (1) a 43-residue-long NH_2-terminal region (F-domain) that is homologous with the finger domain responsible for the fibrin affinity of fibronectin, (2) residues 44–91 (E-domain) which are homologous with human epidermal growth factor, also present in many other serine proteases and cell membrane receptors, (3) two disulfide-rich regions of 82 amino acids each (residues 92–173 and 180–261) (K_1 and K_2 domains) that share a high degree of homology with the kringles of urokinase, plasminogen, prothrombin, Hageman factor, and apolipoprotein a, and (4) a serine proteinase domain (amino acids 276–527) with the active site residues His^{322}, Asp^{371}, and Ser^{478}, which is homologous with other serine proteinases.

The t-PA gene is assembled according to the "exon-shuffling" principle. The different structural domains of the heavy chain (F, E, K_1, K_2) are indeed encoded by a single exon or by two adjacent exons. Because of the striking correlation between the intron-exon distribution of the gene and the putative domain structure of the protein, it was suggested that these domains would harbor autonomous functional entities ("modules"). This concept implies that these structural domains of t-PA are involved in most of its functions and interactions, including its enzymatic activity, binding to fibrin, stimulation of plasminogen activation by fibrin, inhibition by PAI-1, binding to endothelial cells, and in vivo clearance of t-PA. The validity of the "exon-shuffling" concept for t-PA has been investigated by the construction of mutants with precise domain deletions, insertions, or substitutions and the evaluation of the fibrin affinity, the fibrin specificity, and the pharmacokinetic and thrombolytic properties of such mutants. The two-chain form of t-PA arises from cleavage of the Arg^{275}-Ile^{276} peptide bond by endogenous proteinases, most efficiently by plasmin.

The t-PA of saliva from the vampire bat *Desmodus rotundus* (bat-PA) is highly homologous with human t-PA but lacks K_2 and the plasmin cleavage site for conversion to a two-chain form. It was found to be stimulated 45,000-fold by fibrin, and to constitute a potent and fibrin-specific thrombolytic agent in rabbits and dogs with femoral arterial thrombosis.

B.   Fibrin Affinity of t-PA

The structures involved in the fibrin binding of t-PA are fully contained within the NH_2-terminal (heavy) chain, as evidenced by the intact fibrin affinity of the heavy chain isolated after mild reduction of two-chain t-PA. Evidence obtained with domain deletion mutants of t-PA indicated that its affinity for fibrin is mediated via the finger domain and mainly via the second kringle domain.

It has been suggested that in the process of fibrinolysis, binding of t-PA to intact fibrin would initially be mediated by the F domain. Subsequently, upon partial fibrin digestion by plasmin, increased binding of t-PA to newly exposed COOH-terminal lysine residues would occur via the lysine-binding site in the K_2 domain. During degradation of fibrin(ogen) by plasmin, new t-PA–binding sites with markedly lower dissociation constants (2–4 orders of magnitude) are formed, but the increased binding of t-PA does not involve a lysine-binding site.

Some authors have found no difference between the fibrin-binding properties of single-chain and two-chain t-PA, whereas one study reported a significant difference. Binding of t-PA to fibrin appears to be a dynamic interaction, which may be modulated during fibrinolysis by partial degradation of fibrin and by conversion of single-chain to two-chain t-PA.

C. Mechanism of Plasminogen Activation

In the absence of fibrin, t-PA is a poor plasminogen activator, mainly because of a low affinity for its substrate. Single-chain t-PA is less active towards low molecular weight substrates and inhibitors, but its activity towards plasminogen was shown to be comparable to that of the two-chain form. The intrinsic enzymatic activity of single t-PA was confirmed by the construction of rt-PA mutants in which the plasmic cleavage site for conversion to two-chain t-PA was destroyed by site-specific mutagenesis of Arg^{275} to Glu. Such mutants were demonstrated to have lower activity than two-chain t-PA in the absence of fibrin, but full plasminogen-activating activity in the presence of fibrin. Inhibition by PAI-1 was also comparable for the wild-type and mutant t-PA. In contrast to other zymogen precursors of serine proteinases, the single-chain form of t-PA thus appears to be an active enzyme.

In the presence of fibrin, t-PA is a potent plasminogen activator, mainly due to a strongly enhanced affinity for its substrate. The isolated proteinase part of two-chain t-PA, which is fully active, is not stimulated by fibrin, indicating that the structures involved in the fibrin-stimulation are localized in the NH_2-terminal region. The kinetic data suggest that the fibrin-stimulation of plasminogen activation by t-PA occurs by sequential ordered addition of t-PA and plasminogen to fibrin, producing a thermodynamically more stable cyclic ternary complex.

D.   Pharmacokinetics

Single-chain t-PA has a significantly shorter half-life in humans (4.3 minutes, α-phase; 36.5 minutes, β-phase) than two-chain t-PA, the earlier product made available for clinical use (5.2 minutes, α-phase; 46.2 minutes, β-phase). Whether this difference is related to the chain composition or to other factors such as glycosylation remains unclear. When the latter material was studied in healthy human volunteers, the mean clearance (of antigen) was 620 ± 70 ml/min, the volume of distribution at steady state was 8.1 ± 0.8 l and the initial volume of distribution was 4.4 ± 0.5 l.

Animal experiments have indicated that rapid clearance of t-PA occurs via the heavy chain and primarily via hepatocytes. Although a receptor for t-PA has not yet been definitively identified, the rapid uptake probably involves receptor-mediated endocytosis and lysosomal degradation. Large doses of unlabeled t-PA administered concomitantly with radiolabeled t-PA in mice do not affect clearance, suggesting that hepatic binding and catabolism are not saturated by usual therapeutic doses. Two different mechanisms for removal of t-PA have been characterized: a protein-mediated pathway via hepatocytes and a carbohydrate-mediated pathway via endothelial cells in the liver. Recently, studies with rt-PA deletion mutants suggested that interaction of t-PA with hepatocytes would primarily involve kringle 1 (where residue Asn^{117} anchors a high-mannose carbohydrate side chain) but in addition occur via the F and E domains, whereas binding to endothelial cells would occur mainly via the F and E domain.

PAI-1 neutralizes very rapidly single-chain t-PA, two-chain t-PA, and urokinase. To design mutants of t-PA that are resistant to inhibition by PAI-1, Madison et al. have modeled the interactions between the active site of t-PA and PAI-1 based on the known three-dimensional structure of the trypsin–trypsin inhibitor complex. They have identified specific amino acids (residues Lys^{296}-His-Arg-Arg-Ser-Pro-Gly^{302} and Arg^{304}) in t-PA that interact with PAI-1 but not with the substrate plasminogen. Mutants of rt-PA obtained by site-specific mutagenesis in this region were shown to be fully active towards substrates but to display significant resistance to inhibition by PAI-1. In view of the large excess of t-PA over PAI-1 achieved during thrombolytic therapy, resistance of t-PA mutants to PAI-1 may not directly constitute a significant advantage over wild-type t-PA. High PAI-1 levels may, however, contribute to the occurrence of reocclusion, and PAI-1–resistant mutants of rt-PA may be useful for maintenance infusion after initial thrombolysis.

Resistance to PAI-1 has been combined with prolonged half-life in a molecule in which Thr^{103} is substituted by Asn (prolonged half-life) and the sequence Lys^{296}-His-Arg-Arg is mutagenized to Ala-Ala-Ala-Ala (resistance to PAI-1). This mutant was indeed shown to have a reduced plasma clearance and an increased potency on platelet-rich plasma clots (rich in PAI-1) in animal models.

E. Dosage

The recommended dose of alteplase (Activase^R, Actilyse^R) for the treatment of acute myocardial infarction is 100 mg administered as 60 mg in the first hour (of which 6–10 mg is administered as a bolus over the first 1–2 minutes), 20 mg over the second hour, and 20 mg over the third hour. More recently it was proposed to give the same total dose of 100 mg but "front loaded," starting with a bolus of 15 mg, followed by 50 mg in the next 30 minutes and the remaining 35 mg in the following 60 minutes. At present a 15-mg intravenous bolus of alteplase, followed by 0.75 mg/kg over 30 minutes (not to exceed 50 mg), and then 0.50 mg/kg over 60 minutes (not to exceed 35 mg) is being tested in the large-scale GUSTO trial. Whatever the dose regimen used, it is important to coadminister intravenous heparin during and after alteplase treatment. For catheter-directed local thrombolysis with alteplase in patients with recent peripheral arterial occlusion, the dose of 0.05–0.10 mg/kg/h over an 8-hour period is usually recommended.

Duteplase is the generic name for recombinant tissue-type plasminogen activator, produced in its two-chain form by the Burroughs-Wellcome Company. It also differs from recombinant human alteplase due to a substitution of methionine for valine in position 245 in the amino acid sequence and is therefore a variant of the naturally occurring human t-PA. The specific activity of duteplase is approximately 300,000 units per milligram protein, but different production lots may have specific activities that vary as much as ±100,000. For this reason, the dosage of duteplase is given in megaunits per kg body weight (0.6–1.0 MU/kg over 4 hours). In ISIS-3 the lower dose of duteplase (0.6 MU/kg over 4 hours) was used, which corresponds to circa 83% of the thrombolytic activity of 100 mg alteplase, but to a dose of 2 mg/kg (160 mg in the average 80-kg patient).

F. Adverse Effects

Bleeding complications are the most common and feared side effects with any thrombolytic agent, including alteplase. The reported rates of bleeding during treatment with thrombolytic agents depend on the methods of data collection, which can be very elaborate in trials on a limited number of patients, or limited in mega-trials including thousands of patients. Valid conclusions can therefore only be drawn from direct comparisons between drugs in a given trial. In a recent large trial directly comparing alteplase and streptokinase, the reported incidence of cerebral bleeding (confirmed by CT scan and necropsy) was similar for the two thrombolytic agents, but, overall, significantly more strokes were reported in the alteplase group. For both agents there was an excess of strokes in patients above 70 years of age (>70 years: 2.7% alteplase; 1.6% streptokinase; ≤70 years: 0.9% alteplase; 0.8% streptokinase). Significantly more major bleeds occurred in patients allocated to streptokinase. However, the total number of bleeds (minor plus major) was significantly higher with alteplase (4.2 vs. 3.3%). More allergic reactions (0.2 vs. 1.7%) and hypotension (1.7% vs. 3.8%) were seen with streptokinase in this large international trial. In the ISIS-3 trial the incidence of cerebral bleeding was 0.3, 0.5, and 0.6% in patients treated with streptokinase, anistreplase, and duteplase, respectively. To avoid bleeding and other complications, the relative and absolute contradictions to thrombolysis should be carefully observed.

VI. STAPHYLOKINASE

Staphylokinase, a 136-amino-acid protein produced by certain strains of *Staphylococcus aureus*, was shown to have profibrinolytic properties more than four decades ago. Initial evaluation of its thrombolytic properties in dogs had given discouraging results, and further interest in the development of staphylokinase as a thrombolytic agent faded away. More recently, the gene coding for staphylokinase has been cloned and expressed.

A. Mechanism of Plasminogen Activation

Recombinant staphylokinase (STAR), unlike streptokinase, was shown to be able to induce fibrin-specific clot lysis in a human plasma milieu. Both compounds form 1:1 stoichiometric complexes with plasmin(ogen) that activate other plasminogen molecules. Streptokinase and plasminogen produce a complex that exposes the active site in the plasminogen molecule without proteolytic cleavage, whereas generation of plasmin is required for the exposure of the active site in the complex with STAR. In addition, the plasmin(ogen)–streptokinase complex is virtually resistant to inhibition by α_2-antiplasmin, whereas this inhibitor rapidly neutralizes the plasmin–STAR complex. The fibrin specificity of STAR in human plasma has been explained by preferential plasminogen activation at the fibrin surface. This is the result of rapid inhibition of generated plasmin–STAR complex by α_2-antiplasmin in plasma, whereas this inhibition rate is reduced more than 100-fold in the presence of fibrin.

B. Thrombolytic Potency in Animal Models

STAR has a potency for venous clot lysis in hamsters and rabbits comparable to that of streptokinase. In addition, studies in hamsters and dogs suggested that STAR may be relatively more potent than streptokinase towards platelet-rich clots, and potentially less immunogenic. These findings were subsequently confirmed in baboons, where STAR was shown to have a thrombolytic potency towards jugular vein blood clots comparable to that of streptokinase but to be less immunogenic and less allergenic. Repeated administration of STAR, in contrast to streptokinase, did not induce resistance to clot lysis in this model. Furthermore, STAR was significantly more efficient than streptokinase for the dissolution of platelet-rich arterial eversion graft thrombi.

C. Initial Results in Patients

These encouraging results have formed the basis for the evaluation, on a pilot scale, of the pharmacokinetic, thrombolytic, and immunogenic properties of STAR in patients with acute myocardial infarction. In 4 of 5 patients with acute myocardial infarction, 10 mg STAR given intravenously over 30 minutes was found to induce angiographically documented coronary artery recanalization within 40 minutes. Plasma fibrinogen and α_2-antiplasmin levels were unaffected and allergic reactions were not observed. In these patients, no neutralizing antibodies against STAR could be demonstrated at baseline and up to 6 days after infusion. However, neutralizing antibodies, which did not cross-react with streptokinase, were consistently demonstrable in plasma at 14–35 days. Thus, with respect to immunogenicity, the initial observations in humans are not as encouraging as the experience in baboons.

Although the small number of patients studied precludes valid estimation of the frequency of coronary recanalization with STAR and of the adequacy of the dose used, this feasibility study suggests that intravenous infusion of 10 mg STAR may produce fibrin-specific coronary thrombolysis. Definition of the relative therapeutic benefit, or lack thereof, will require more detailed initial dose-finding studies followed by randomized clinical trials against other thrombolytic agents.

PERTINENT REFERENCES

Bennett W F, Paoni N F, Keyt B A, Botstein D, Jones A J S, Presta L, Wurm F M, Zoller M J: High resolution analysis of functional determinants on human tissue-type plasminogen activator. *J Biol Chem* 1991;266:5191–5201.

Christensen L R, MacLeod M: Streptococcal fibrinolysis: a proteolytic reaction due to a serum enzyme activated by streptococcal fibrinolysin. *J Gen Physiol* 1945;28:363–383.

Collen D, De Cock F, Stassen J M: Comparative immunogenicity and thrombolytic properties towards arterial and venous thrombi of streptokinase and recombinant staphylokinase in baboons. *Circulation* 1993;87:996–1006.

Collen D, Van de Werf F: Coronary thrombolysis with recombinant staphylokinase in patients with evolving myocardial infarction. *Circulation* (in press).

Gardell S J, Duong L T, Diehl R E, York J D, Hare T R, Registrer R B, Jacobs J W, Dixon R A F, Friedman P A: Isolation, characterization, and cDNA cloning of a vampire bat salivary plasminogen activator. *J Biol Chem* 1989;264:17947–17952.

Goa K L, Henwood J M, Stolz J F, Langley M S, Clissold S P: Intravenous streptokinase. A reappraisal of its therapeutic use in acute myocardial infarction. *Drugs* 1990;39:693–719.

Günzler W A, Steffens G J, Ötting F, Buse G, Flohe L: Structural relationship between human high and low molecular mass urokinase. *Hoppe Seyler's Z Physiol Chem* 1982;363:133–141.

Holmes W E, Pennica D, Blaber M, Rey M W, Guenzler W A, Steffens G, Heyneker H L: Cloning and expression of the gene for pro-urokinase in *Escherichia coli. Biotechnology* 1985;3:923–929.

Hoylaerts M, Rijken D C, Lijnen H R, Collen D: Kinetics of the activation of plasminogen by human tissue plasminogen activator. Role of fibrin. *J Biol Chem* 1982;257:2912–2919.

Jalihal S, Morris G K: Antistreptokinase titres after intravenous streptokinase. *Lancet* 1990;335:184–185.

Krätzschmar J, Haendler B, Langer G, Boidol W, Bringmann P, Alagon A, Donner P, Schleuning W D: The plasminogen activator family from the salivary gland of the vampire bat Desmodus rotundus: cloning and expression. *Gene* 1991;105:229–237.

Kruithof E K O, Tran-Thang C, Ransijn A, Bachmann F: Demonstration of a fast-acting inhibitor of plasminogen activators in human plasma. *Blood* 1984;64:907–913.

Lack C H: Staphylokinase: an activator of plasma protease. *Nature* 1948; 161:559–560.

Lewis J H, Kerber C W, Wilson J H: Effects of fibrinolytic agents and heparin on intravascular clot lysis. *Am J Physiol* 1964;207:1044–1048.

Lijnen H R, Van Hoef B, De Cock F, Collen D: The mechanism of plasminogen activation and fibrin dissolution by single chain urokinase-type plasminogen activator in a plasma milieu in vitro. *Blood* 1989;73:1864–1872.

Lijnen H R, Van Hoef B, De Cock F, Okada K, Ueshima S, Matsuo O, Collen D: On the mechanism of fibrin-specific plasminogen activation by staphylokinase. *J Biol Chem* 1991;266:11826–11832.

Madison E L, Goldsmith E J, Gerard R D, Gething M J H, Sambrook J F, Bassel-Duby R S: Amino acid residues that affect interaction of tissue-type plasminogen activator with plasminogen activator inhibitor 1. *Proc Natl Acad Sci USA* 1990;87:3530–3533.

Matsuo O, Okada K, Fukao H, Tomioka Y, Ueshima S, Watanuki M, Sakai M: Thrombolytic properties of staphylokinase. *Blood* 1990;76:925–929.

McClintock D K, Englert M E, Dziobkowski C, Snedeker E H, Bell P H: Two distinct pathways of the streptokinase-mediated activation of highly purified human plasminogen. *Biochemistry* 1974;13:5334–5344.

Patthy L: Evolution of the proteases of blood coagulation and fibrinolysis by assembly from modules. *Cell* 1985;41:657–663.

Pennica D, Holmes W E, Kohr W J, Harkins R N, Vehar G A, Ward C A, Bennett W F, Yelverton E, Seeburg P H, Heyneker H L, Goeddel D V, Collen D: Cloning and expression of human tissue-type plasminogen activator cDNA in E. coli. *Nature* 1983;301:214–221.

PRIMI Trial Study Group: Randomised double-blind trial of recombinant pro-urokinase against streptokinase in acute myocardial infarction. *Lancet* 1989;1:863–868.

Smith R A G, Dupe R J, English P D, Green J: Fibrinolysis with acylenzymes: a new approach to thrombolytic therapy. *Nature* 1981; 290:505–508.

The International Study Group: In-hospital mortality and clinical course of 20,891 patients with suspected acute myocardial infarction randomised between alteplase and streptokinase with or without heparin. *Lancet* 1990;336:71–75.

Third International Study of Infarct Survival Collaborative Group: ISIS-3: a randomized comparison of streptokinase versus tissue plasminogen activator versus anistreplase and of aspirin plus heparin versus aspirin alone among 41,299 cases of suspected acute myocardial infarction. *Lancet* 1992;339:753–770.

van Zonneveld A J, Veerman H, Pannekoek H: On the interaction of the finger and the kringle-2 domain of tissue-type plasminogen activator with fibrin. Inhibition of kringle-2 binding of fibrin by E-amino caproic acid. *J Biol Chem* 1986;261:14214–14218.

Verstraete M, Bounameaux H, De Cock F, Van de Werf, Collen D: Pharmacokinetics and systemic fibrinogenolytic effects of recombinant human tissue-type plasminogen activator (rt-PA) in humans. *J Pharmacol Exp Ther* 1985;235:506–512.

White W F, Barlow G H, Mozen M M: The isolation and characterization of plasminogen activators (urokinase) from human urine. *Biochemistry* 1966;5:2160–2169.

3

The Nature of Atherosclerotic Lesions Giving Rise to Acute Coronary Thrombosis

Erling Falk and Ik-Kyung Jang
Harvard Medical School and Massachusetts General Hospital
Boston, Massachusetts

I. INTRODUCTION

Atherosclerosis is the main cause of coronary thrombosis. Although atherosclerotic changes develop early in life, it usually takes several decades before this process begins to manifest clinically. In patients with stable angina and in a small group of patients with unstable angina, symptoms occur as a result of increase in oxygen demand. However, acute coronary syndromes, such as unstable angina and acute myocardial infarction, are usually caused by rupture of coronary atherosclerotic plaque with superimposed thrombus and subsequent decrease in oxygen supply.

The risk of a rupture/thrombus-related acute heart attack is clearly related to plaque composition and vulnerability (type of lesion) rather than degree of stenosis (size of lesion). Therefore, this chapter will focus first on the characteristic pathoanatomic features of stable, vulnerable, and ruptured atherosclerotic plaques and then discuss the consequences of plaque rupture with particular emphasis on mechanisms of luminal thrombus formation.

II. ATHEROSCLEROTIC PLAQUE

A. Plaque Composition and Vulnerability

Atherosclerotic plaques differ in composition, consistency, and vulnerability. As the name atherosclerosis implies, *atheromatous gruel* (lipid-rich and soft) and *sclerotic tissue* (collagen-rich and hard) are the two main components of plaque. However, there is a large variability in relative composition of individual plaques. Although these two plaque components are usually considered to represent different stages of the same disease, their pathogenesis and relationship are poorly understood. Although hard, collagenous tissue usually constitutes the most voluminous component of coronary plaques, it is stable and thus rather innocuous. In contrast, soft atheromatous gruel is dangerous because it softens plaques and thus determines their vulnerability. Thus, vulnerability is determined by the composition of a plaque, rather than the size of a plaque. Typically, a vulnerable plaque consists of a pool of soft extracellular lipid (the gruel) separated from the vascular lumen by a thin fibrous cap (Fig. 1). This fibrous cap varies greatly in thickness, strength, stiffness, and cellularity, but it is often its "shoulder regions," the junctions between the cap and the adjacent more normal intima, that are thinnest and most heavily infiltrated by macrophage foam cells. These shoulder regions are probably also points of maximal stress, and therefore are at high risk for rupture.

Therefore, the question arises: Is plaque rupture due solely to ongoing disease activity within the plaque causing progressive weakening (vulnerability), or do factors external to the plaque (triggers) also contribute? Muller et al. proposed the "circadian-triggering" concept: a plaque becomes vulnerable because of internal changes and then even a minor stress may trigger onset, most frequently between 6 a.m. and noon. Triggers for plaque rupture may be hemodynamic and me-

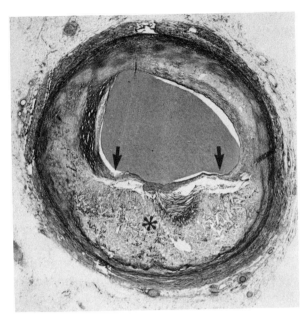

Figure 1 A typical vulnerable plaque consisting of a pool of soft extracellular lipid, the "gruel" (asterisk), separated from the vascular lumen by a thin cap of fibrous tissue. The lumen is filled by contrast medium. The thin and vulnerable "shoulder regions" are marked with arrows. These regions are not only weak points but probably also points of maximal stress, therefore prone to rupture.

chanical stresses due to "surges in sympathetic activity," resulting in increase in blood pressure, heart rate, myocardial contractility, coronary flow, and coronary tone. Thrombogenic factors may also be partly responsible for the circadian rhythm in clinical disease onset. Plaque vulnerability seems, however, to play a much more important role in rupture than triggers, because only vulnerable plaques are prone to rupture, and most acute myocardial infarctions occur during *normal* daily activities without an obvious precipitating cause. Even exercise stress test of patients with advanced coronary artery disease rarely "triggers" an acute myocardial infarction, despite the much greater hemodynamic changes usually associated with such an activity than the morning "surge."

B. Plaque Growth

Two processes are involved in the atherosclerotic plaque growth. *Slow progression* is caused by lipid accumulation, vascular smooth muscle cell proliferation, and extracellular matrix synthesis, but the individual significance of and interaction among lipids and cells (endothelium, macrophages, smooth muscle cells, platelets, and lymphocytes) during human atherogenesis are poorly understood. However, *rapid progression* is mainly caused by local thrombosis with subsequent organization and cell proliferation, or by intraplaque hemorrhage, as a consequence of plaque rupture. Autopsy studies suggest that coronary atherosclerotic plaque rupture occurs frequently during plaque evolution. Most ruptures are sealed by a small mural thrombus without causing significant hemodynamic changes, i.e., they are clinically silent. Clinical symptoms occur only if a flow-limiting lesion evolves, usually due to an obstructive luminal thrombus with or without associated vasospasm.

C. Fate of Plaque Rupture

There seem to be three major determinants for the outcome of a plaque rupture, i.e., whether a small mural or an occlusive thrombus evolves: (1) the exposed thrombogenic substrates, (2) local flow disturbances, and (3) the *actual* thrombotic propensity (Fig. 2).

Thrombogenic Substrates

Experimentally, the thrombotic response after vascular injury depends on the amount and characteristics of exposed thrombogenic material. A recent coronary angioscopic study indicated a similar substrate-thrombosis relation in humans: mild intimal irregularities with mural thrombus were found in unstable angina, while more extensive injury with occlusive thrombus were present in acute myocardial infarction. Tissue

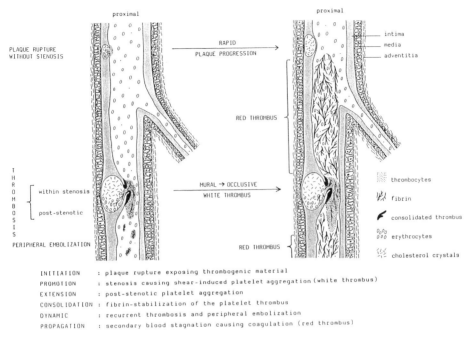

INITIATION	: plaque rupture exposing thrombogenic material
PROMOTION	: stenosis causing shear-induced platelet aggregation (white thrombus)
EXTENSION	: post-stenotic platelet aggregation
CONSOLIDATION	: fibrin-stabilization of the platelet thrombus
DYNAMIC	: recurrent thrombosis and peripheral embolization
PROPAGATION	: secondary blood stagnation causing coagulation (red thrombus)

Figure 2   Coronary thrombosis: pathogenesis.

factor, collagen, and lipids including lipoprotein(a) seem to be key substrates in human thrombus formation.

Stenosis/Flow

The degree of preexisting atherosclerosis stenosis determines, to some extent, the outcome of a plaque rupture: local flow disturbances around stenotic lesions seem to promote arterial thrombosis, probably via shear-induced platelet activation. Experimentally, a platelet thrombus may indeed form and grow within a severe stenosis, predominantly at the apex where blood velocity and shear forces are highest. Unlike venous thrombosis, arterial thrombosis is not primarily associated with blood stagnation; many atherosclerotic stenoses underlying infarct-related thrombi are hemodynamically insignificant, i.e., slow flow has not preceded thrombus formation. Whereas mild or moderate stenoses most frequently progress to infarct-related occlusion, severe stenoses frequently occlude, often clinically silent due to well-developed collateral vessels.

Thrombotic Propensity

Platelets and fibrin as well as endogenous fibrinolytic activity are also important in the development of acute myocardial infarction. People at risk of plaque rupture (stable angina) or thought to have ruptured coronary plaques (unstable angina and acute myocardial infarction) may benefit from antithrombotic therapy with antiplatelet agents and/or anticoagulants. Thus, in the case of plaque rupture, the actual thrombotic-thrombolytic equilibrium may play a decisive role for the outcome.

Experimental data suggest that some plasma lipoproteins, epinephrine, cigarette smoke, and exercise promote platelet aggregation and arterial thrombosis.

III. CORONARY THROMBOSIS: PATHOGENESIS AND DYNAMICS

In the majority of patients with acute coronary syndromes, thrombi are precipitated by the sudden rupture of a plaque surface exposing thrombogenic material to the flowing blood (Fig. 3). Careful analysis of the athero-thrombotic lesion may be helpful in understanding the role of individual blood components in thrombus formation, particularly the relationship between platelets and fibrin at the site of primary flow obstruction, the dynamic changes occurring during thrombus evolution, and subsequent thrombus propagation due to blood stagnation in the case of total occlusion.

A. First Platelets, Then Fibrin

Light-microscopic studies have shown that fresh coronary thrombi usually consist mainly of platelets with a small amount of fibrin. With time, fibrin enmeshes the initial platelet-rich thrombus concealing the individual platelets in a homogeneous mass (Fig. 4). Thus, even in fibrin-rich–looking thrombus, the core is always platelet-rich. Like the initial thrombotic occlusion, rethrombosis is also platelet-mediated.

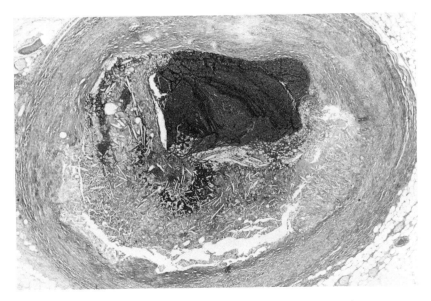

Figure 3 Thrombosed coronary artery showing atheromatous gruel extruded through the ruptured surface into the lumen (asterisk). The gruel is embedded in the luminal thrombus, clearly indicating the temporal sequence of events: plaque rupture must have immediately preceded luminal thrombus formation.

Early platelet-rich thrombus is, however, very unstable and may easily be swept away by the flowing blood. The embolization may be followed by new thrombus formation, leading to "cyclic changes of blood flow" until the thrombus becomes stabilized by fibrin. Such a temporal interplay between platelets and fibrin explains why both antiplatelet agents and anticoagulants may benefit patients at risk for coronary thrombosis, and also why fresh thrombi are more easily lysed than older, consolidated thrombi.

B. Dynamic Thrombosis

More than 80% of coronary thrombi have a layered structure, indicating episodic growth by repeated mural deposits over time (Fig. 4). As the thrombus grows, local resistance to blood

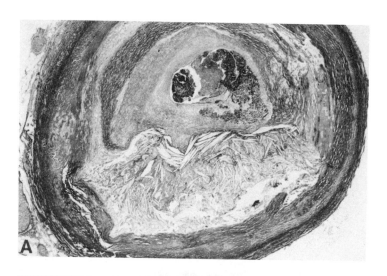

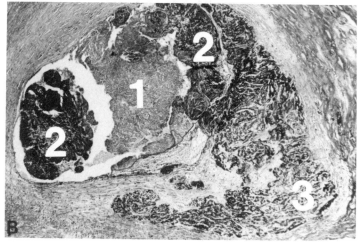

Figure 4   (A) Occlusive thrombus with a layered structure indicating episodic growth. (B) At higher magnification, it is clearly seen that the most recent part of the thrombus, located centrally (1), consists of individually discernible platelets with very little fibrin, while older parts, close to the vessel wall (2 and 3), are homogeneous, without structure. These "fibrinous" looking older parts of the thrombus are, however, also platelet-rich. Light microscopically, the platelets are just concealed due to fibrin enmeshment.

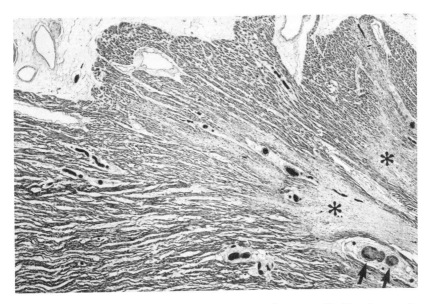

Figure 5 Small thromboemboli impacted in small distal vessels (arrows) associated with microinfarcts (asterisks); these were found in the perfusion area distal to an evolving coronary thrombosis, indicating thrombus fragmentation with peripheral embolization.

flow and the pressure gradient across the lesion increase, which may cause an "unstable" thrombus to break and embolize. The residual thrombus is extremely thrombogenic and may give rise to new occlusive thrombosis. This episodic thrombus growth and distal embolization is evidenced by the frequent finding of small thrombus fragments impacted in intramyocardial arteries, often associated with microinfarcts (Fig. 5). This phenomenon causes "cyclic flow variations" and may manifest clinically as unstable angina pectoris. A free-floating tail of thrombus may extend downstream from the stenosis, often growing much larger than the mural thrombus within the stenosis.

Another contributing factor is local vascular spasm. Platelets release vasoactive substances, such as thromboxane A_2 and serotonin, and induce local spasm. The spasm again increases shear forces, endothelial damage, and platelet deposition, resulting in a vicious cycle.

C. Thrombus Propagation

If the platelet-rich thrombus at the rupture site evolves into an occlusive thrombus, the blood proximal and distal to the occlusion may stagnate and coagulate, i.e., "clot" (Fig. 6). This type of thrombus, similar to a venous thrombus formed in stagnant blood, is composed primarily of fibrin-bound erythrocytes. Depending on side branches and collateral flow, the extent of thrombus propagation varies greatly both downstream and upstream. Particularly in venous bypass grafts (lacking side branches) and in the right coronary artery (with few major side branches), this secondarily formed clot may contribute significantly to the "thrombotic burden." If not too large, the clot is probably more easily lysed than the primary platelet-rich thrombus at the rupture site.

IV. CLINICO-PATHOLOGICAL CORRELATION

A. Risk Factors

Hyperlipidemia, hypertension, smoking, age, male sex, and diabetes are well-known risk factors for atherosclerotic coronary artery disease. Postmortem studies have shown that there is a clear association between these factors (except smoking) and the amount (volume) of plaques in coronary arteries. However, little is known about an association between risk factors and specific plaque components. There are some indications that smoking correlates most strongly with the thrombotic (rapidly preventable and reversible) plaque component, serum lipids with macrophage foam cells (fatty streaks), and blood pressure particularly with the fibrous component. Surprisingly, hyperlipoproteinemia does not seem to correlate in particular with lipid-rich (vulnerable) plaques. In general, conventional risk factors are not very helpful in predicting the character of coronary lesions.

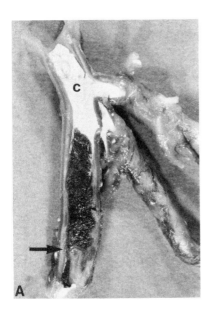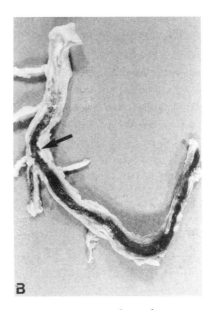

Figure 6 A red erythrocyte/fibrin-rich stagnation thrombus may form secondary to the reduced flow caused by the primary white platelet-rich thrombus at the rupture site. (A) Thrombosed coronary artery has been cut open longitudinally (left anterior descending artery) showing a red stagnation thrombus rich in erythrocytes (similar to a venous thrombus formed in stagnant blood), propagating upstream to the first diagonal branch. (B) Thrombosed right coronary artery has been cut open longitudinally, showing extensive downstream thrombus propagation causing side branch occlusion; a smaller upstream thrombus propagation without side branch occlusion is also seen. Arrow = primary platelet-rich thrombus at ruptured plaque; c = contrast medium.

B. Clinical Disease

Unlike patient-related factors, the actual symptomatic status correlates strongly with the morphological features of the culprit lesion. Particularly, the progression from stable to unstable coronary artery disease is clearly related to plaque vulnerability, plaque rupture, and/or luminal thrombosis (plaque type), rather than to extent of disease (plaque volume).

Stable Angina Pectoris

In patients with stable angina, the composition and eccentricity of atherosclerotic plaques vary greatly from individual to individual and from vessel to vessel. Most patients have a mixture of different plaque types in varying proportion, and the characteristics of one plaque may often differ from those of adjacent plaque. The majority of plaques responsible for stable angina are collagen-rich (lipid-poor). Patients with this type of plaque are probably at low risk of experiencing a thrombus-related acute heart attack.

Acute Coronary Syndromes

As mentioned above, acute coronary syndromes are usually caused by a local obstructive thrombus. Depending upon the severity and duration of obstruction and the degree of collateral flow, these athero-thrombotic lesions may give rise to unstable angina, non–Q-wave infarction, and Q-wave infarction. The patho-anatomical substrate responsible for sudden coronary death is often similar to that of unstable angina.

V. IMPLICATIONS FOR TREATMENT

Plaque rupture is a phenomenon in which the cause differs from patient to patient and from plaque to plaque within the same person. Generally, the dynamic interaction between vulnerability of a plaque and external stresses determines the particular moment and site of rupture. Therefore, the risk of plaque rupture may be reduced by modifying two different factors: vulnerability or triggers. The former may predispose the plaque to rupture, whereas the latter may precipitate it.

A. Plaque Stabilization

Clinical and experimental data indicate that the biology of the atherosclerotic vessel (i.e., vasomotion, growth potential, and rupture risk) may change much earlier than the regression of plaque volume. Plaque components associated with vulnerability (soft lipid and macrophages) are more mobile, with greater potential to regress than the usually much more volu-minous solid components (collagen and crystalline choles-terol). Therefore, the vulnerability and rupture risk may change much faster than the volume of the entire plaque, which may explain the results of recent lipid-lowering clinical trials: the incidence of rupture/thrombus-related clinical events decreased despite only minor angiographic improvements. A lipid-lowering regimen apparently stabilizes atherosclerotic plaques, leaving them less vulnerable to rupture even before detectable volume regression.

Another approach is "trigger reduction," with calcium channel blockers and/or beta blockers, for example, which may delay the time to or decrease the extent of a plaque rupture. Although the mechanism by which angiotensin-converting en-zyme inhibitors reduce the incidence of acute myocardial in-farction in patients with compromised left ventricular function is not known, they may theoretically influence both plaque bi-ology and triggers. Or they may reduce the myocardial dam-age by promoting collateral/microvascular development.

Unfortunately, coronary angiography is unable to predict the vulnerability and rupture risk of coronary lesions. Particu-larly, the size of the plaque (degree of stenosis) is not helpful. Therefore, to prevent rupture/thrombosis-related acute heart attacks, therapy needs to address the entire coronary tree (sys-temic), not just the obstructive lesions. In the future, new imaging techniques may help identify soft, rupture-prone le-sions, thus guiding the choice of treatment.

B. Evolving, Dynamic Thrombosis

Thrombosis and thrombolysis are dynamic processes occur-ring simultaneously in patients with acute coronary syn-dromes. Thus, the goal of rapid and sustained reperfusion may be reached most effectively by targeting both processes: in-hibiting thrombosis and enhancing thrombolysis. The ISIS-2 trial gave the first clear vision that antithrombotic therapy is crucial in the management of patients with acute myocardial infarction. Aspirin alone reduced mortality to the same extent as streptokinase alone, and the combination of both agents was additive. Aspirin may have prevented reocclusion following streptokinase-induced or endogenous thrombolysis, but the fact that a significant number of patients had unstable angina rather than acute infarction may have influenced the result, as it is known that aspirin is effective in patients with unstable angina.

C. Rethrombosis

Platelets play a key role in early thrombotic reocclusion after initial successful recanalization. Rethrombosis probably depends on the same factors (though dissimilar qualitatively and/or quantitatively) as those responsible for the initial event, i.e., (1) the residual thrombogenic substrate, especially residual thrombus, (2) local flow disturbances (residual stenosis/flow), and (3) the acute thrombotic-thrombolytic equilibrium. Recent clinical studies indicate that the latter, the systemic thrombotic propensity, is indeed very important in reocclusion. A severe stenosis will often be present immediately after otherwise successful thrombolysis, probably due to preexisting atherosclerosis and residual thrombus. Particularly, if severe, the residual stenosis may reocclude rapidly and marked irregularity of the infarct-related lesion seems to predispose to early clinical instability. These unstable features may resolve over a few days, probably due to continuing endogenous thrombolysis, while subsequent remodeling may improve the result further.

D. Failed Thrombolysis

Persistent occlusion despite pharmacological thrombolysis remains a problem. Current thrombolytic regimens fail to recanalize a substantial proportion of infarct-related arteries, although thrombus usually underlies persistent occlusions. The mechanisms of resistance to thrombolysis are not known, but the relative abundance of platelets in relation to erythro-

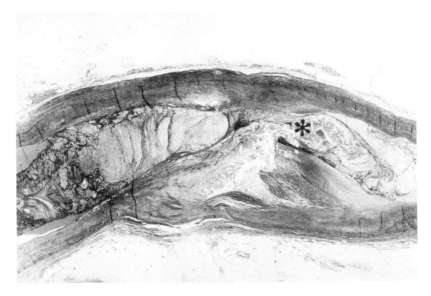

Figure 7 Right coronary artery has been cut open longitudinally, showing plaque rupture with extrusion of atheromatous "gruel" with cholesterol crystals (asterisk) from the plaque into the narrowed lumen, resulting in nonthrombotic vascular occlusion. Erythrocyte/fibrin-rich stagnation thrombus is seen proximal to the occluding "gruel."

cyte/fibrin may explain the apparently intrinsic resistance of some thrombi. Experimental data indicate clearly that platelet-rich thrombi formed on a strong thrombogenic surface are more resistant to lysis than erythrocyte/fibrin-rich "clots." Thrombus formed within severe stenoses is also platelet-rich and may be difficult to lyse, explaining the lower recanalization rate seen in infarct patients with preceding chronic stable angina, indicating an underlying severe atherosclerotic stenosis.

Other causes of unsuccessful thrombolysis could be too large a thrombotic burden due to extensive stagnant thrombus (see Fig. 6B) or nonthrombotic mechanical obstructions such as major plaque "disasters" with dissecting plaque hemorrhages, intimal flaps, or extruded atheromatous plaque material (Fig. 7). Vasospasm probably does not play a major role in the persistence of occlusion.

VI. CONCLUSIONS

Rupture of an atherosclerotic plaque is the main cause of acute coronary syndromes. In most patients, the responsible lesions are moderately stenotic and lipid-rich. In a smaller proportion of patients (20–30%), minor superficial damage on a severely stenotic plaque causes these syndromes. The thrombus that forms at the rupture site usually waxes and wanes over a period of time causing intermittent flow obstruction; thrombosis and thrombolysis are dynamic processes occurring simultaneously. The severity and duration of obstruction and the degree of collateral development determine the clinical manifestation: unstable angina, non–Q-wave infarction, Q-wave infarction, or sudden ischemic death. Optimal treatment for the individual patient should differ according to the underlying athero-thrombotic lesion. Unfortunately, the clinical presentation is usually not helpful in determining *the specific* patho-anatomic substrate present in the individual patient. However, antithrombotic therapy is universally recommended in acute coronary syndromes.

PERTINENT REFERENCES

Badimon L, Badimon J J: Mechanisms of arterial thrombosis in nonparallel streamlines: platelet thrombi grow on the apex of stenotic severely injured vessel wall. Experimental study in the pig model. *J Clin Invest* 1989;84:1134–1144.

Braunwald E: Coronary artery patency in patients with myocardial infarction (editorial). *JACC* 1990;16:1550–1552.

Brown B G, Gallery C A, Badger R S, Kennedy J W, Mathey D, Bolson E L, Dodge H T: Incomplete lysis of thrombus in the moderate underlying atherosclerotic lesion during intracoronary infusion of streptokinase for acute myocardial infarction: quantitative angiographic observations. *Circulation* 1986;73:653–661.

Chesebro J H, Fuster V: Dynamic thrombosis and thrombolysis. Role of antithrombins (editorial). *Circulation* 1991;83:1815–1817.

Cohen M, Sherman W, Rentrop K P, Gorlin R: Determinants of collateral filling observed during sudden controlled coronary artery occlusion in human subjects. *J Am Coll Cardiol* 1989;13:297–303.

Davies M J: Successful and unsuccessful coronary thrombolysis (editorial). *Br Heart J* 1989;61:381–384.

Falk E: Unstable angina with fatal outcome: dynamic coronary thrombosis leading to infarction and/or sudden death. Autopsy evidence of recurrent mural thrombosis with peripheral embolization culminating in total vascular occlusion. *Circulation* 1985;71:699–708.

Falk E: Why do plaques rupture? *Circulation* 1992;86(suppl III):30–42.

Folts J: An in vivo model of experimental arterial stenosis, intimal damage, and periodic thrombosis. *Circulation* 1991;83(suppl IV):3–14.

Fuster V, Badimon L, Badimon J J, Chesebro J H: The pathogenesis of coronary artery disease and the acute coronary syndromes. *N Engl J Med* 1992;326:242–250, 310–318.

Goto S, Ikeda Y, Murata M, Handa M, Takahashi E, Yoshioka A, Fujimura Y, Fukuyama M, Handa S, Ogawa S: Epinephrine augments von Willebrand factor-dependent shear-induced platelet aggregation. *Circulation* 1992;86:1859–1863.

Jang I K, Gold H K, Ziskind A A, Fallon J T, Holt R E, Leinbach R C, May J W, Collen D: Differential sensitivity of erythrocyte-rich and platelet-rich arterial thrombi to lysis with recombinant tissue-type plasminogen activator. A possible explanation for resistance to coronary thrombolysis. *Circulation* 1989;79:920—928.

Jang I K, Gold H K, Leinbach R C, Fallon J T, Collen D: In vivo thrombin inhibition enhances and sustains arterial recanalization with recombinant tissue-type plasminogen activator. *Circ Res* 1990;67:1552–1561.

Jorgensen L, Rowsell H C, Hovig T, Mustard J F: Resolution and organization of platelet-rich mural thrombi in carotid arteries of swine. *Am J Pathol* 1967;51:681–719.

Mizuno K, Miyamoto A, Satomura K, Kurita A, Arai T, Sakurada M, Yanagida S, Nakamura H: Angioscopic coronary macromorphology in patients with acute coronary disorders. *Lancet* 1991;337:809–812.

Mizuno K, Satomura K, Miyamoto A, et al. Angioscopic evaluation of coronary-artery thrombi in acute coronary syndrome. *N Engl J Med* 1992;326:287–291.

Muller J E, Tofler G H, Stone P H: Circadian variation and triggers of onset of acute cardiovascular disease. *Circulation* 1989;79:733–743.

Muller J E, Tofler G H: Circadian variation and cardiovascular disease (editorial). *N Engl J Med* 1991;325:1038–1039.

Roux S, Christeller S, Ludin E: Effects of aspirin on coronary reocclusion and recurrent ischemia after thrombolysis: a meta-analysis. *J Am Coll Cardiol* 1992;19:671–677.

Sabia P J, Powers E R, Ragosta M, Sarembock I J, Burwell L R, Kaul S: An association between collateral blood flow and myocardial viability in patients with recent myocardial infarction. *N Engl J Med* 1992;327:1825–1831.

Shah P K: Pathophysiology of unstable angina. *Cardiology Clinics* 1991;9:11–26.

Sobel B E, Hirsh J: Principles and practice of coronary thrombolysis and conjunctive treatment. *Am J Cardiol* 1991;68:382–388.

Stary H C: Composition and classification of human atherosclerotic lesions (review). *Virchows Archiv Pathol Anat Histopathol* 1992;421:277–290.

Taeymans Y, Theroux P, Lesperance J, Waters D: Quantitative angiographic morphology of the coronary artery lesions at risk of thrombotic occlusion. *Circulation* 1992;85:78–85.

Waters D, Lam J Y T: Is thrombolytic therapy striking out in unstable angina? (editorial). *Circulation* 1992;86:1642–1644.

Zeiher A M, Schachinger V, Weitzel S H, Wollschlager H, Just H: Intracoronary thrombus formation causes focal vasoconstriction of epicardial arteries in patients with coronary artery disease. *Circulation* 1991;83:1519–1525.

4

The Objectives of Coronary Thrombolysis

David de Bono
University of Leicester and Glenfield General Hospital
Leicester, United Kingdom

I. INTRODUCTION

The ultimate objective of coronary thrombolysis is to restore the state of health that existed prior to coronary thrombosis. There are three components to this: preservation of life, preservation of myocardial integrity, and preservation of coronary patency. In practice, achievement of these objectives must be accomplished with the minimum risk of adverse side effects, particularly those with long-term consequences such as stroke. This chapter will explore the extent to which the objectives are interdependent, will discuss how far they have been attained or are attainable, and will consider the implications both for current therapy and for future trials.

II. CORONARY THROMBOLYSIS WORKS BY OPENING THROMBOSED CORONARY ARTERIES: TRUE OR FALSE?

The historical debate concerning the relationship of coronary thrombosis to myocardial infarction has already been considered in Chapter 1. There is no longer serious dispute that the vast majority of myocardial infarcts result from coronary thrombosis and that this usually occurs on the basis of a cracked or ruptured atheromatous plaque. All currently used thrombolytic agents have been shown to recanalize thrombosed coronary arteries clinically and in animal models. The moment when flow is restored is frequently marked by transient arrhythmias and electrocardiographic repolarization changes, and sometimes by functional improvement. There is a consistent survival benefit in patients with patent infarct-related coronary arteries compared to those with occluded arteries, irrespective of whether patency was achieved spontaneously, by thrombolytic therapy or by angioplasty.

In animal models, studies of the extent of myocardial necrosis at different time intervals after coronary occlusion provided an apparent parallel to clinical thrombolysis with their demonstration of a quantitative relationship between myocardial necrosis and time between coronary occlusion and recanalization. This appeared to be mirrored clinically in the GISSI-1 trial, in which a steep time-dependent relationship between the institution of thrombolysis and survival was demonstrated. It should be noted, however, that whereas animal studies suggested no further myocardial salvage after 3 hours of total ischemia, clinical benefit in GISSI-1 was seen at 9 hours and in ISIS-2 at 24 hours after the onset of symptoms. The wider therapeutic window in clinical trials was attributed to intermittent rather than total occlusion, to the uncertainty of pinpointing the onset of ischemia, or to other factors such as preconditioning.

III. WHAT IS AN "OPEN ARTERY"?

Coronary arteriography is capable of displaying the shape and dimensions of the coronary lumen with some accuracy, but is less good at measuring coronary flow. TIMI investigators distinguished between "complete perfusion" (grade 3) in which an infarct-related vessel opacified as rapidly as unaffected vessels of similar size, and incomplete perfusion, in which perfusion as assessed by the inflow of contrast was less rapid than in

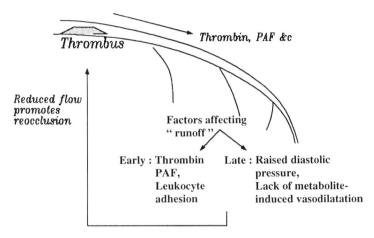

Figure 1 Interdependence of patency at the original site of thrombosis and "runoff" determined by microvascular patency and tone.

equivalent unaffected vessels. It is now clear that grade 3, but not grade 2, perfusion is associated with myocardial salvage, and assessments of patency or reperfusion based on combining grade 3 and grade 2 perfusion are overoptimistic. Even if flow through large coronary vessels is rapid, perfusion of small intramyocardial vessels may be diminished after proximal thrombotic occlusion and recanalization. This "no-reflow" phenomenon has variously been attributed to endothelial damage, to plugging of capillaries with leukocytes, to edema, and to the vasoplastic effects of thrombin, thromboxane, and platelet aggregating factor (PAF) released from the proximal thrombus. It is possible, and indeed likely, that adjunctive therapy with appropriate inhibitors will improve tissue perfusion to an extent not immediately apparent from observations on large vessel patency, although their effects may be reflected in reduced reocclusion rates (Fig. 1).

IV. POTENTIAL PROBLEMS WITH THE SIMPLE OPEN-ARTERY HYPOTHESIS

If coronary thrombolysis works by opening occluded coronary arteries, then agents or regimens that produce prompter and more reliable opening would be expected to produce better survival and more myocardial salvage. The TIMI-1 trial and ECSG-2 trial of recombinant tissue plasminogen activator (alteplase) against streptokinase both indicated superior early coronary patency rates with alteplase. However, tissue plasminogen activator, whether as alteplase (GISSI-2, International Study Group) or duteplase (ISIS-3), has not been shown to be superior to streptokinase in large-scale mortality end-point trials.

Another problem with the open artery → myocardial salvage → survival hypothesis is that the close relationship between arterial patency and myocardial preservation shown in early trials with a very short delay between symptom onset and therapy is much harder to demonstrate in larger multicenter trials. White and colleagues showed no difference in left ventricular function between patients treated with alteplase and streptokinase, and more surprisingly, the ECSG-IV study showed only modest differences in left ventricular function or enzymatic infarct size in surviving patients treated with alteplase or placebo. The ECSG-V study showed no difference in left ventricular function between patients treated with alteplase or with a more aggressive regimen involving early angioplasty, and even when allowance was made for unsuccessful angioplasty, differences were small. Van de Werf has pondered the apparent paradox that trials have tended to show *either* improved left ventricular function *or* better survival, but seldom both.

V. MODIFICATIONS TO THE SIMPLE OPEN ARTERY HYPOTHESIS

The most obvious answer to the criticism that neither GISSI-2/ISG nor ISIS-3 showed the advantage to tissue plasminogen activator that would have been anticipated from TIMI-1 is that neither employed precisely the same supporting regimen (intravenous heparin, aspirin) and that this might have affected both the initial patency rate and also the extent to which patency was sustained. Several studies reporting after GISSI-2 and ISIS-3 were designed have emphasized the importance of effective anticoagulation in maintaining patency after tissue plasminogen activator thrombolysis and have implied that early and clinically silent reocclusion may have negated any advantage of alteplase or duteplase in the GISSI-2 or ISIS-3 trials. Previous angiographic studies were either too small to be capable of detecting any survival benefit or were incapable of assessing the time course of patency because angiograms were performed at a single time point. The current (spring 1993) GUSTO trial addresses these issues by comparing streptokinase and alteplase in the presence of different ancillary regimens and by performing angiograms (in a trial subgroup) at different intervals after therapy. Meanwhile, the open artery hypothesis has to be made more specific by relating outcome to early and *sustained* coronary patency.

VI. DISPARITY BETWEEN SURVIVAL AND MYOCARDIAL SALVAGE: REAL OR ARTIFACT?

The issue concerning the apparent disparity between myocardial salvage and survival needs separate consideration. Initially, the prospect of some measure of "outcome" less onerous than total mortality seemed attractive. Measurement of left ventricular ejection fraction requires meticulous attention to detail if it is to be reproducible between centers. The Auckland, New Zealand Group has suggested that left ventricular end-systolic volume may be the most reliable measurement. Yet difficulties in correlating improvement in ventricular function with patency and survival have led to doubts, and to the suggestion that left ventricular function may not be a practicable "surrogate" for survival. To some extent, the problem is one of analysis. Should nonsurviving patients be excluded from analysis of ventricular function or infarct size, or should they be included and allocated an "imputed" value based on the worst values of surviving patients? Even if the latter solution is

Table 1 Advantages and Disadvantages of Left Ventricular Function as a Measure of Thrombolytic Outcome

Advantages	Disadvantages
Left ventricular function correlates with late survival and functional capacity	Missing patients, likely to be those with extreme values or who have died
Several invasive and noninvasive methods available	Can be major problems with interlab reproducibility, especially for noninvasive methods
Continuous variable for statistical analysis	Highly nonlinear relation between left ventricular function and survival. Most points lie close to mean, but outliers important

adopted, differences between thrombolytic-treated and control patients may remain small. In any trial conducted in multiple centers, intercenter variations in measurement, particularly when noninvasive techniques are used, make it difficult to assess differences between treatment groups (Table 1). Left ventricular function does not necessarily remain constant after infarction but changes with time to different extents according to the site of infarction and with the use of different medications.

Even allowing for these uncertainties, there is a definite impression that there is a quantitative, and possibly qualitative, difference in the patency–left ventricular function survival relationship between patients who receive very early restoration of patency and patients in whom reperfusion is delayed beyond, perhaps 3 hours. In the former, there is a good chance of preserving ventricular function as well as a major survival benefit; in the latter there is still a worthwhile improvement in survival, but permanent ventricular impairment is likely and there is a disparity between survival and functional data. In order to explain this, it is important to remember that both the increase in mortality risk with loss of ventricular function and the loss of myocardium with increasing ischemia time are highly nonlinear functions.

Early in the course of ischemia, there is progressive irreversible muscle loss, but a patient with a previously healthy heart can tolerate this without risk of dying from pump failure. Later, muscle loss takes place over a much slower time course, but death from pump failure becomes progressively more likely.

A further and more controversial factor that may affect the relationship between vessel patency and myocardial salvage is reperfusion injury. It is suggested that under certain circumstances the abrupt restoration of blood flow to critically ischemic muscle can actually accelerate muscle damage. A variety of mechanisms have been suggested, including oxygen free radical–mediated damage, complement activation, and leukocyte-mediated damage. (The topic is discussed in detail in Chapter 15.)

VII. THE RISKS AND CONSEQUENCES OF REOCCLUSION

There is an important distinction between reocclusion as assessed by angiography and reinfarction as diagnosed on the basis of clinical symptoms and enzymatic and electrocardiographic changes. Early reocclusion may be clinically indistinguishable from the effects of the original thrombosis; late reocclusion may be clinically silent because a collateral circulation has developed or because there is in fact no viable muscle supplied by the occluded vessel. As a general rule, reocclusion is perceived as a greater clinical problem in studies that have adopted an earlier and more aggressive approach to reperfusion, especially if this has involved angioplasty or early angiography. The very low early reinfarction rates in large clinical trials conducted principally in general hospitals almost certainly reflect the difficulty of diagnosing the problem rather than its absence. Late assessment of vessel patency is no answer, as slow spontaneous restoration of patency may occur irrespective of early reocclusion. Serial angiography is the best way of following the time course of patency, but is difficult now to justify. Staged angiography, as in the GUSTO trial, is the next best alternative. Practically, the more widespread use of multilead ST segment monitoring may lead both to better noninvasive detection of failure to reperfuse and to better detection of reocclusion.

VIII. CONCLUSIONS

Coronary thrombolysis has unequivocally been shown to improve survival, but at best mortality in large-scale trials has been no more than halved. We do not know for certain whether this reflects a conceptual limitation to thrombolytic therapy or the imperfection of current techniques. Some of the ways in which our concept of objectives of coronary thrombolysis have changed in the light of evolving knowledge are summarized in Figure 2. The idea that early restoration of patency is a crucial part of the mechanism by which thrombolytic therapy achieves its benefits remains valid, but maintenance of patency is also important, and the possibility that in some patients the acute restoration of bloodflow may be followed by further myocardial damage cannot be excluded. The overall effect of thrombolytic therapy on preservation of left ventricular function has been disappointing, but this conceals a combination of very effective preservation with early thrombolysis and mediocre preservation with delayed thrombolysis. Long-term coronary patency is reflected in diminished infarct expansion, but it is arguable whether late patency preserves viable myocardium or vice versa. Despite its success, coronary thrombolysis is still a long way from reaching all its objectives, and the technical achievement of large-scale clinical trials has to be matched by the imagination and perceptiveness of the questions they ask.

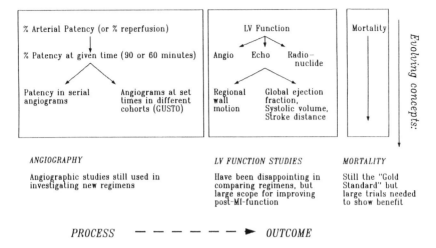

Figure 2   How concepts about the objectives of coronary thrombolysis have changed in the light of evolving knowledge.

PERTINENT REFERENCES

Arnold A E R, Serruys P W, Rutsch W, et al.: Reasons for the lack of benefit of immediate angioplasty during recombinant tissue plasminogen activator therapy for acute myocardial infarction: a regional wall motion analysis. *J Am Coll Cardiol* 1991;17:11–20.

Been M, de Bono D P, Muir A L, Boulton F E, Fears R, Standring R, Ferres H: Clinical effects and pharmocokinetics of intravenous APSAC—anisoylated plasminogen-streptokinase activator complex (BRL26921)—in acute myocardial infarction. *Int J Cariol* 1986;11:53–61.

Bleich S D, Nichols T C, Schumacher R R, et al.: Effect of heparin on coronary arterial patency after thrombolysis with tissue plasminogen activator in acute myocardial infraction. *Am J Cardiol* 1990;66:1412–1417.

Califf R M, Harrelson-Woodlief L, Topol E J: Left ventricular ejection fraction may not be useful as an end point of thrombolytic therapy comparative trials. *Circulation* 1990;82:1847–1853.

Califf R M, O'Neill W W, Stack R S, et al.: Failure of simple clinical measurements to predict perfusion status after intravenous thrombolysis. *Ann Intern Med* 1988;108:658–662.

Chesebro J H, Knatterud G, Roberts R, et al.: Thrombolysis in myocardial infarction (TIMI) trial, phase I: a comparison between intravenous tissue
  plasminogen activator and intravenous streptokinase. *Circulation*
  1987;76:142–154.

Cigarroa R G, Lange R A, Hillis L D: Prognosis after acute myocardial infarction in patients with and without residual anterograde coronary
  blood flow. *Am J Cardiol* 1989;64:155–160.

Davies M J, Thomas A C: Plaque fissuring: the cause of acute myocardial infarction, sudden ischaemic death, and crescendo angina. Br Heart J
  1985;53:363–373.

de Bono D P, Simoons M R, Tijssen J, et al.: Effect of early intravenous heparin on coronary patency, infarct size, and bleeding complications after
  alteplase thrombolysis: results of a randomised double blind European
  Cooperative Study Group trial. *Br Heart J* 1992;67:122–128.

De Feyter P J, van Eenige M J, van der Wall E E, et al.: Effects of spontaneous
  and streptokinase-induced recanalisation on left ventricular function after myocardial infarction. *Circulation* 1983;67:1039–1044.

De Wood M A, Spores J, Notske R, Mouser L T, Burroughs R, Golden M S,
  Lang H T: Prevalence of total coronary occlusion during the early hours
  of transmural myocardial infarction. *N Engl J Med* 1980;303:897–902.

Gruppo Italiano per lo Studio della Sopravivvenza nell'Infarto Miocardico:
  GISSI-2: A factorial randomised trial of alteplase versus streptokinase
  and heparin versus no heparin among 12,490 patients with acute myocardial infarction. *Lancet* 1990;336:65–71.

Gruppo Italiano per lo Studio della Streptochinasi nell'Infarto Miocardico
  (GISSI): Effectiveness of intravenous thrombolytic treatment in acute
  myocardial infarction. *Lancet* 1986;i:397–402.

Hsia J, Hamilton W P, Kleiman N, Roberts R, Chaitman B R, Ross A M: A
  comparison between heparin and low-dose aspirin as adjunctive therapy with tissue plasminogen activator for acute myocardial infarction. *N
  Engl J Med* 1990;323:1433–1437.

The International Study Group: In-hospital mortality and clinical course of
  20,891 patients with suspected acute myocardial infarction randomised
  between alteplase and streptokinase with or without heparin. *Lancet*
  1990;336:71–75.

ISIS-2 Collaborative Group: Randomised trial of intravenous streptokinase,
  oral aspirin, both or neither among 17,187 cases of suspected acute myocardial infarction: ISIS-2. *Lancet* 1988;ii:349–360.

ISIS-3 (Third International Study of Infarct Survival) Collaborative Group.
  ISIS-3: A randomised comparison of streptokinase vs tissue plasminogen

activator vs anistreplase and of aspirin plus heparin vs aspirin alone among 41229 cases of suspected acute myocardial infarction. *Lancet* 1992;339:753–770.

Koren G, Weiss A T, Hasin Y, et al.: Prevention of myocardial damage in acute myocardial ischemia by early treatment with intravenous streptokinase. *N Engl J Med* 1985;313:1384–1389.

Krucoff M W, Wagner N B, Pope J E, et al.: The portable programmable microprocessor-driven real-time 12-lead electrocardiographic monitor: a preliminary report of a new device for the noninvasive detection of successful reperfusion or silent coronary reocclusion. *Am J Cardiol* 1990;65:143–148.

Kwon K, Freedman S B, Wilcox I, et al.: The unstable ST segment early after thrombolysis for acute infarction and its usefulness as a marker of recurrent coronary occlusion. *Am J Cardiol* 1991;67:109–115.

Mathey D G, Schofer J, Sheehan F H, Becker H, Tilsner V, Dodge H T: Intravenous urokinase in acute myocardial infarction. *Am J Cardiol* 1985;55:878–882.

Norris R M, White H D: Therapeutic trials in coronary thrombosis should measure left ventricular function as primary end-point of treatment. *Lancet* 1988;1:104–106.

Rapold H J, de Bono D P, Arnold A E R, Arnout J, De Cock F, Collen D, Verstraete M: Plasma fibrinopeptide A levels in patients with acute myocardial infarction treated with alteplase: correlation with concomitant heparin, coronary artery patency, and recurrent ischemia. *Circulation* 1992;85:928–954.

Reimer K A, Lowe J E, Rasmussen M M, Jennings R B: The wave front phenomenon of ischemic cell death: 1. Myocardial infarct size vs duration of coronary occlusion in dogs. *Circulation* 1977;56:786–794.

Serruys P W, Arnold A E R, Brower R W, et al.: Effect of continued rt-PA administration on the residual stenosis after initially successful recanalization in acute myocardial infarction—a quantitative angiographic study of a randomized trial. *Eur Heart J.* 1987;8:1172–1181.

Serruys P W, Simoons M L, Suryapranata H, et al.: Preservation of global and regional left ventricular function after early thrombolysis in acute myocardial infarction. *J Am Coll Cardiol* 1986;7:729–742.

Simoons M L, Arnold A E R, Betriu A, et al.: Thrombolysis with tissue plasminogen activator in acute myocardial infarction: no additional benefit from immediate percutaneous coronary angioplasty. *Lancet* 1988;i:197–203.

Van de Werf F: Discrepancies between the effects of coronary reperfusion on survival and left ventricular function. *Lancet* 1989;2:1367–1369.

Van de Werf F, Arnold A E R for the European Cooperative Study Group: Intravenous tissue plasminogen activator and size of infarct, left ventricular function, and survival in acute myocardial infarction. *Br Med J* 1988;297:1374–1379.

Verstraete M, Arnold A E R, Brower R W, et al.: Acute coronary thrombolysis with recombinant human tissue type plasminogen activator: initial patency and effect of a maintenance infusion. *Am J Cardiol* 1987;60:231–237.

Verstraete M, Bernard R, Bory M, et al.: Randomised trial of intravenous recombinant tissue type plasminogen activator versus streptokinase in acute myocardial infarction. *Lancet* 1985;i:842–847.

White H D, Norris R M, Brown M A, Brandt P W T, Whitlock R M L, Wild C J: Left ventricular end-systolic volume as the major determinant of survival after recovery from myocardial infarction. *Circulation* 1987;76:44–51.

White H D, Rivers J T, Maslowski A H, et al.: Effect of intravenous streptokinase as compared with that of tissue type plasminogen activator on left ventricular function after first myocardial infarction. *N Engl J Med* 1989;320:817–821.

5

The Impact of Time to Treatment on the Efficacy of Coronary Thrombolysis

Burton E. Sobel
Washington University School of Medicine and Barnes Hospital
St. Louis, Missouri

I. INTRODUCTION

Despite compelling evidence that early and sustained coronary recanalization is the mechanism by which coronary thrombolysis confers benefit to the heart, the relevance of early recanalization to clinical benefit has been debated intensely. Skeptics have sometimes summarily dismissed the pertinence of observations in studies of laboratory animals that are consistent with the principle that infarction is dynamic and can be arrested by early reperfusion, thereby salvaging jeopardized ischemic myocardium. They have also questioned whether improved left ventricular function, diminution of subsequent recurrent ischemia, and enhanced survival depend on salvage of myocardium and the recanalization responsible for it. Nevertheless, it is becoming clear that these principles are fundamental.

II. EARLY OBSERVATIONS

The potential value of coronary thrombolysis was realized only when a rationale had evolved in which salvage of ischemic myocardium was central. The conventional wisdom of the 1950s dictated that acute myocardial infarction resulted either in death or in survival, with no gray area between. However, after electrical defibrillation had become available and was employed widely in the then new coronary care units, survival increased dramatically, with hospital mortality declining from 30 to 15% in patients hospitalized with bona fide transmural infarction. It soon became evident that the status of survivors ranged from profound affliction with severe pump failure, cardiogenic shock, and imminent demise to apparent good health. The enigmatic diversity of outcome and the paucity of information explaining its causes led Braunwald and colleagues to formulate and ultimately validate the hypothesis that outcome after acute myocardial infarction in patients who survived the initial insult was dependent upon the extent of irreversibly injured myocardium. A corollary was that jeopardized, ischemic myocardium could be salvaged by reduction of myocardial oxygen requirements, augmentation of myocardial oxygen supply, or both during a temporal window in which ischemic myocardium would have otherwise become irreversibly injured.

In studies in experimental animals, several interventions designed to reduce myocardial oxygen requirements were shown to be capable of preserving jeopardized ischemic myocardium despite the presence of an induced coronary occlusion. Soon after, it became clear that the interval during which salvage could be implemented was markedly circumscribed and that irreversible myocardial injury occurred quickly when perfusion was interrupted for intervals as brief as 20–60 minutes. This profound temporal dependence probably explains the failure of clinical studies designed to salvage myocardium by reducing myocardial oxygen requirements to demonstrate benefits proportional to those seen in experimental animals in which the intervention could be implemented much more rapidly with respect to the time of onset of ischemia.

In dogs with experimentally induced coronary thrombosis, salvage of myocardium was striking when reperfusion was induced within a few hours. By contrast, reperfusion induced substantially later exerted no apparent benefit. Thus, investigators soon recognized the remarkable dependence of the extent and severity of irreversible ischemic injury on the duration of ischemia and the remarkable temporal dependence of benefit inducible by recanalization on the rapidity of its implementation.

III. RELATIONSHIPS BETWEEN SALVAGE OF MYOCARDIUM AND CLINICAL BENEFIT

These concepts, developed initially in studies in laboratory animals, were soon applied to patients. In the landmark GISSI-1 trial, the reduction of mortality in patients treated with streptokinase compared with placebo was particularly striking among those in whom the interval between the onset of chest pain and the time of onset of treatment was brief. Thus, when treatment could be initiated in the first hour after the onset of the apparent index infarction, the reduction in mortality attributable to early recanalization was 47%. By contrast, no significant reduction in mortality was evident in patients who could be treated only 6 hours or more after the onset of chest pain. Analogous observations were soon made in the European cooperative trial of intravenous tissue-type plasminogen activator (t-PA) compared with placebo. In that study, overall mortality 3 months after the onset of the index infarction was reduced by more than 33% (not statistically significant). However, in patients who were treated within 3 hours of the onset of symptoms, the reduction was particularly striking (59%). A similar dependence of benefit on the brevity of ischemia preceding treatment was noted in the ISIS-2 trial of intravenous streptokinase compared with placebo. Again, the most striking reduction of mortality was evident in patients who were treated very early. Thus, reduction was 56% in patients treated within the first hour after the onset of chest pain but only 39% in the trial overall.

In concert, observations from studies in laboratory animals and patients are consistent with the hypothesis that early and sustained restitution of myocardial perfusion is the critical determinant of benefit conferred by coronary thrombolysis. Thus, whether one considers restoration of depressed function in regions of myocardium subserved by thrombotically occluded coronary arteries, regional myocardial metabolism reflected by oxidation of fatty acids measured with positron emission tomography, or survival itself, the conclusion is the same.

IV. THE CONUNDRUM OF POTENTIAL BENEFITS OF LATE RECANALIZATION

On the basis of the etiology of infarction and its sequelae, it is certainly not surprising that early recanalization maintains myocardial viability, restores regional wall motion, and improves prognosis—conclusions compatible with the now well-recognized wavefront of myocardial necrosis that progresses over time. However, it appears that even late recanalization can confer benefit. Patients who are discharged from the hospital with a spontaneously patent infarct-related artery fare better than those whose infarct-related artery is found to have remained persistently occluded. Yet, this observation does not prove that therapeutically induced late recanalization will necessarily be beneficial. Some investigators have suggested that prognosis is indeed improved when infarct artery patency is restored even long after the onset of an index infarction. Nevertheless, these observations as well as the results in studies of the natural history of infarction demonstrating a more favorable outcome in patients who are discharged with a patent infarct-related artery are subject to ambiguous interpretation. For example, it may well be the case that patients in whom late, therapeutically induced recanalization appears to bestow benefit are those in whom occult spontaneous recanalization has occurred intermittently early after the onset of infarction, while jeopardized, ischemic myocardium can still be salvaged. Thus, the late, therapeutically induced recanalization may simply consolidate benefits conferred by unrecognized, earlier spontaneous recanalization in this subset of patients. Regrettably, it will never be possible, because of ethical considerations, to perform a study that can definitively address this question. To do so, one would have to identify patients in whom infarct-related artery occlusion was documented to be present and persistent for many hours after the onset of infarction, to randomize the identified patients without inducing immediate recanalization into a treatment and placebo group, and to pharmacologically induce coronary thrombolysis only in the treatment group at selected intervals late after the onset of infarction after a long interval during which uninterrupted thrombotic coronary occlusion was documented to persist. Such a design is untenable. If one recognized persistent occlusion in a patient in whom salvage of myocardium subserved by the infarct-related artery might still be possible, it would be incumbent upon the investigator to restore perfusion immediately in order to preclude unmitigated myocardial cell death.

Despite the conundrum of whether or not exclusively late recanalization is beneficial, several mechanisms have been proposed to explain its possible benefits. Among these is the provision of conduits for the development of collateral blood flow, facilitation of healing and remodeling of irreversibly injured ventricular myocardium, reduction of arrhythmogenicity secondary to maintenance of survival of jeopardized myocardium adjacent to zones of completed infarction, diminution of the severity of ventricular aneurysm formation, amelioration of ventricular dilatation and hence diminution of wall stress with consequent improvement in the balance between myocardial oxygen availability and oxygen supply, and improved electrophysiological stability of cells in peri-infarct zones.

Those who advocate late coronary thrombolysis recognize that the quantitative impact of this intervention is more modest than the quantitative impact of early recanalization. Thus, compared with the reductions of mortality as great as 50% in patients treated within 1 hour of the onset of infarction with fibrinolytic drugs compared with placebo (GISSI-1) and absolute mortality rates as low as 1% in patients treated with t-PA and i.v. heparin within 90 minutes in a prehospital treatment trial (MITI), absolute mortality rates in patients treated late with fibrinolytic drugs compared with placebo differ only slightly. Accordingly, whether or not late recanalization per se in the absence of recognized or unrecognized occult earlier spontaneous recanalization can confer benefit, no one would claim that the primary objective should be exclusively late rather than early coronary thrombolysis.

V. AMBIGUITIES IN THE INTERPRETATIONS OF RESULTS OF CLINICAL TRIALS

Unfortunately, much of the debate regarding clinical trial results has been characterized by imprecise delineation of and inadequate recognition of the seminal importance of the timing of coronary thrombolysis. Thus, although it is well accepted that fibrin-selective fibrinolytic agents (such as t-PA and prourokinase) induce coronary recanalization more rapidly and more often compared with first-generation, nonselective fibrinolytic agents such as streptokinase and urokinase, some have claimed that the clinical implications of the differences are modest or trivial. Such claims rest largely on results of three types of studies.

In one type of study, late patency of the infarct-related artery (e.g., after 7–10 days) is considered to be the criterion for comparison. It is well known that as many as 50–70% of infarct-related arteries will recanalize spontaneously, without any treatment of the patient with a fibrinolytic drug. Accordingly, differences in patency that would be evident earlier in patients treated with one as opposed to another agent diminish with time—a phenomenon called "catch-up." However, it is the induction of patency early that salvages myocardium. Accordingly, even though catch-up obscures drug-dependent differences when only late angiography is used for evaluation of efficacy, the unrecognized difference in early patency is what matters in studies relying upon late angiography as the sole or primary end point. The presence of catch-up does not belie the clinical importance of differences in the induction of early patency.

In the second type of study, drug-dependent differences are evaluated in terms of late global ventricular function and found to be lacking. However, clinically effective thrombolysis often does not change global ventricular function despite improving the regional function of jeopardized ischemic myocardium because the initially compensatory hyperfunction in normal myocardium, driven by adrenergic stimulation, regresses as impairment in the jeopardized zones is attenuated. Furthermore, average global ventricular function in successfully treated patients may be low because of survival of patients with markedly impaired ventricles who would otherwise have succumbed and inclusion of data from them in the analysis of ventricular function in the entire group (the ventricular function/mortality paradox discussed by Dr. Van de Werf).

In the third type of study that has failed to delineate drug-dependent differences that may well have been present, mortality has been a primary end point, yet no significant differences were seen no matter what type of fibrinolytic agent was used. However, studies such as the GISSI-2 and ISIS-3 mega-trials in which fibrinolytic drug–dependent differences in mortality were not observed suffer from several potential weaknesses that may explain the lack of observation of a difference. One is the inclusion of many patients treated late after the apparent onset of infarction (the median time to treatment in ISIS-3 was 4 hr). A second is the lack of adequately aggressive, prompt anticoagulation with bolus followed by constant infusion of intravenous heparin, necessary to sustain recanalization and capture the benefits of early restoration of patency seen with fibrin-selective compared with nonselective drugs. Differential benefit conferred by earlier, more frequent induction of patency, or both, may therefore have been obviated by a high incidence of therapeutic failure attributable to lack of persistence of recanalization because of thrombotic reocclusion, particularly in patients treated with fibrin-selective agents in whom generation of fibrinogen degradation products that confer some anticoagulant properties is modest. Conversely, in smaller mechanistic trials in which fibrin-selective compared with nonselective agents have been evaluated head-to-head in randomized patients, the increased rapidity and frequency of recanalization associated with fibrin-selective agents has been paralleled by an overall reduction in mortality, highly significant when assessed with conventional statistical methods in a meta analysis.

Thus, it appears that the apparent controversies in the literature can be readily reconciled. Fibrin-selective agents open more infarct-related arteries within the first 60–90 minutes after the onset of treatment than nonselective agents, a fact that is no longer arguable. Early restoration of patency confers benefit, as shown in studies of laboratory animals and patients. Such benefits, when sustained by anticoagulation sufficient to prevent early reocclusion of recanalized vessels, translate into clinical benefit evident in results of many clinical trials. Those studies in which prompt, early recanalization has not been shown to confer clinical benefit are, perhaps, distorted by the inclusion of large numbers of patients who could be treated only late after the onset of index infarctions or by inclusion of many patients in whom early recanalization has been compromised by early thrombotic reocclusion as a result of inadequate anticoagulation.

VI. CONCLUSIONS

There is perhaps no more powerful determinant of the benefit of coronary thrombolysis than the rapidity of its implementation. Recent clinical trials including the MITI and EMIP investigations have demonstrated conclusively that mortality is substantially lower in patients treated with fibrinolytic drugs early after the onset of infarction (e.g., in the prehospital phase) compared with those treated later. The reduced mortality accompanying early treatment is entirely consistent with an extensive body of knowledge acquired over several decades in studies in laboratory animals and patients. Improved patient education to reduce the delay time between the onset of incipient or evolving infarction and entrance into the medical surveillance system, physician education to reduce the interval between presentation of a patient with evolving infarction and the onset of treatment, and education of hospital administrators and personnel responsible for emergency department facilities to reduce delay time to treatment as well are powerful tools for extending the proven benefits of coronary thrombolysis to a larger number of patients at risk. With vigorous, prompt, and judicious implementation of coronary thrombolysis for patients with evolving myocardial infarction accompanied by vigorous anticoagulation to sustain the benefits conferred and avoid early thrombotic reocclusion, the overall mortality associated with acute myocardial infarction in patients 75 years of age or younger can be reduced to the range of 5–6% in marked contrast to the 30% that was common in hospitalized patients only a few decades ago and the 10% common after the implementation of electrical defibrillation in coronary care units.

It has been said that "time is muscle" (S. J. Sarnoff, personal communication). The implication of this epigrammatic statement is obvious. Early recanalization should be the primary objective of pharmacologically induced coronary thrombolysis. Net clinical benefit bestowed by this intervention will of course be contingent upon diverse additional factors, including maintenance of patency with vigorous anticoagulation, definitive amelioration of thrombogenic lesions that would otherwise give rise to recurrent coronary thrombosis, infarction or restenosis, and arrest of progressive coronary atherosclerotic vascular disease to avoid progressive compromise of the coronary vasculature and recurrent infarction after initially successful coronary thrombolysis.

PERTINENT REFERENCES

Bergmann S R, Fox K A A, Geltman E M, Sobel B E: Positron emission tomography of the heart. *Prog Cardiovasc Dis* 1985;28:165–194.

Bergmann S R, Fox K A A, Ter-Pogossian M M, Sobel B E, Collen D: Clot-selective coronary thrombolysis with tissue-type plasminogen activator. *Science* 1983;220:1181–1183.

Bergmann S R, Lerch R A, Fox K A A, Ludbrook P A, Welch M J, Ter-Pogossian M M, Sobel B E: Temporal dependence of beneficial effects of coronary thrombolysis characterized by positron tomography. *Am J Med* 1982;73:573–581.

Boissel J-P: European Myocardial Infarction Project (EMIP): short-term mortality and nonfatal outcomes. Presented at the National Meeting of the American College of Cardiology, Dallas, April 15, 1992.

Braunwald E: Myocardial perfusion, limitation of infarct size, reduction of left ventricular dysfunction, and improved survival: should the paradigm be expanded? *Circulation* 1989;79:441–444.

Chesebro J H, Knatterud G, Roberts R, Borer J, Cohen L S, Dalen J, Dodge H T, Francis C K, Hillis D, Ludbrook P A, Markis J E, Mueller H, Passamani E R, Powers E R, Rao A K, Robertson T, Ross A, Ryan T J, Sobel B E, Willerson J, Williams D O, Zaret B L, Braunwald E: Thrombolysis in myocardial infarction (TIMI) trial, phase I: a comparison between intravenous tissue plasminogen activator and intravenous streptokinase. *Circulation* 1987;76:142–154.

Cigarroa R G, Lange R A, Hillis L D: Prognosis after acute myocardial infarction in patients with and without residual anterograde coronary blood flow. *Am J Cardiol* 1989; 64:155–160.

Collen D: Trials comparing the available thrombolytic agents. *Coronary Artery Dis* 1992;3:117–122.

Fortin D F, Califf R M: Long-term survival from acute myocardial infarction: salutary effect of an open coronary vessel. *Am J Med* 1990;88:9N–15N.

Gruppo Italiano Per Lo Studio Della Streptochinasi Nell'infarto Miocardico (GISSI): Effectiveness of intravenous thrombolytic treatment in acute myocardial infarction. *Lancet* 1986;1:397–401.

Gruppo Italiano Per Lo Studio Della Sopravvivenza Nell'infarto Miocardico: GISSI 2: A factorial randomised trial of alteplase versus streptokinase and heparin versus no heparin among 12,490 patients with acute myocardial infarction. *Lancet* 1990;336:65–71.

Gutovitz A L, Sobel B E, Roberts R: Progressive nature of myocardial injury in selected patients with cardiogenic shock. *Am J Cardiol* 1978;41:469–475.

Hsia J, Hamilton W P, Kleiman N, Roberts R, Chaitman B R, Ross A M, Heparin-Aspirin Reperfusion Trial (HART) Investigators: A comparison between heparin and low-dose aspirin as adjunctive therapy with tissue plasminogen activator for acute myocardial infarction. *N Engl J Med* 1990;323:1433–1437.

International Study Group: In-hospital mortality and clinical course of 20,891 patients with suspected acute myocardial infarction randomised between alteplase and streptokinase with or without heparin. *Lancet* 1990; 336:71–75.

ISIS-2 Collaborative Group: Randomised trial of intravenous streptokinase, oral aspirin, both, or neither among 17,187 cases of suspected acute myocardial infarction: ISIS-2, *Lancet* 1988;2:349–360.

ISIS-3: A randomized comparison of streptokinase vs tissue plasminogen activator vs anistreplase and of aspirin plus heparin vs aspirin alone among 41,299 cases of suspected acute myocardial infarction. *Lancet* 1992;339:753–770.

Maroko P R, Kjekshus J K, Sobel B E, Watanabe T, Covell J W, Ross J, Jr., Braunwald E: Factors influencing infarct size following experimental coronary artery occlusions. *Circulation* 1971;43:67–82.

Reimer K A, Lowe J E, Rasmussen M M, Jennings R B: The wave front phenomenon of ischemic cell death: I. Myocardial infarct size versus duration of coronary occlusion in dogs. *Circulation* 1977;56:786–794.

Roberts R, Croft C, Gold H K, Hartwell T D, Jaffe A S, Muller J E, Mullin S M, Parker C, Passamani E R, Poole W K, Raabe D S, Jr., Rude R E, Stone P H, Turi Z G, Sobel B E, Willerson J T, Braunwald E, MILIS Study Group: Effect of propranolol on myocardial-infarct size in a randomized, blinded, multicenter trial. *N Engl J Med* 1984;311:218–225.

Shell W E, Sobel B E: Protection of jeopardized ischemic myocardium by reduction of ventricular afterload. *N Engl J Med* 1974;291:481–486.

Sobel B E: Infarct size, prognosis, and causal contiguity. *Circulation* 1976;53 (suppl I):146–148.

Sobel B E: Safety and efficacy of tissue-type plasminogen activator produced by recombinant DNA technology (rt-PA). *J Am Coll Cardiol* 1987;10: 40B–44B.

Sobel B E: Conjunctive therapy for thrombolysis. *Coronary Artery Dis* 1992; 3:987–989.

Sobel B E, Bresnahan G F, Shell W E, Yoder R D: Estimation of infarct size in man and its relation to prognosis. *Circulation* 1972;46:640–648.

Sobel B E, Collen D: Questions unresolved by the Third International Study of Infarct Survival. *Am J Cardiol* 1992;70:385–389.

Sobel B E, Hirsh J: Principles and practice of coronary thrombolysis and conjuctive treatment. *Am J Cardiol* 1991;68:382–388.

Sobel B E, Shell W E: Jeopardized, blighted, and necrotic myocardium. *Circulation* 1973;47:215–216.

Tiefenbrunn A J, Sobel B E: Factors contributing to the emergence of coronary thrombolysis. *Cardiol Clin* 1987;5:49–53.

Tiefenbrunn A J, Sobel B E: The impact of coronary thrombolysis on myocardial infarction. *Fibrinolysis* 1989;3:1–15.

Tiefenbrunn A J, Sobel B E: Thrombolysis and myocardial infarction. *Fibrinolysis* 1991;5:1–15.

Tiefenbrunn A J, Sobel B E: Timing of coronary recanalization. Paradigms, paradoxes, and pertinence. *Circulation* 1992;85:2311–2315.

TIMI Study Group: Special report: the Thrombolysis in Myocardial Infarction (TIMI) trial. *N Engl J Med* 1985;312:932–936.

Van de Werf F, Arnold A E R: Intravenous tissue plasminogen activator and size of infarct, left ventricular function, and survival in acute myocardial infarction. *Br Med J* 1988;297:1374–1379.

Van de Werf F, Ludbrook P A, Bergmann S R, Tiefenbrunn A J, Fox K A A, de Geest H, Verstraete M, Collen D, Sobel B E: Coronary thrombolysis with tissue-type plasminogen activator in patients with evolving myocardial infarction. *N Engl J Med* 1984;310:609–613.

Weaver W D: Myocardial Infarction Triage and Intervention (MITI) trial of pre-hospital initiated thrombolysis—results. Presented at the American College of Cardiology National Meeting, Dallas, April 14, 1992.

Wilcox R, LATE Study Group: The LATE study: late assessment of thrombolytic efficacy: double-blind placebo controlled trial of Alteplase given 6-24 hours after onset of symptoms of acute myocardial infarction. Presented at the 14th Congress of the European Society of Cardiology, Barcelona, August 30–September 3, 1992.

6

Procoagulant Effects of Fibrinolytic Agents

Paul R. Eisenberg
Washington University School of Medicine
St. Louis, Missouri

I. INTRODUCTION

The importance of inhibition of procoagulant activity to the success of coronary thrombolysis has only recently been documented. It is now known that maximal reduction of mortality in patients treated with streptokinase for myocardial infarction requires inhibition of platelet activation with aspirin and that the death rate may be reduced further by use of conjunctive anticoagulation with subcutaneous heparin in addition to aspirin. In patients treated with tissue-type plasminogen activator (t-PA), even more aggressive conjunctive anticoagulation with intravenous heparin is necessary to achieve maximal rates of sustained coronary patency. Presumably, the benefits conferred by these conjunctive antithrombotic regimens are primarily attributable to inhibition of recurrent coronary thrombosis.

The mechanisms responsible for recurrent thrombosis after coronary thrombolysis have not been completely characterized but appear to involve increases in procoagulant activity induced by pharmacological activation of plasminogen as well as local expression of procoagulant activity associated with the recanalization of a thrombotic vessel. There is considerable evidence that thrombin is elaborated in response to pharmacological thrombolysis. Thrombin activity increases rapidly after administration of fibrinolytic agents, and these increases are markedly attenuated by conjunctive administration of intravenous heparin. However, because coronary reocclusion occurs after completion of the infusion of the plasminogen activator despite administration of heparin, it is unlikely that the early increases in thrombin activity are the primary determinant of recurrent thrombosis. Ultimately, reocclusion of the recanalized thrombotic vessel depends on the intensity of local procoagulant activity expressed by factors associated with the residual thrombus and the underlying coronary atherosclerotic lesion. However, local procoagulant activity may be modulated by circulating factors. Thus, recurrent thrombosis after coronary thrombolysis depends on a complex interaction between multiple processes, including procoagulant factors associated with the atherosclerotic plaque, procoagulant activity induced by the residual thrombus, the extent to which pharmacological thrombolysis attenuates or promotes procoagulant activity, differences in the extent of procoagulant activity induced by plasminogen activators with different mechanisms of action, and temporal changes in the balance of procoagulant and fibrinolytic activity during and after administration of the plasminogen activator.

Factors leading to an increase in procoagulant activity in response to pharmacological thrombolysis as a consequence of a number of factors include plasmin-mediated activation of coagulation factors, exposure of procoagulant factors bound to the residual thrombus, and platelet activation. Although each of these mechanisms may promote increased procoagulant activity during thrombolysis, the most important determinant of recurrent thrombosis appears to be the extent to which thrombin activity is increased. The dependence of recurrent thrombosis on thrombin is not surprising, because elaboration of thrombin is the ultimate consequence of activation of the coagulation system, inducing the formation of fibrin, activation of platelets, and increased activity of factors IXa and Xa by thrombin-mediated activation of cofactors VIII and V (Fig. 1). Results of experimental and clinical studies indicate that potent inhibition of thrombin activity may accelerate the rapidity of coronary thrombolysis and prevent reocclusion. In dogs, conjunctive administration of the direct-acting thrombin inhibitor hirudin decreased the incidence of recurrent thrombosis after coronary thrombolysis to a greater extent than intravenous heparin, aspirin, or a potent inhibitor of platelet aggregation. Preliminary results of the fifth Thrombolysis in Myocardial Infarction Study (TIMI-5) are consistent with the efficacy of hirudin in preventing recurrent coronary occlusion, and thus support the hypothesis that the extent of thrombin activity after thrombolysis is a critical determinant of recurrent thrombosis. Despite the proven importance of inhibition of thrombin to coronary thrombolysis, the mechanisms responsible for increases in thrombin activity in patients treated with coronary thrombolysis have not been well defined.

II. MECHANISMS RESPONSIBLE FOR CORONARY THROMBOSIS

Coronary thrombosis occurs in response to disruption of the endothelium overlying atherosclerotic plaques. Fissuring or rupture of atherosclerotic plaques exposes tissue factor, a potent procoagulant that accelerates factor VIIa–mediated activation of factors IX and X, to circulating coagulation factors. Exposure of adhesive glycoproteins in the matrix with plaque rupture promotes platelet adhesion, activation, and aggregation. Activation of the coagulation system with elaboration of thrombin is crucial in the formation of the thrombus because it induces deposition of fibrin and activation of platelets. The tissue factor/VIIa complex, which induces activation of factors IX and X, probably assembles on membranes of the macrophages or smooth muscle cells within the atherosclerotic plaque (Fig. 1). Subsequently, maximal procoagulant activity requires formation of factor Xa/Va and IXa/VIIIa complexes on phos-

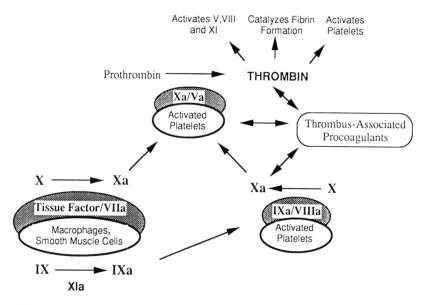

Figure 1   The interaction between procoagulant factors associated with atherosclerotic plaque rupture and those associated with a thrombus. Rupture of atherosclerotic plaques or deep arterial injury initiates coagulation by the tissue factor pathway, in which tissue factor/VIIa complex on cell membranes catalyzes the activation of factors IX and X. Macrophages and smooth muscle cells in atherosclerotic plaques appear to express tissue factor, and therefore may support formation of tissue factor/VIIa complexes. Factor Xa catalyzes the activation of prothrombin when bound with its cofactor Va on cell membranes, likely those of activated platelets or platelet microparticles. Thrombin augments procoagulant activity by activating the cofactors VIII and V, and possibly factor XI, and inducing platelet activation and fibrin formation. The forming thrombus promotes coagulation by binding of thrombin to fibrin within the thrombus and by expressing Xa activity, either due to binding of Xa to fibrin or expression of Xa/Va complex activity by activated platelets in the thrombus. Persistence of these thrombus-associated procoagulants and tissue factor/VIIa complex on the underlying atherosclerotic plaque may promote procoagulant activity after coronary thrombolysis.

pholipid membranes, most likely on platelets aggregating at the site of injury. The formation of thrombin is pivotal because thrombin activates factors VIII and V and promotes platelet activation and aggregation. Thus, thrombin not only mediates fibrin deposition, but potentiates procoagulant activity and platelet aggregation. Thrombin also promotes stabilization of the fibrin mesh by binding to fibrin and activating factor XIII. Factor XIIIa induces cross-linking of fibrin, as well as binding of α_2-antiplasmin to fibrin, which stabilizes the clot and provides a modest degree of resistance to fibrinolytic activity, judging from the acceleration rate of clot lysis when t-PA is given in conjunction with antibodies that interfere with the activity of factor XIIIa or clot-bound α-antiplasmin.

Thrombin binds to fibrin at a secondary binding site (anion-binding exocite) distinct from the catalytic site involved in cleavage of the fibrinopeptides from fibrinogen. Thrombin appears to remain bound to the cross-linked fibrin within the thrombus and is protected from inactivation by antithrombin III while it is bound to fibrin. Because thrombin bound to fibrin appears to retain catalytic activity toward fibrinogen and may activate factors V, VIII, and platelets, clot-associated thrombin activity may play an important role in recurrent thrombosis. Proteolysis of fibrin by plasmin releases bound thrombin, which may further increase its procoagulant potential. In addition to promoting procoagulant activity at the site of thrombosis, thrombin exerts anticoagulant effects by binding to thrombomodulin on endothelium. Thrombin bound to thrombomodulin promotes activation of protein C, a serine protease that inactivates factors VIIIa and Va, thus attenuating procoagulant activity. Administration of recombinant activated protein C has recently been shown to prevent thrombosis in arterial shunts in baboons, a finding that is consistent with the importance of the activity of the IXa/VIIIa and Xa/Va complexes in arterial thrombosis.

In addition to thrombin bound to fibrin, factor Xa appears to contribute to procoagulant activity of arterial thrombi. Clot-associated factor Xa activity appears to be attributable to the presence of Xa/Va complex on platelets in whole blood thrombi, and possibly to binding of Xa to fibrin. Factor Xa is protected from antithrombin III–mediated inhibition in the presence of fibrin and when bound to phospholipid membranes in the complex with Va. Thus, during clot lysis, thrombus-associated thrombin and Xa induce procoagulant activity that is relatively resistant to inhibition by antithrombin III or heparin–antithrombin III.

Because proteolysis of fibrin by plasmin both exposes and releases clot-associated thrombin and Xa, the extent of clot lysis may regulate the intensity of clot-associated procoagulant activity. In addition, more extensive clot lysis reduces the severity of residual stenosis, which in turn decreases shear forces that promote recurrent platelet-rich thrombosis. Thus, fibrinolytic agents that induce complete and rapid clot lysis are likely, at least initially, to attenuate the extent of local procoagulant activity more effectively than agents that induce slower rates of clot lysis. This balance between procoagulant and fibrinolytic activity may in part account for the more rapid rates of clot lysis observed with fibrin-specific agents such as t-PA compared with streptokinase or urokinase; i.e., the net rate of clot lysis compared with clot formation is greater for agents that preferentially activate plasminogen bound to fibrin. However, as long as a residual thrombus is present, the potential for clot-associated procoagulants to induce recurrent thrombosis remains.

III. ANTICOAGULANT EFFECTS OF PHARMACOLOGICAL ACTIVATION OF PLASMINOGEN

Plasmin is a potent, relatively nonspecific protease that may induce proteolysis of a number of substrates in addition to fibrin and fibrinogen. Physiological clot lysis is regulated by the preferential activation of plasminogen bound to fibrin by t-PA and the rapid inhibition of free plasmin by α_2-antiplasmin. Pharmacological activation of plasminogen is associated with varying degrees of depletion of circulating α_2-antiplasmin and consequent free plasmin activity. With the first-generation fibrinolytic agents streptokinase and urokinase, extensive free plasmin activity induces proteolysis of multiple plasma proteins, including fibrinogen and coagulation factors. This lytic state is generally thought to result in predominantly anticoagulant effects due to degradation of fibrinogen and elaboration of fibrinogen degradation products. Circulating fibrinogen degradation products inhibit thrombosis by interfering with fibrin polymerization and platelet aggregation. Proteolysis of coagulation factors may also contribute to the anticoagulant activity of the lytic state by decreasing the concentration of functional coagulant factors. At the doses required to induce rapid coronary thrombolysis, second-generation fibrinolytic agents such as t-PA also induce systemic plasmin activity, but to a lesser extent than that with streptokinase. In addition, streptokinase induces more prolonged systemic lytic activity than t-PA, because of the longer half-life of the streptokinase–plasminogen complex (4–6 hours) compared with that of t-PA (3–5 minutes). As a consequence, in patients given t-PA, the extent of fibrinogen degradation is less marked and the fibrinogen degradation products elaborated (e.g., fragment X) are of higher molecular weight. Although the relative potencies of fibrinogen degradation products of differing molecular weights in inducing anticoagulant or antiplatelet effects have not been well defined, it is likely the degree of inhibition of fibrin polymerization and platelet deposition is related to extent of fibrinogen degradation. The anticoagulant effects of marked fibrinogenolysis likely account for the lower incidence of coronary reocclusion in patients in the TAMI-5 trial randomly assigned to an aggressive treatment strategy of catheterization, coronary angioplasty, and a combination of t-PA and urokinase than the incidence in patients treated with either agent alone.

IV. PLASMIN-MEDIATED ACTIVATION OF THE COAGULATION SYSTEM

A. Potential Mechanisms

Incubation of t-PA, streptokinase, or urokinase with nonanticoagulated plasma or whole blood induces marked increases in the concentration of fibrinopeptide A (FPA), a marker of thrombin-induced fibrin formation. The increases in thrombin activity that occur appear to be attributable to plasmin-mediated activation of the coagulation system. Increases in FPA are less marked in nonanticoagulated blood incubated with 100 IU/ml streptokinase or 2.5 μg/ml t-PA than in that incubated with 1000 IU/ml of streptokinase, suggesting that the extent of thrombin induced by plasminogen activation is directly related to the intensity of free plasmin activity. Increases in FPA are markedly attenuated in blood incubated with streptokinase or t-PA in the presence of heparin. The inhibitory effect of heparin may be due to inhibition of thrombin activity induced by plasmin-mediated activation of the coagulation system, inhibition of elaboration of thrombin, or both.

Potential mechanisms for activation of the coagulation system in response to pharmacological plasminogen activation were recently characterized in plasma with a two-stage assay designed to detect procoagulant activity even in the presence of extensive fibrinogen degradation. In the first stage of the assay, citrated plasma was recalcified and incubated with various concentrations of t-PA, streptokinase, or urokinase. To detect procoagulant activity induced by activation of plasminogen, an aliquot of the first-stage plasma was added to recalcified second-stage citrated plasma, and the clotting time of the second-stage plasma was measured. When first-stage plasma incubated with fibrinolytic agents was added to second-stage plasma, the clotting time was significantly accelerated after addition of first-stage plasma that was recalcified but not incubated with a fibrinolytic agent. Clotting times of the second-stage plasma were more markedly accelerated by addition of first-stage plasma incubated with streptokinase and urokinase than by addition of plasma incubated with t-PA and was more accelerated with higher than with lower concentrations of each agent. These results confirm the relationship between the extent of plasminogen activation and the intensity of procoagulant activity induced. Furthermore, inhibition of plasmin activity with aprotinin, a plasmin inhibitor, essentially abolished the increases in thrombin activity induced by incubation with t-PA or streptokinase.

To determine which coagulation factors were necessary for procoagulant activity to be induced by plasmin, streptokinase was incubated with plasma deficient in specific coagulation factors. The activation of factor X induced by streptokinase was apparently due to activation by the factor IXa/VIIIa complex, judging from the marked attenuation of procoagulant activity observed in plasma deficient in these factors when incubated with streptokinase. In contrast, marked procoagulant activity was observed in plasma deficient in factor VII during incubation with streptokinase. Whether the increased activity of the factor IXa/VIIIa complex reflects a direct effect of plasmin on these factors or whether it reflects plasmin-mediated activation of factor XII, as has been observed in purified systems, remains to be defined. Plasmin also transiently activates factor V, a cofactor that when activated markedly accelerates the activation of prothrombin by factor Xa/Va complex. Thus, there is considerable evidence based on in vitro studies that pharmacological activation of plasminogen induces plasmin-mediated activation of the coagulation system in direct proportion to the extent of free plasmin activity.

B. Increased Procoagulant Activity During Pharmacological Thrombolysis

Increases in thrombin activity potentially due to plasmin-mediated activation of the coagulation system have been documented in patients given t-PA or streptokinase for acute myocardial infarction. In patients treated with streptokinase without conjunctive intravenous heparin, plasma concentrations of FPA increase immediately after initiation of the streptokinase infusion and decrease promptly after administration of a 5000 U intravenous bolus of heparin. Similar results have been reported in patients treated with t-PA. The increased concentrations of FPA reflect thrombin activity, judging from the prompt decrease in the concentrations of FPA after administration of heparin, as well as the less marked increases in FPA observed in patients treated with either streptokinase or t-PA and conjunctive intravenous heparin.

The question of whether the increased concentrations of FPA observed in plasma of patients treated with fibrinolytic agents reflect de novo thrombin formation or exposure of preformed thrombin bound to fibrin during clot lysis was recently addressed in patients treated with t-PA by measuring changes in the plasma concentrations of prothrombin fragment 1.2, a polypeptide released when prothrombin is activated by factor Xa. In the absence of conjunctive intravenous heparin therapy, fragment 1.2 concentrations increased after initiation of the t-PA infusion; concentrations decreased significantly after a 5000-U bolus of heparin. Concentrations of thrombin–antithrombin III complexes in plasma also increased in patients treated with fibrinolytic agents, consistent with increased levels of thrombin accessible to inhibition by antithrombin III. Thus, the results of clinical trials are consistent with activation of the coagulation system during pharmacological thrombolysis. Although multiple factors may promote increased procoagulant activity during coronary thrombolysis, the prompt increase in thrombin activity after initiation of the infusion of fibrinolytic agents is consistent with plasmin-mediated activation of the coagulation system. Conjunctive administration of heparin appears to significantly attenuate the thrombin activity induced by pharmacological activation of plasminogen.

C. Determinants of Recurrent Thrombosis in Response to Plasmin-Mediated Activation of the Coagulation System

Administration of fibrinolytic agents is not thought to induce clinically evident thrombosis, despite apparent plasmin-mediated activation of the coagulation system. Because both the intensity of procoagulant activity and the extent of fibrinogen degradation are attributable to the elaboration of free plasmin, it is likely that fibrin polymerization is in part inhibited by fibrinogen degradation products and/or rapid proteolysis of polymerized fibrin. For example, low levels of thrombin activity have been shown to elaborate soluble fibrin polymers, which in the presence of high concentrations of t-PA undergo proteolysis to yield the soluble cross-linked fibrin degradation product D-dimer. Thus, clinically apparent thrombosis may not develop with pharmacological plasminogen activation because there is sufficient simultaneous fibrinolytic activity to degrade fibrin formed as a consequence of increased thrombin activity. However, in both clinical and experimental studies thrombus formation has occasionally been observed early after initiation of infusion of fibrinolytic agents, possibly as a consequence of plasmin-mediated activation of the coagulation system.

The results of a recent study by Gruber et al. illustrate the potential importance of the balance of procoagulant and fibrinolytic activity in determining the extent of clot lysis in response to administration of fibrinolytic agents. These investigators characterized the effects of low and intermediate doses of activated protein C, urokinase, or both in combination in attenuating thrombosis on Dacron grafts in baboons. Although both procoagulant and fibrinolytic activity increased in response to infusion of low or intermediate doses of urokinase, reflected by increases in plasma concentrations of FPA and D-dimer, deposition of fibrin on the grafts was attenuated in a dose-dependent manner. However, low- and high-dose combinations of activated protein C (APC) and urokinase, despite inducing similar degrees of fibrinolytic activity, markedly attenuated the increases in FPA and decreased fibrin deposition to a greater extent than observed with either dose of urokinase alone. Thus, the antithrombotic efficacy of urokinase was significantly potentiated by the inhibition of increases in procoagulant activity. Although the mechanisms responsible for the efficacy of activated protein C in attenuating increases in FPA in response to pharmacological activation of plasminogen were not specifically defined in this study, the results are consistent with inhibition of plasmin-mediated activation of the coagulation system as defined in studies in vitro.

V. PLATELET ACTIVATION IN RESPONSE TO PHARMACOLOGICAL THROMBOLYSIS

Pharmacological thrombolysis may induce both activation of platelets and inhibition of platelet aggregation. Activation of platelets appears to occur early after the administration of fibrinolytic agents and is more marked with streptokinase than with t-PA. Although plasmin has been shown to directly induce activation of platelets in purified systems, the concentrations of plasmin required are severalfold higher than those achieved during pharmacological thrombolysis. At concentrations similar to those achieved during pharmacological thrombolysis, t-PA and SK do not induce activation of platelets in plasma in vitro. Nonetheless, in patients given t-PA or streptokinase, marked platelet activation appears to occur immediately after initiation of infusion of the fibrinolytic agents, judging from increases in the concentrations in urine of metabolites of thromboxane A_2. Pretreatment with aspirin markedly attenuates the increases in the concentrations of thromboxane metabolites in urine in response to streptokinase, but conjunctive administration of intravenous heparin does not appear to prevent platelet activation.

One potential mechanism for platelet activation in patients treated with fibrinolytic agents is the elaboration of thrombin in response to plasmin-mediated activation of the coagulation system. Thrombin is a potent platelet agonist, and inhibition of thrombin has been shown to prevent arterial platelet-rich thrombosis. In a recent study, incubation of recalcified platelet-rich plasma with 1000 IU/ml streptokinase or 1 caseinolytic unit/ml of plasmin induced thrombin-mediated activation of platelets. Elaboration of thrombin was attributable to plasmin-mediated activation of the coagulation system. Incubation of recalcified platelet-rich plasma with streptokinase or plasmin in the presence of the thrombin inhibitor hirudin markedly attenuated activation of platelets. Hirudin has also been shown to be more effective than heparin, aspirin, or potent inhibition of the platelet fibrinogen receptor in preventing recurrent thrombosis after coronary thrombolysis in dogs. However, activation of platelets has been observed during coronary thrombolysis with t-PA in dogs despite inhibition of thrombin with another direct-acting inhibitor, argatroban, judging from increases in the concentration of urinary metabolites of thromboxane A_2. Thus, while elaboration of thrombin is likely to induce activation of platelets during pharmacological thrombolysis, other mechanisms for activation of platelets may play a role (see Chapter 7).

VI. INFLUENCE OF PROCOAGULANT ACTIVITY ON THE FIBRINOLYTIC EFFICACY OF PLASMINOGEN ACTIVATORS

In addition to promoting recurrent thrombosis, increased procoagulant activity and platelet activation during pharmacologic thrombolysis may influence the success of thrombolysis by decreasing the fibrinolytic efficacy of fibrin-specific plasminogen activators and attenuating physiologic fibrinolytic activity. For example, increased plasma concentrations of fibrinogen degradation products decrease the fibrin specificity of t-PA by stimulating the catalytic activity of t-PA toward circulating plasminogen. Activation of circulating plasminogen induces degradation of fibrinogen, promotes plasmin-mediated activation of the coagulation system, and consequently has the potential of decreasing the efficacy of t-PA in inducing clot lysis.

VII. ATTENUATION OF PHYSIOLOGICAL FIBRINOLYTIC ACTIVITY AFTER PHARMACOLOGICAL THROMBOLYSIS

Activation of platelets during thrombolysis may also attenuate the fibrinolytic efficacy of t-PA by increasing the plasma activity of circulating plasminogen activator inhibitor-1 (PAI-1). Increases in PAI-1 are mediated both by its secretion from platelets and the secretion of growth factors that induce increased synthesis of PAI-1 by endothelial cells. Secretion of

PAI-1 from platelets, while insufficient to attenuate the activity of high concentrations of t-PA during its infusion, may attenuate t-PA–induced lysis of platelet-rich thrombus. Sustained increases in circulating PAI-1 may attenuate physiological fibrinolytic activity after pharmacological fibrinolytic activity wanes. In patients treated for myocardial infarction, increases in the activity of PAI-1 24–48 hours after infusion of t-PA may increase the risk of recurrent infarction. In addition, attenuated activity of factor XII–dependent plasminogen activation (i.e., intrinsic plasminogen activation system) has been documented after pharmacological thrombolysis and also may increase the potential for recurrent infarction. The exact mechanisms responsible for the attenuated activity of the intrinsic plasminogen activation system after pharmacological thrombolysis are unknown, but are related to the extent of free plasmin activity induced by pharmacological activation of plasminogen, and may therefore be related to plasmin-mediated activation of the coagulation system. Thus, increases in procoagulant activity in response to pharmacological activation of plasminogen may induce recurrent thrombosis not only by increasing thrombin activity and platelet activation early after infusion of the fibrinolytic agent, but also by attenuating physiological fibrinolytic activity late after coronary thrombolysis.

VIII. DIFFERENTIAL EFFECTS OF SPECIFIC PLASMINOGEN ACTIVATORS ON THE BALANCE OF PROCOAGULANT AND FIBRINOLYTIC ACTIVITY IN RESPONSE TO PHARMACOLOGICAL THROMBOLYSIS

When pharmacological activation of plasminogen is initiated, procoagulant activity may be more intense than fibrinolytic activity. With administration of streptokinase or urokinase in the absence of conjunctive intravenous heparin, marked increases in thrombin activity may occur, but the intense free plasmin activity induced by streptokinase and urokinase rapidly results in sufficient degradation of fibrinogen to attenuate fibrin formation and platelet aggregation (Table 1). Thus, within 30–60

Table 1 Temporal Changes in Procoagulant and Fibrinolytic Activity Induced by Administration of Selected Fibrinolytic Agents

Agent	0–60 min after initiation of plasminogen activator		2–8 h after initiation of plasminogen activator		2–24 h after initiation of plasminogen activator	
	Procoagulant activity	Fibrinolytic activity	Procoagulant activity	Fibrinolytic activity	Procoagulant activity	Fibrinolytic activity
SK/UK	+ + + +	+ + +	+ + (reflects attenuation of procoagulant activity by fibrin(ogen) degradation products)	+ + +	+ +	–
t-PA	+ + +	+ + + +	+ +	+	+ +	+

minutes after initiation of an infusion of streptokinase there is significant anticoagulant activity induced as a consequence of marked fibrinogen degradation. In contrast, in patients treated with t-PA the increases in thrombin activity induced are more modest than those observed in patients treated with streptokinase, although because of the lesser degree of fibrinogen degradation there is a greater potential for recurrent thrombosis. The immediate increases in thrombin activity induced by fibrinolytic agents are markedly attenuated by heparin, and in experimental studies conjunctive administration of heparin with t-PA or streptokinase has been shown to accelerate the rate of clot lysis. However, a beneficial effect of inhibiting early increases in procoagulant activity was not observed in the TAMI-5 study, in which conjunctive administration of heparin with a 3-hour infusion of t-PA did not improve the 90-minute patency rate over that with t-PA alone. Thus, it can be argued that in patients treated for myocardial infarction the fibrinolytic activity induced by initiation of pharmacological thrombolysis is sufficiently intense within the first few hours to balance the procoagulant activity. Even if this hypothesis is correct, however, early increases in procoagulant activity may activate platelets and increase the concentration of activated coagulation factors associated with the residual thrombosis; this may have important consequences on the subsequent tendency to recurrent thrombosis by promotion of procoagulant activity at the site of recanalized thrombus and attenuation of physiological fibrinolytic activity, as discussed above (Table 1).

The pharmacological properties of a given plasminogen activator also determine the extent to which procoagulant activity promotes recurrent thrombosis. Streptokinase induces significant fibrinogen degradation (and its attendant anticoagulant effects) and elaboration of fibrinogen degradation products for 3–6 hours after completion of the infusion, during which time fibrinolytic activity is potentiated. Nonetheless, the relatively slow rate of clot lysis and the more marked early increases in procoagulant activity with streptokinase may result in expression of significant procoagulant activity by the residual thrombus in the recanalized vessel. Thus, as the anticoagulant effects of fibrinogen degradation wane, the potential for recurrent thrombosis increases (Table 1). The relative balance of procoagulant and fibrinolytic activity induced by administration of anisoylated streptokinase–plasminogen complex (anistreplase) or urokinase is less well characterized. The extent of fibrinogen degradation may be less marked with these agents, but at doses sufficient to induce coronary thrombolysis it is likely that the factors influencing the tendency for recurrent thrombosis are similar to those of streptokinase.

The extent of fibrinogen degradation induced by fibrin-specific agents is significantly less marked than that induced by streptokinase or urokinase in most patients. In patients treated with t-PA, degradation of fibrinogen essentially ceases after completion of the infusion because of the rapid clearance of the drug from the circulation. However, characteristics of t-PA that make recurrent thrombosis more likely may be balanced by the greater degree of clot lysis, and hence less procoagulant activity attributable to the residual thrombus, with t-PA than with streptokinase. Nonetheless, the rate of infarct-related artery patency decreases between 90 minutes and 24 hours after infusion of t-PA, despite the use of heparin, and it decreases markedly by 24 hours in patients not treated with conjunctive heparin at all.

The tendency for recurrent thrombosis may be further potentiated by the inhibition of physiologic fibrinolytic activity 24–48 hours after administration of fibrinolytic agents. Platelet activation induced by pharmacological activation of plasminogen, either directly or as a consequence of plasmin-mediated activation of the coagulation system, may play a role in the late suppression of fibrinolytic activity by inducing increases in circulating PAI-1 activity. In addition, factor XII–dependent fibrinolytic activity is attenuated. Thus, early procoagulant events may influence the later likelihood of recurrent thrombosis (Table 1).

IX. SUMMARY

Pharmacological thrombolysis is invariably associated with increases in procoagulant activity. The extent of procoagulant activity induced and the tendency for recurrent thrombosis to occur depend on the specific plasminogen activator used and the adequacy and timing of conjunctive anticoagulant regimens. Although conjunctive anticoagulation inhibits much of the procoagulant activity induced by pharmacological thrombolysis, clot-associated procoagulant activity is relatively resistant to inhibition by heparin–antithrombin III and may promote recurrent thrombosis. Furthermore, increases in procoagulant activity in response to pharmacological activation of plasminogen may have other important effects that influence the outcome of coronary thrombolysis, including activation of platelets, secretion of growth factors by platelets, activation of the endothelium, and inhibition of physiological fibrinolytic activity.

ACKNOWLEDGMENTS

Supported in part by SCOR in Coronary and Vascular Diseases (Grant HL-17646), National Heart, Lung and Blood Institute, National Institutes of Health, Bethesda, MD.

PERTINENT REFERENCES

Bach R R: Initiation of coagulation by tissue factor. *CRC Crit Rev Biochem* 1988;23:339–368.

Bleich S D, Nicholas T C, Schumacher R R, Cooke D H, Tate D A, Teichman S L: Effect of heparin on coronary arterial patency after thrombolysis with tissue plasminogen activator in acute myocardial infarction. *Am J Cardiol* 1990; 66:1412–1417.

Califf R M, Topol E J, Stack R S, Ellis S G, George B S, Kereiakes D J, Samaha J K, Worley S J, Anderson J L, Harrelson-Woodlief L, Wall T C, Phillips H R, Abbotsmith C W, Candela R J, Flanagan W H, Sasahara A A, Mantell S J, Lee K L, TAMI Study Group: Evaluation of combination thrombolytic therapy and timing of cardiac catheterization in acute myocardial infarction. Results of Thrombolysis and Angioplasty in Myocardial Infarction-phase 5 randomized trial. *Circulation* 1991;83:1543–1556.

Collen D: On the regulation and control of fibrinolysis. *Thromb Haemost* 1980;43:77–89.

Coller B: Platelets and thrombolytic therapy. *N Engl J Med* 1990;322:33–42.

de Bono D P, Simoons M L, Tijssen J, Arnold A E R, Betriu A, Burgersdijk C, Lopez Bescos L, Mueller E, Pfisterer M, Van de Werf F, Zijlstra F, Verstraete M for the European Cooperative Study Group: Effect of early intravenous heparin on coronary patency, infarct size, and bleeding complications after alteplase thrombolysis: results of a randomized double blind European Cooperative Study Group trial *Br Heart J* 1992;67: 122–128.

de Fouw N J, de Jong Y F, Haverkate F, Bertina R M: The influence of thrombin and platelets on fibrin clot lysis rates in vitro: a study using a clot lysis system consisting of purified human proteins. *Fibrinolysis* 1988; 2:235–244.

Eisenberg P R, Miletich J P: Induction of marked thrombin activity by pharmacologic concentrations of plasminogen activators in nonanticoagulated whole blood. *Thromb Res* 1989;55:635–643.

Eisenberg P R, Miletich J P, Sobel B E: Factors responsible for the differential procoagulant effects of diverse plasminogen activators in plasma. *Fibrinolysis* 1991;5:217–224.

Eisenberg P R, Sherman L A, Jaffe A S: Paradoxic elevation of fibrinopeptide A after streptokinase: Evidence for continued thrombosis despite intensive fibrinolysis. *J Am Coll Cardiol* 1987;10:527–529.

Eisenberg P R, Siegel J E, Abendshein D R, Miletich J P: Importance of factor Xa in determining the procoagulant activity of whole-blood clots. *J Clin Invest* (in press).

Eisenberg P R, Sobel B E, Jaffe A S: Activation of prothrombin accompanying thrombolysis with recombinant tissue-type plasminogen activator. *J Am Coll Cardiol* 1992;19:1065–1069.

Esmon N L, Owen W G, Esmon C T: Isolation of a membrane-bound cofactor for thrombin-catalyzed activation of protein C. *J Biol Chem* 1982;257: 859–864.

Fitzgerald D J, Catella F, Roy L, FitzGerald G A: Marked platelet activation in vivo after intravenous streptokinase in patients with acute myocardial infarction. *Circulation* 1988;77:142–150.

Fitzgerald D J, Fitzgerald G A: Role of thrombin and thromboxane A2 in reocclusion following coronary thrombolysis with tissue-type plasminogen activator. *Proc Natl Acad Sci USA* 1989;86:7585–7589.

Fitzgerald D J, Hanson M, FitzGerald G A: Systemic lysis protects against the effects of platelet activation during coronary thrombolysis. *J Clin Invest* 1991;88:1589–1595.

Fitzgerald D J, Wright F, FitzGerald G A: Increased thromboxane biosynthesis during coronary thrombolysis. Evidence that platelet activation and thromboxane A2 modulate the response to tissue-type plasminogen activator in vivo. *Circ Res* 1989;65:83–94.

Francis C W, Doughney K B, Brenner B, Klingbiel K, Marder V J: Increased immunoreactivity of plasma after fibrinolytic activation in an anti-DD ELISA system: role of soluble crosslinked fibrin polymers. *Circulation* 1989;79:666–673.

Fujii S, Abendschein D R, Sobel B E: Augmentation of plasminogen activator inhibitor type 1. Activity in plasma by thrombosis and by thrombolysis. *J Am Coll Cardiol* 1991;18:1547–1554.

Fujii S, Hopkins W E, Sobel B E: Mechanisms contributing to increased synthesis of plasminogen activator inhibitor type 1 in endothelial cell constituents of platelets and their implications for thrombolysis. *Circulation* 1991;83:645–651.

Gold H K, Leinbach R C, Garabedian H D, Yasuda T, Johns J A, Grossbard E B, Palacios I, Collen D: Acute coronary reocclusion after thrombolysis with recombinant human tissue-type plasminogen activator: Prevention by a maintenance infusion. *Circulation* 1986;73:347–352.

Gouin I, Lecompte T, Morel M C, Lebrazi J, Modderman P W, Kaplan C, Samama M M: In vitro effect of plasmin on human platelet function in plasma. Inhibition of aggregation caused by fibrinogenolysis. *Circulation* 1992;85:935–941.

Gruber A, Griffin J H, Harker L A, Hanson S R: Inhibition of platelet-dependent thrombus formation by human activated protein C in a primate model. *Blood* 1989;73:639–642.

Gruber A, Harker L A, Hanson S R, Kelly A B, Griffin J H: Antithrombotic effects of combining activated protein C and urokinase in non-human primates. *Circulation* 1991;84:2454–2462.

Gulba D C, Barthels M, Westhoff-Bleck M, Jost S, Rafflenbeul W, Daniel W G, Hecker H, Lichtlen P R: Increased thrombin levels during thrombolytic therapy in acute myocardial infarction. *Circulation* 1991;83:937–944.

Hanson S R, Harker L A: Interruption of acute platelet-dependent thrombosis by the synthetic antithrombin D-phenylalanyl-prolyl-L-arginyl chloromethyl ketone. *Proc Natl Acad Sci USA* 1988;85:3184–3188.

Haskel E J, Prager N A, Sobel B E, Abendschein D R: Relative efficacy of antithrombin compared with antiplatelet agents in accelerating coronary thrombolysis and preventing early reocclusion. *Circulation* 1991;83:1048–1056.

Hawiger J. Adhesive interactions of platelets and their blockade. *Ann NY Acad Sci* 1991;614:270–278.

Heras M, Chesebro J H, Penny W J, Bailey K R, Badimon L, Fuster V: Effects of thrombin inhibition on the development of acute platelet-thrombus deposition during angioplasty in pigs. Heparin versus recombinant hirudin, a specific thrombin inhibitor. *Circulation* 1989;79:657–665.

Hogg P J, Jackson C M: Fibrin monomer protects thrombin from inactivation by heparin-antithrombin III: implications for heparin efficacy. *Proc Natl Acad Sci USA* 1989;86:3619–3623.

Hsia J, Hamilton W P, Kleiman N S, Roberts R, Chaitman B R, Ross A M: A comparison between heparin and low-dose aspirin as adjunctive therapy with tissue plasminogen activator for acute myocardial infarction. *N Engl J Med* 1990;323:1433–1437.

ISIS-2 Study Group: ISIS-2 (Second International Study of Infarct Survival). Randomized trial of intravenous streptokinase, oral aspirin, both, or neither among 17,187 cases of suspected myocardial infarction:ISIS-2. *Lancet* 1988;2:349–360.

ISIS-3 (Third International Study of Infarct Survival) Collaborative Group: ISIS-3: A randomized comparison of streptokinase vs tissue plasminogen activator vs anistreplase and of aspirin plus heparin vs aspirin alone among 41,299 cases of suspected acute myocardial infarction. *Lancet* 1992;339:753–770.

Kaminski M, McDonagh J: Studies on the mechanism of thrombin: Interaction with fibrin. *J Biol Chem* 1983;258:10530–10535.

Larrieu M J, Rigollot C, Marder V J: Comparitive effects of fibrinogen degradation products D and E on coagulation. *Br J Haematol* 1973;22:719–733.

Lee C D, Mann K G: The activation/inactivation of human coagulation factor V by plasmin. *Blood* 1989;73:185–190.

Liu C Y, Nossel H L, Kaplan K: The binding of thrombin by fibrin. *J Biol Chem* 1979;254:10421–10425.

Lucore C L, Sobel B E: Interactions of tissue-type plasminogen activator with plasma inhibitors and their pharmacologic significance. *Circulation* 1988; 77:660–669.

Lukacova D, Matsueda G R, Haber E, Reed G L: Inhibition of factor XIII activation by an anti-peptide monoclonal antibody. *Biochemistry* 1991;30: 10164–70.

Mann K G, Nesheim M E, Church W R, Haley P, Krishnaswamy S: Surface-dependent reactions of the vitamin K-dependent enzyme complexes. *Blood* 1990;76:1–16.

Marlar R A, Kleiss A J, Griffin J H: Mechanism of action of human activated protein C, a thrombin-dependent anticoagulant enzyme. *Blood* 1982;59: 1067–1072.

Mentzer R L, Budzynski A Z, Sherry S: High-dose, brief-duration intravenous infusion of streptokinase in acute myocardial infarction: description of effects in the circulation. *Am J Cardiol* 1986;57:1220–1226.

Munkvad S, Jespersen J, Gram J, Kluft C: Depression of factor XII-dependent fibrinolytic activity characterizes patients with early myocardial reinfarction after recombinant tissue-type plasminogen-activator therapy. *J Am Coll Cardiol* 1991;18:454–458.

Nachman R L, Leung L L K, Kloczewiak M, Hawiger J: Complex formation of platelet membrane glycoproteins IIb and IIIa with the fibrinogen D domain. *J Biol Chem* 1984;259:8584–8588.

Owen J, Friedman K D, Grossman B A, Wilkins C, Berke A D, Powers E R: Thrombolytic therapy with tissue plasminogen activator or streptokinase induces transient thrombin activity. *Blood* 1988;72:616–620.

Owen J, Friedman K D, Grossman B A, Wilkins C, Powers E R: Quantification of fragment X formation during thrombolytic therapy with streptokinase and tissue plasminogen activator. *J Clin Invest* 1987;79: 1642–1647.

Rapold H J: Promotion of thrombin activity by thrombolytic therapy without simultaneous anticoagulation. *Lancet* 1990;335:481–482.

Rapold H J, de Bono D, Arnold A E R, Arnout J, De Cock F, Collen D, Verstraete M: Plasma fibrinopeptide A levels in patients with acute myocardial infarction treated with alteplase. *Circulation* 1992;85:928–934.

Reed G L I, Matsueda G R, Haber E: Synergistic fibrinolysis: combined effects of plasminogen activators and an antibody that inhibits alpha 2-antiplasmin. *Proc Natl Acad Sci USA* 1990;87:1114–1118.

Schafer A I, Maas A K, Ware A, Johnson P C, Rittenhouse S E, Salzman E W: Platelet protein phosphorylation, elevation of cytosolic calcium, and inositol phospholipid breakdown in platelet activation induced by plasmin. *J Clin Invest* 1986;78:73–79.

Thorsen L I, Brosstad F, Gogstad G, Sletten K, Solum N O: Competitions between fibrinogen with its degradation products for interactions with the platelet-fibrinogen receptor. *Thromb Res* 1986;44:611–623.

Weitz J I, Hudoba M, Massel D, Maraganore J, Hirsh J: Clot-bound thrombin is protected from inhibition by heparin-antithrombin III but is susceptible to inactivation by antithrombin III-independent inhibitors. *J Clin Invest* 1990;86:385–391

Wilner G D, Danitz M P, Mudd M S, Hsieh K, Fenton J W: Selective immobo-
lization of alpha-thrombin by surface-bound fibrin. *J Lab Clin Med* 1981;
97:403–411.

Winters K J, Eisenberg P R, Jaffe A S, Santoro S A: Dependence of plasmin-
mediated degradation of platelet adhesive receptors on temperature and
Ca^{++}. *Blood* 1990;76:1546–1557.

Winters K J, Santoro S A, Miletich J P, Eisenberg P R: Relative importance of
thrombin compared with plasmin-mediated platelet activation in response to plasminogen activation with streptokinase. *Circulation* 1991;
84:1552–1560.

Yasuda T, Gold H K, Yaoita H, Leinbach R C, Guerrero J L, Jang I, Holt R,
Fallon J T, Collen D: Comparative effects of aspirin, a synthetic thrombin
inhibitor and a monoclonal antiplatelet glycoprotein IIb/IIIa antibody on
coronary artery reperfusion, reocclusion and bleeding with recombinant
tissue-type plasminogen activator in a canine preparation. *J Am Coll Cardiol* 1990;16:714–722.

7

The Role of Platelets in Thrombolysis, Thrombosis, and Thrombolytic Therapy

Edward F. Plow
Center for Thrombosis and Vascular Biology
The Cleveland Clinic Foundation
Cleveland, Ohio

I. INTRODUCTION

That fibrinolytic agents have a major beneficial impact on the outcome of coronary thrombosis and myocardial infarction has been clearly established in numerous and large clinical trials. With the objective of most recent clinical trials heavily focused upon selecting the most effective thrombolytic drug, the fact that none of the clinically available fibrinolytics—streptokinase (SK), tissue plasminogen activator (t-PA), or urokinase (u-PA)—is optimal has become obscured. Yet three well-established sets of observations emphasize the potential for significant improvement in thrombolytic therapy. First, a large group of patients (25%) fail to respond to the current regimens of thrombolytic therapy. Second, reocclusion occurs after initial recanalization in a significant percentage of patients (20–30%). Third, although the incidence of severe bleeding complications in association with thrombolytic therapy is low, safety has no end point, and risk minimization must always continue.

In considering the issues of efficiency, reoccurrence, and safety, the relationship between platelets and thrombolytic therapy is of pivotal importance. A number of studies have established that platelet-rich thrombi are considerably more resistant to lysis by thrombolytic agents than fibrin-rich thrombi. The thrombi, which reocclude coronary arteries after initial successful thrombolysis, are enriched in platelets and can form even in the face of aggressive anticoagulation. Thus, the presence of platelet-rich thrombi may account for or contribute to the failure of patients to respond to thrombolytic therapy. Further evidence for the role of platelets in thrombolysis are studies showing that targeting fibrinolytic agents to platelets has a positive effect on thrombolysis. Finally, the major impact that the antiplatelet drug aspirin had on survival in the ISIS-II trial further emphasizes the intimate interrelationship between platelet function and thrombolysis.

In vitro studies have shown that antiplatelet agents can accelerate the lysis of platelet-rich thrombi. In experimental animal models, a variety of antiplatelet drugs have had beneficial effects on thrombolysis. These include thromboxane synthase inhibitors, thromboxane A_2, and serotonin receptor antagonists and an antibody to a platelet membrane glycoprotein. The beneficial effects ascribed to these agents have been multiple and have included a reduction in the dose of thrombolytic agent required for recanalization, a decrease in the time to reperfusion and the quality of reperfusion, and a prevention of reocclusion. Taken together, these observations provide a groundwork for considering conjunctive therapy with antiplatelet and thrombolytic agents. However, by their mode of action, antiplatelet agents influence the hemostatic contributions of platelets, and increased bleeding risks may be encountered. With this background in mind, this chapter seeks to briefly outline our current understanding of the basic molecular and cellular mechanisms by which platelets contribute to thrombolysis and thrombosis. It is clear that platelets play a pivotal role in these processes, and their contributions are complex and multifaceted.

II. PLATELETS AND THROMBOLYSIS

In the relationship between platelets and thrombolysis, multiple and counterbalancing effects come into play. These include (1) platelet secretion of both profibrinolytic and antifibrinolytic components, (2) assembly of fibrinolytic components on the platelet surface, resulting in enhanced plasmin generation, which may be either pro- or antifibrinolytic, (3) the prothrombotic and antithrombotic influences of plasmin on platelet function, and (4) the effects of platelets on the physical properties of thrombi. These topics are discussed separately below.

A. Platelet Release of Fibrinolytic Components

The influence of platelets on fibrinolysis has long been recognized. Platelets contain a number of fibrinolytic components. Many of these reside within alpha granules and are secreted when platelets are stimulated by agonists. Intracellular constituents also may become available as a consequence of the lysis of platelets within a thrombus. In general, the concentration of the fibrinolytic constituents present within platelets is low relative to their levels in plasma. However, some relevant constituents, such as plasminogen activator inhibitor-1 (PAI-1) and thrombospondin, are enriched within platelets. Moreover, as the platelets accumulate within the thrombus, the released constituents may reach levels sufficient to influence thrombolysis within the local microenvironment. This consideration is particularly pertinent for platelet constituents, such as plasminogen and alpha$_2$-antiplasmin, which are preferentially retained within the thrombus by virtue of their binding to platelet and/or fibrin surfaces.

A listing of the fibrinolytic proteins within platelet alpha granules is provided in Table 1. Two mechanisms have been defined for entry of such proteins into alpha granules: (1) biosynthesis within megakaryocytes or (2) endocytosis by platelets or megakaryocytes. Table 1 encompasses a broad cross section of molecules that influence fibrinolysis and includes both profibrinolytic and antifibrinolytic activities. These molecules

Table 1   Major Intraplatelet Modulators
of Fibrinolysis

Profibrinolytic
  Plasminogen
  Urokinase
  Tissue plasminogen activator
Antifibrinolytic
  Plasminogen activator inhibitor-1
  α_2-Antiplasmin
  Protease-nexin
Modulators
  Factor XIII
  Thrombospondin
  Fibronectin
  Histidine-rich glycoprotein

---

range from plasminogen activators to inhibitors of these activators to molecules that influence the character of fibrin within
a thrombus, such as factor XIII or thombospondin. The general
consensus is that the antifibrinolytic activity predominates in
platelet lysates or releasates. This conclusion is consistent with
the overall resistance of platelet-rich thrombi to thrombolysis
both in vitro and in vivo. Of the antifibrinolytic molecules, recent attention has focused on the contribution of PAI-1 to the
resistance of platelet-rich thrombi to lysis.

B. The Platelet Surface and Fibrinolysis

In contrast to the predominance of antiproteolytic activity
within the intracellular compartments, the cell surface of the
platelets promotes plasmin generation. As depicted in Figure 1, platelets can assemble all three major categories of plasminogen activators on their surface. Direct binding of u-PA
and t-PA to platelets has been demonstrated. These activators
bind to different sites on the cell surface, and platelet activation
is not a requisite for their interaction. Both u-PA and t-PA bind
saturably, suggesting the presence of a discrete number of

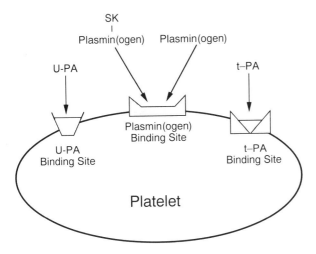

Figure 1   Interactions of the fibrinolytic system at the platelet surface. The plasminogen activators, t-PA and u-PA, bind directly and at
independent sites on the platelet surface. Streptokinase (SK) binds as
the SK-plasmin(ogen) complex. Plasminogen and plasmin bind to the
same site on the platelet surface. These latter sites are dependent
upon GPIIb-IIIa and fibrin(ogen).

binding sites. t-PA and u-PA receptors have been identified on
variety of cells. The characteristics of t-PA or u-PA binding to
platelets, either in terms of affinity or recognition specificity,
indicate that the binding sites for each activator are distinct
from those described on other cells. SK does not bind directly
to platelets. However, as discussed below, plasmin(ogen) does
bind to platelets, and SK can "piggyback" onto the cell surface
by virtue of its interaction with plasminogen. As fibrin binds to
the surface of platelets, it is anticipated that t-PA bound to fibrin would also be tethered to the surface, but the published
data have not demonstrated this possibility.

Plasminogen also binds in a specific and saturable manner
to platelets. Platelet activation by thrombin, but not by other
agonists, enhances plasminogen binding three- to ninefold.
Plasminogen binding to nonstimulated platelets is dependent

upon GPIIb-IIIa, the major platelet membrane glycoprotein; and the number of plasminogen binding sites on resting platelets, approximately 40,000, is consistent with the number of GPIIb-IIIa molecules of the cell surface. Fibrin, which can be acquired from the fibrinogen in the plasma or from within the platelet alpha granules, also associates with GPIIb-IIIa and accounts for the incremental increase in plasminogen-binding sites on thrombin-stimulated platelets. Plasminogen also binds to a variety of adhesive proteins, which associate with the platelet surface. Thrombospondin and fibronectin fall into this category. Accordingly, the "piggybacking" of plasminogen onto the platelet surface via carrier proteins can be postulated, but the experimental conditions to demonstrate this mechanism have not been established.

A primary consequence of plasminogen binding to platelets is to enhance its activation. Augmented plasmin formation on the platelet surface is observed with all three types of plasminogen activator (t-PA, u-PA, and SK), but this enhancement may be most dramatic for t-PA. This effect may explain the in vitro observation that platelet-rich thrombi are more susceptible to t-PA than to SK. In addition to accelerating plasminogen activation, the platelet surface also stabilizes plasmin activity. Plasmin bound to cell surfaces is protected from $alpha_2$-antiplasmin. This protection is similar to that afforded plasmin bound to the fibrin surface.

Based upon the kinetic advantages afforded by the combination of augmented plasminogen activation and the protection of plasmin from $alpha_2$-antiplasmin, it is calculated that the platelet surface enhances proteolytic potential at least 500-fold compared to the soluble phase. However, this enhancement need not be prothrombolytic. The binding of plasminogen and plasmin, as well as the plasminogen activators, to the cell surface may compete with their binding to the fibrin surface and, thus, limit their free diffusion throughout the thrombus. Thus, in a paradoxical fashion, the favored generation of plasmin on the platelet surface may, in fact, contribute to the resistance of platelet-rich thrombi to thrombolysis.

C. The Effects of Plasmin on Platelets

Plasmin has been shown to affect platelet function in multiple and confounding ways. Several studies have shown that plasmin can activate platelets, as assessed by alterations in typical intracellular signaling markers. As a consequence, platelet aggregation and secretion can ensue. There is consistent evidence for platelet activation during thrombolytic therapy, although it has not been shown that the responsible stimulus is plasmin.

Other studies have shown that plasmin can blunt platelet responses. Direct proteolysis of adhesion receptors on the cell surface by plasmin contributes to these inhibitory effects. Most sensitive to proteolysis is GPIb, although a redistribution from between cell-surface GPIb and an internal pool tends to minimize net changes. GPIIb-IIIa also can be cleaved by plasmin, but its susceptibility to proteolysis depends upon experimental conditions, and it is uncertain whether such proteolysis occurs during thrombolytic therapy.

Some of the effects of plasmin on platelet function may be indirect. With the dependence of platelet aggregation upon fibrinogen, the extent of fibrinogen depletion during thrombolytic therapy would blunt this response. Even with an agent such as t-PA, which induces limited fibrinogenolysis, partial proteolysis of fibrinogen occurs, and the major fibrinogen fragment generated (Fragment X) supports platelet aggregation only poorly. With more extensive fibrinogen breakdown, the degradation products produced not only fail to support platelet aggregation but also inhibit the response.

D. Effects of Platelets on the Physical Characteristics of Thrombi

In addition to the molecular and cellular considerations delineated above, the influence of platelets on the physical properties of thrombi may be of equal (and perhaps even of greater) importance in regulating thrombolysis. A fibrin clot is composed largely of water. Therefore, protein molecules—

plasminogen activators, plasminogen, etc.—diffuse readily throughout the clot. Platelets retract clots. In addition to decreased diffusion through a retracted clot, extrusion of profibrinolytic proteins may occur. Consistent with this scenario, compaction of platelet-poor clots to mimic the effect of platelet-induced clot retraction renders them resistant to lysis. Platelet-induced clot retraction is mediated by linkage between the actin-rich cytoskeleton of the cell with the membrane receptor GPIIb-IIIa when it becomes occupied by fibrin(ogen). In addition, as noted above, certain proteins secreted from platelets can influence the physical characteristics of clots.

E. Perspective

In vitro and vivo studies emphasize that the incorporation of platelets into a thrombus imparts resistance to lysis. Thus, there is a natural inclination to dismiss the potential profibrinolytic contributions of platelets and to focus their antifibrinolytic activities. Some cautions must be raised regarding this emphasis. Most in vitro experiments are conducted with a preformed thrombus under nonflowing conditions. Just as blood flow and shear have crucial effects on thrombus formation, they are also likely to influence thrombolysis. Thrombus formation, particularly in the face of ongoing thrombolytic therapy, is a dynamic process with a continuous accrual and turnover of fibrin and platelets. The fibrinolytic role of the platelets within the thrombus may change as the character of the thrombus changes over time. Thus, at early stages of thrombolysis, the profibrinolytic properties may be influential and are supplanted by antithrombolytic effects. Moreover, while in vivo studies show that lysis-resistant thrombi are platelet-rich, it cannot be excluded that a population of platelet-rich thrombi are particularly susceptible to lysis. These complexities are not raised as an argument against the use of antiplatelet agents as adjuncts to thrombolytic therapy. Indeed, a variety of antiplatelet agents have had very encouraging effects on thrombolysis in experimental models and in humans.

Table 2 Major Platelet Adhesion Receptors and Their Ligands

Receptor	Ligands
$\alpha_2\beta_1$ (GPIa-IIa)	Collagen
$\alpha_5\beta_1$ (GPIc-IIIa)	Fibronectin
$\alpha_6\beta_1$	Laminin
$\alpha_{IIb}\beta_3$ (GPIIb-IIIa)	Fibrinogen, fibronectin, von Willebrand's factor, vitronectin
$\alpha_v\beta_3$ (vitronectin receptor)	Vitronectin, fibrinogen
GPIb	von Willebrand's factor
GPIV	Collagen, thrombospondin

However, caution must be taken. Therapeutic manipulation of the platelets may not only increase bleeding risks (as discussed below) but also may blunt their positive contributions to thrombolysis.

III. PLATELETS AND THROMBOSIS

The role of platelets in thrombus formation can be divided into two sequential steps: (1) platelet adhesion and (2) platelet aggregation.

A. Platelet Adhesion

The initial involvement of platelets in thrombus formation entails their adhesion to sites of vascular wall perturbation or injury. The adhesive reaction is mediated by cell surface receptors, which recognize constituents within the exposed subendothelial matrix. The receptors and ligands involved in mediating platelet adhesion are summarized in Table 2. The receptors are multiple, and their ligands are diverse. Several of the membrane proteins are members of the integrin family of adhesion receptors. Integrins are α-β heterodimers, composed of two nonidentical and noncovalently linked subunits. There

are at least 19 members of the integrin family, and posttran-
scriptional and postranslational modifications further expand
the diversity of the family. Three members of the β_1 integrin
subfamily are present on platelets; these (α_2, α_5, and α_6) share
a common β_1 subunit, which combines with distinct α subunits
to form receptors with unique recognition specificities. These
β_1 integrins are found on a variety of other cell types as well.
Both representatives of the β_3 subfamily GPIIb-IIIa ($\alpha_{IIb}\beta_3$) and
the vitronectin receptor ($\alpha_v\beta_3$) are present on platelets.

GPIb, a nonintegrin, functions as a receptor for von Willebrand's factor (vWF). Based on the bleeding tendencies in patients deficient in vWF or GPIb (Bernard-Soulier syndrome),
this receptor-ligand pair plays a major role in mediating platelet adhesion. Recognition of vWF by GPIb is shear dependent;
vWF-mediated platelet adhesion is particularly important in
vessels of small caliber.

B. Platelet Aggregation

In addition to their adhesion to the vessel wall, the involvement of platelets in thrombus formation depends on their capacity to interact with one another. Like platelet adhesion,
platelet aggregation also is receptor mediated; unlike platelet
adhesion, in which multiple receptors are involved, occupancy
of a single receptor on the platelet surface elicits the aggregation response. The cell membrane glycoprotein GPIIb-IIIa,
schematically depicted in Figure 2, mediates platelet aggregation. As noted above, GPIIb-IIIa is an integrin of the β_3
subfamily. This membrane protein is multifunctional, as it
can mediate platelet adhesion as well as aggregation, and is
also involved in assembly of the fibrinolytic system as a
plasminogen-binding site.

Multiple adhesive ligands, including fibrinogen, fibronectin, vWF, and vitronectin, can interact with GPIIb-IIIa. These
ligands appear to occupy a common binding site of GPIIb-IIIa.
Occupancy of the receptor by fibrinogen leads to platelet aggregation. Under conditions of high shear, occupancy of
GPIIb-IIIa by vWF also may result in platelet aggregation. The

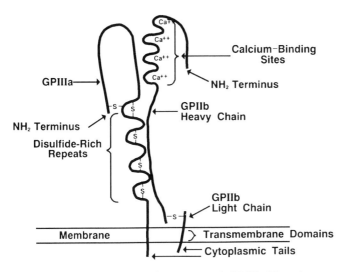

Figure 2   Schematic depiction of GPIIb-IIIa. As a typical integrin adhesion receptor, GPIIb-IIIa ($\alpha_{IIb}\beta_3$) consists of two subunits, which associate noncovalently. GPIIb is proteolytically processed into a heavy and light chain. The ligand-binding site for fibrinogen and other ligands resides in the amino-terminal aspect of the receptor, in close proximity to the second divalent cation-binding site in the GPIIb subunit. The short cytoplasmic tails are involved in regulating activation to the receptor for ligand-binding function and also mediate binding to the intracellular cytoskeleton, an interaction essential for platelet-mediated clot retraction. (From D'Souza et al., 1991, with permission.)

interaction of fibronectin and vitronectin with GPIIb-IIIa does not support aggregation; binding of these adhesive ligands to GPIIb-IIIa may be important in platelet adhesion to the subendothelium.

As platelets circulate in the blood, they are continuously exposed to high concentrations of GPIIb-IIIa ligands; yet receptor occupancy and platelet aggregation do not occur spontaneously. Ligand binding to GPIIb-IIIa is a regulated event. The event that allows the receptor to become competent to bind ligand is platelet activation. A variety of physiologically relevant agonists, including thrombin, collagen, epinephrine,

ADP, and certain prostaglandin derivatives, are capable of stimulating platelets and activating the receptor. The latter two agonists are carried within platelets and are released when platelets are stimulated. Thus, initial stimulation of platelets releases agonists, which are capable of recruiting additional platelets in thrombus formation. The various agonists interact with multiple receptors on the platelet surface to generate an array of intracellular signals. By a still undefined mechanism, these events converge to induce conformational changes in the receptor such that it becomes competent to bind ligands. Once occupied by an appropriate ligand, fibrinogen or vWF, platelet aggregation ensues very rapidly. Reocclusion of vessels with platelet-rich thrombi following initial successful thrombolytic therapy also will depend upon occupancy of GPIIb-IIIa. Reocclusion should be less of a problem with thrombolytic agents that deplete circulating fibrinogen than with fibrin-targeted agents. However, the turbulence of blood flow created by residual thrombus within a lesion may accentuate the role of vWF as a GPIIb-IIIa ligand.

IV. THERAPEUTIC CONSIDERATIONS

The exposure of specific platelet-adhesive ligands at a site of vascular injury is determined by the characteristics of the lesion (e.g., depth, location), the adsorption of plasma factors, and the biosynthetic output of the cells within the microenvironment. Thus, a multiplicity of adhesive interactions is possible. Such complexity makes it unlikely that any single agent would effectively block all platelet-adhesive reactions. Moreover, since platelet adhesion is the initial line of defense against excessive bleeding, there is a perception, though not necessarily justified, that interference with platelet adhesion would result in severe bleeding complications. For these reasons, inhibition of platelet adhesion has not been pursued vigorously as a target for antithrombotic drugs. In contrast, the dependence of platelet aggregation, regardless of the inducing agonist, upon GPIIb-IIIa has made this receptor a very attractive target for antithrombotic therapy. A number of antagonists of ligand binding to GPIIb-IIIa have been identified. These have included antibodies to the receptor and a variety of ligand mimetics. Included in the latter category are snake venoms (the disintegrins), small peptides, and mimetics of these peptides. Several GPIIb-IIIa antagonists are in clinical testing and hold considerable promise as antithrombotic drugs.

Of the GPIIb-IIIa antagonists, the monoclonal antibody 7E3, or more specifically a humanized fragment of the antibody, is furthest in clinical testing and development. Promising initial results have been obtained with 7E3 in patients with unstable angina and coronary angioplasty. The distinction among the various GPIIb-IIIa antagonists as antithrombotic agents will ultimately reside in their potency, specificity, pharmokinetic properties, oral availability, and cost. Since clinical trials to test combinations of therapeutics, a GPIIb-IIIa antagonist and a thrombolytic agent, are highly complex and costly, GPIIb-IIIa antagonists are likely to find utility in indications other than thrombolytic therapy first.

With regard to thrombolysis, 7E3 did have a profound effect when given in conjunction with t-PA in a canine model of thrombosis. These encouraging results provide a basis for testing 7E3 and other GPIIb-IIIa antagonists as conjunctive agents in thrombolytic therapy.

Rather than interfering directly with ligand binding to GPIIb-IIIa, antagonists that prevent activation of the receptor may also be efficacious. Falling within this category are antagonists of the prostanoid system, ADP antagonists, PAF inhibitors, serotonin and epinephrine antagonists, and thrombin receptor antagonists. Since there are multiple and independent pathways for stimulation of platelets and activation of GPIIb-IIIa, blockade of any single pathway is unlikely to be effective as a general approach to prevent thrombosis. However, the mechanism of rethrombosis following thrombolytic therapy may be dominated by a single activation pathway, and blockade of a specific platelet activation pathway may be effective.

A central issue in considering the efficacy of any platelet inhibitor, including a GIIb-IIIa antagonist, is the risk of bleeding. Genetic defects in platelet adhesive and aggregation functions are associated with episodic bleeding. Thus, therapeutic interference with platelet function will predictably be associated with increased bleeding. This risk will undoubtedly be accentuated in thrombolytic therapy, which has, in itself, an inherent bleeding risk. The critical questions, of course, are whether the bleeding will be life threatening and require significant additional intervention. Unfortunately, the answers to these questions are not predictable. Nor can the characteristics of the most effective platelet conjunctive agent be specified. Of the GPIIb-IIIa antagonists currently under development, some, such as a monoclonal antibody, would have a long-lasting effect, while others would be short-acting and reversible. The latter category may be associated with fewer bleeding complications but may not be less effective in preventing rethrombosis.

PERTINENT REFERENCES

Adelman B, Michelson A D, Loscalzo J, Greenberg J, Handin R I: Plasmin effect on platelet glycoprotein IB-von Willebrand factor interactions. *Blood* 1985;65:32–40.

Adnot S, Ferry N, Hanoune J, Lacombe M L: Plasmin: a possible physiological modulator of human platelet adenylate cyclase system. *Clin Sci* 1987;72:467–473.

Ashton J H, Ogletree M L, Michel I M, et al.: Cooperative mediation by serotonin S_2 and thromboxane A_2/prostaglandin H_2 receptor activation cooperatively mediate cyclic flow variations in dogs with severe coronary artery stenosis. *Circulation* 1987;76:952–959.

Ashton J H, Benedict C R, Fitzgerald C, et al.: Serotonin as a mediator of cyclic flow variations in stenosed canine coronary arteries. *Circulation* 1986;73:572–578.

Bale M D, Mosher D F: Effects of thrombospondin on fibrin polymerization and structure. *J Biol Chem* 1986;261:862–868.

Bode C, Meinhardt G, Runge M S, et al.: Platelet-targeted fibrinolysis enhances clot lysis and inhibits platelet aggregation. *Circulation* 1991;84: 805–813.

Braaten, J V, Handt S, Jerome W G, Kirkpatrick J, Lewis J C, Hantgan R R: Regulation of fibrinolysis by platelet-released plasminogen activator inhibitor 1: light scattering and ultrastructural examination of lysis of a model platelet-fibrin thrombus. *Blood* 1993;81:1290–1299.

Carroll R C, Butler R G, Morris P A, Gerrard J M: Separable assembly of platelet pseudopodal and contractile cytoskeletons. *Cell* 1982;30:385–393.

Carroll R C, Radcliffe R D, Taylor F B, Jr., Gerrard J M. Plasminogen, plasminogen activator, and platelets in the regulation of clot lysis. *J Lab Clin Med* 1982;100:986–996.

Chesebro J H, Knatterud G, Roberts R, et al.: Thrombolysis in myocardial infarction (TIMI) trial, phase I: a comparison between intravenous tissue plasminogen activator and intravenous streptokinase. *Circulation* 1987; 76:142–154.

Collen D, Stump D C, Gold H K: Thrombolytic therapy. *Annu Rev Med* 1988;39:405–423.

Coller B S: Platelets and thrombolytic therapy. *N Engl J Med* 1990;322:33–42.

Coller B S, Peerschke E I, Scudder L E, Sullivan C A: A murine monoclonal antibody that completely blocks the binding of fibrinogen to platelets produces a thrombasthenic-like state in normal platelets and binds to glycoproteins IIb and/or IIIa. *J Clin Invest* 1983;72:325–338.

Deguchi K, Murashima S, Shirakawa S, et al.: The potentiating effect of platelet on plasminogen activation by tissue plasminogen activator. *Thromb Res* 1985;40:853–861.

Dewerchin M, Lijnen H R, Stassen J M, et al.: Effect of chemical conjugation of recombinant single-chain urokinase-type plasminogen activator with monoclonal antiplatelet antibodies on platelet aggregation and on plasma clot lysis in vitro and in vivo. *Blood* 1991;78:1005–1018.

D'Souza S E, Ginsberg M H, Plow E F: Arginyl-glycyl-aspartic acid (RGD): a cell adhesion motif. *Trends Biochem Sci* 1991;16:246–250.

Ellis S G, Tcheng J E, Navetta F I, et al.: Safety and antiplatelet effect of murine monoclonal antibody 7E3 Fab directed against platelet glycoprotein IIb/IIIa in patients undergoing elective coronary angioplasty. *Coronary Artery Dis* 1993;4:167–176.

Erickson L A, Ginsberg M H, Loskutoff D J: Detection and partial characterization of an inhibitor of plasminogen activator in human platelets. *J Clin Invest* 1984;74:1465–1472.

Fitzgerald D J, Catella F, Roy L, FitzGerald G A: Marked platelet activation in vivo after intravenous streptokinase in patients with acute myocardial infarction. *Circulation* 1988;77:142–150.

Fitzgerald D J, Wright F, FitzGerald G A: Increased thromboxane biosynthesis during coronary thrombolysis: evidence that platelet activation and thromboxane A_2 modulate the response to tissue-type plasminogen activator in vivo. *Circ Res* 1989;65:83–94.

Fox J E B, Boyles J K, Reynolds C C, Phillips D R: Actin filament content and organization in unstimulated platelets. *J Cell Biol* 1984;98:1985–1991.

Francis C W, Marder V J: Rapid formation of large molecular weight α-polymers in cross-linked fibrin induced by high factor XIII concentration: role of platelet factor XIII. *J Clin Invest* 1987;80:1459–1465.

George J N, Nurden A T, Phillips D R: Molecular defects in interactions of platelets with the vessel wall. *N Engl J Med* 1984;311:1084–1098.

Gold H K, Coller B S, Yasuda T, et al.: Rapid and sustained coronary artery recanalization with combined bolus injection of recombinant tissue-type plasminogen activator and monoclonal antiplatelet GPIIb/IIIa antibody in a canine preparation. *Circulation* 1988;77:670–677.

Golino P, Ashton J H, Glas-Greenwalt P, McNatt J, Buja L M, Willerson J T: Mediation of reocclusion by thromboxane A_2 and serotonin after thrombolysis with tissue-type plasminogen activator in a canine preparation of coronary thrombosis. *Circulation* 1988;77:678–684.

Golino P, Ashton J H, McNatt J, et al.: Simultaneous administration of thromboxane A_2- and serotonin S_2-receptor antagonists markedly enhances thrombolysis and prevents or delays reocclusion after tissue-type plasminogen activator in a canine model of coronary thrombosis. *Circulation* 1989;79:911–919.

Gouin I, Lecompte T, Morel M-C, et al.: In vitro effect of plasmin on human platelet function in plasma. *Circulation* 1992;85:935–941.

Gould R J, Polokoff M A, Friedman P A, et al.: Disintegrins: a family of integrin inhibitory proteins from viper venoms. *Proc Soc Exp Biol Med* 1990;195:168–171.

Gould R J, Zhang G, Manno P D, Nutt R F, Lynch R J, Friedman P A: L-367,073 is a selective inhibitor of platelet aggregation, acting at platelet integrin glycoprotein IIb/IIIa. *Thromb Haemost* 1991;65:842 (abstract).

Gruppo Italiano per lo Studio della Sopravvivenza Nell'Infarto Miocardico: GISSI-2: a factorial randomized trial of alteplase versus streptokinase and heparin versus no heparin among 12,490 patients with acute myocardial infarction. *Lancet* 1990;336:65–71.

Guccione M A, Kinlough-Rathbone R L, Packham M A, et al.: Effects of plasmin on rabbit platelets. *Thromb Haemost* 1985;53:8–14.

Hall S W, Humphries J E, Gonias S L: Inhibition of cell surface receptor-bound plasmin by α_2-antiplasmin and α_2-macroglobulin. *J Biol Chem* 1991;266:12329–12336.

Handagama P J, George J N, Shuman M A, McEver R P, Bainton D F: Incorporation of a circulating protein into megakaryocyte and platelet granules. *Proc Natl Acad Sci USA* 1987;84:861–865.

Haskel E J, Adams S P, Feigen L P, et al.: Prevention of reoccluding platelet-rich thrombi in canine femoral arteries with a novel peptide antagonist of platelet glycoprotein IIb/IIIa receptors. *Circulation* 1989;80:1775–1782.

Houdijk W P M, Sakariassen K S, Nievelstein P F E M, Sixma J J: Role of factor VIII-von Willebrand factor and fibronectin in the interaction of platelets in flowing blood with monomeric and fibrillar human collagen types I and III. *J. Clin Invest* 1985;75:531–540.

Humphries J E, Hall S W, VandenBerg S R, Gonias S L: Streptokinase-plasmin complex binds to plasminogen receptors on rat hepatocytes and human endothelium. *Fibrinolysis* 1991;5:171–176.

Hynes R O: Integrins: a family of cell surface receptors. *Cell* 1987;48:549–554.

International Study Group: In-hospital mortality and clinical course of 20,891 patients with suspected acute myocardial infarction randomized between alteplase and streptokinase with or without heparin. *Lancet* 1990; 336:71–75.

Jang I K, Gold H K, Ziskind A A, et al.: Differential sensitivity of erythrocyte-rich and platelet-rich arerial thrombi to lysis with recombinant tissue-type plasminogen activator. A possible explanation for resistance to coronary thrombolysis. *Circulation* 1989;79:920–928.

Jeanneau C, Sultan Y: Tissue plasminogen activator in human megakaryocytes and platelets: immunocytochemical localization, immunoblotting and zymographic analysis. *Thromb Haemost* 1988;59:529–534.

Joist J H: Platelets and fibrinolysis. *Thromb Haemostas* 1977;38:955–962.

Kloczewiak M, Timmons S, Hawiger J: Recognition site for the platelet receptor is present on the 15-residue carboxy-terminal fragment of the gamma chain of human fibrinogen and is not involved in the fibrin polymerization reaction. *Thromb Res* 1983;29:249–255.

Kruithof E K, Tran-Thang C, Bachmann F: Studies on the release of plasminogen activator inhibitor by human platelets. *Thrombos Haemostas* 1986;55:201–205.

Kunicki T J, Nugent D J, Staats S, Orchekowski R P, Wayner E A, Carter W G: The human fibroblast class II extracellular matrix receptor (ECMR II) mediates platelet adhesion to collagen and is identical to the platelet glycoprotein IIa-IIa complex. *Blood* 1987;70(Suppl 1):353a.

Kunitada S, Fitzgerald G A, Fitzgerald D J: Inhibition of clot lysis and decreased binding of tissue-type plasminogen activator as a consequence of clot retraction. *Blood* 1992;79:1420–1427.

Lam S C-T, Dieter J P, Strebel L C, et al.: Rapid dissociation of platelet-rich fibrin clots in vitro by a combination of plasminogen activators and antiplatelet agents. *J Pharmacol Exp Ther* 1991;259:1371–1378.

Lam S C, Plow E F, D'Souza S E, Cheresh D A, Frelinger A L, III, Ginsberg M H: Isolation and characterization of a platelet membrane protein related to the vitronectin receptor. *J Biol Chem* 1989;264:3742–3749.

Lawler J, Hynes R O: The structure of human thrombospondin, and adhesive glycoprotein with multiple calcium-binding sites and homologies with several different proteins. *J Cell Biol* 1986;103:1635–1648.

Loscalzo J, Vaughan D E: Tissue plasminogen activator promotes platelet disaggregation in plasma. *J Clin Invest* 1987;79:1749–1755.

Lu H R, Gold H K, Wu Z, et al.: Acceleration and persistence of recombinant tissue plasminogen activator-induced arterial eversion graft recanalization with a single bolus injection of F(ab')$_2$ fragments of the antiplatelet glycoprotein IIb/IIIa antibody 7E3. *Coronary Artery Dis* 1991;2:1039–1046.

Michelson A D, Barnard M R: Plasmin-induced redistribution of platelet glycoprotein Ib. *Blood* 1990;76:2005–2010.

Mickelson J K, Simpson P J, Gallas M T, Lucchesi B R: Thromboxane synthase inhibition with CGS 13080 improves coronary blood flow after streptokinase-induced thrombolysis. *Am Heart J* 1987;113:1345–1352.

Miles L A, Ginsberg M H, White J G, Plow E F: Plasminogen interacts with human platelets through two distinct mechanisms. *J Clin Invest* 1986; 77:2001–2009.

Miles L A, Plow E F: Binding and activation of plasminogen on the platelet surface. *J Biol Chem* 1985;260:4303–4311.

Muller D W M, Topol E J: *Textbook of interventional cardiology*, Update 4, 4th ed., Philadelphia, W. B. Saunders Co., 1992, pp. 59–74.

Niewiarowski S, Budzynski A Z, Lipinski B: Significance of the intact polypeptide chains of human fibrinogen in ADP-induced platelet aggregation. *Blood* 1977;49(4):635–644.

Niewiarowski S, Gurewich V, Senyi A F, Mustard J F: The effect of fibrinolysis on platelet function. *Thromb Diath Haemorrh Suppl* 1971;47:99–111.

Niewiarowski S, Senyi A F, Gillies P: Plasmin-induced platelet aggregation and platelet release reaction. *J Clin Invest* 1973;52:1647–1659.

Owen J, Friedman K D, Grossman B A, Wilkens C, Berke A D, Powers E R: Quantitation of fragment X formation during thrombolytic therapy with streptokinase and tissue plasminogen activator. *J Clin Invest* 1987; 79:1642–1647.

Park S, Harker L A, Marzec U M, Levin E G: Demonstration of single chain urokinase-type plasminogen activator on human platelet membrane. *Blood* 1989;73:1421–1425.

Phillips D R, Charo I F, Scarborough R M: GPIIb-IIIa: the responsive integrin. *Cell* 1991;65:359–362.

Plow E F, Collen D: The presence and release of alpha2-antiplasmin from human platelets. *Blood* 1981;58:1069–1074.

Plow E F, Felez J, Miles L A: Cellular regulation of fibrinolysis. *Thromb Haemost* 1991;66:32–36.

Plow E F, Freaney D E, Plescia J, Miles L A: The plasminogen system and cell surfaces: evidence for plasminogen and urokinase receptors on the same cell type. *J Cell Biol* 1986;103:2411–2420.

Plow E F, Ginsberg M H: Cellular adhesion: GPIIb-IIIa as a prototypic adhesion receptor, in Coller B S, (ed): *Progress in Hemostasis and thrombosis*, Vol. 9. Philadelphia, W. B. Saunders, 1989, pp. 117–156.

Plow E F, Marguerie G A, Ginsberg M: Fibrinogen, fibrinogen receptors and the peptides that inhibit these interactions. *Biochem Pharmacol* 1987; 36:4035–4040.

Plow E F, McEver R P, Coller B S, Woods V L, Marguerie G A, Ginsberg M H: Related binding mechanisms for fibrinogen, fibronectin, von Willebrand factor and thrombospondin on thrombin-stimulated human platelets. *Blood* 1985;66:724–727.

Randomised trial of intravenous streptokinase, oral aspirin, both, or neither among 17,187 cases of suspected acute myocardial infarction: ISIS-2. *Lancet* 1988;2:349–360.

Sabovic M, Lijnen H R, Keber D, Collen D: Effect of retraction on the lysis of human clots with fibrin specific and non-fibrin specific plasminogen activators. *Thromb Haemost* 1989;62:1083–1087.

Sabovic M, Lijnen H R, Keber D, Collen D: Correlation between progressive adsorption of plaminogen to blood clots and their sensitivity to lysis. *Thromb Haemost* 1990;64:450–454.

Salonen E M, Sakeseki O, Vartio T, Vaheri A, Neilsen L S, Zeuthen J: Plasminogen and tissue-type plasminogen activator bind to immobilized fibronectin. *J Biol Chem* 1985;260:12302–12307.

Santoro S A, Rajpara S M, Staatz W D, Woods V L, Jr.: Isolation and characterization of a platelet surface collagen binding complex related to VLA-2. *Biochem Biophys Res Commun* 1988;153:217–223.

Scarborough R M, Hsu M A, Teng W, et al. Potent and integrin specific KGD-containing platelet antagonists designed from the GPIIb-IIIa specific antagonist barbourin. *Thromb Haemost* 1991;65:843 (abstract).

Schafer A I, Ademan B: Plasmin inhibition of platelet function and of arachidonic acid metabolism. *J. Clin Invest* 1985;75:456–461.

Schafer A I, Maas A K, Ware J A, Johnson P C, Rittenhouse S E, Salzman E W: Platelet protein phosphorylation, elevation of cytosolic calcium, and inositol phospholipid breakdown in platelet activation induced by plasmin. *J Clin Invest* 1986;78:73–79.

Shebuski R J, Stabilito I J, Sitko G R, Polokoff M H: Acceleration of recombinant tissue-type plasminogen activator-induced thrombolysis and prevention of reocclusion by the combination of heparin and the Arg-Gly-Asp-containing peptide bitistatin in a canine model of coronary thrombosis. *Circulation* 1990;82:169–177.

Shebuski R J, Storer B L, Fujita T: Effect of thromboxane synthase inhibition on the thrombolytic action of tissue-type plasminogen activator in a rabbit model of peripheral arterial thrombosis. *Thromb Res* 1988;52:381–392.

Silverstein R L, Leung L L K, Harpel P C, Nachman R L: Complex formation of platelet thrombospondin with plasminogen. *J Clin Invest* 1984;74: 1625–1633.

Simoons M L, European Cooperative Study Group: Randomized trial of monoclonal platelet antibody for refractory unstable angina pectoris. European Congress of Cardiology, Barcelona, Spain, 1992.

Sonnenberg A, Modderman P W, Hoøervorst F: Laminin receptor on platelets is the integrin VLA-6. *Nature* 1989;336:487–489.

Solum N O, Rigollot C, Budzynski A Z, Marder V J: A quantitative evaluation of the inhibition of platelet aggregation by low molecular weight degradation products of fibrinogen. *Br J Haematol* 1973;24:419–434.

Stricker R B, Wong D, Tak Shiu D, Reyes P T, Shuman M A: Activation of plasminogen by tissue plasminogen activator on normal and thrombasthenic platelets: Effects on surface proteins and platelet aggregation. *Blood* 1986;68:275–280.

Taylor F B, Jr., Muller-Eberhard H J: Qualitative description of factors involved in the retraction and lysis of dilute whole blood clots and in the aggregation and retraction of platelets. *J Clin Invest* 1970;49:2068–2085.

Taylor F B, Jr., Carroll R C, Gerrard J, Esmon C T, Radcliffe R D: Lysis of clots prepared from whole blood and plasma. *Fed Proc* 1981;40:2092–2098.

Tcheng J E, Kleiman N S, Miller M J, Sane D S, Wang A L, Weisman H F: Chimeric antiplatelet GPIIb/IIIa receptor antibody (C-7E3) in elective PTCA: safety and platelet function inhibition. *Circulation* 1992;84 (Suppl.II):590a (abstract).

Thorsen S, Brakman F, Astrup T: Influence of platelets on fibrinolysis: A critical review, in Ambrose J L, (ed): *Hematologic reviews*, Vol. 3, New York, Marcel Dekker, Inc., 1972, pp. 123–179.

Topol E J, Califf R M, George B S, et al.: Coronary arterial thrombolysis with combined infusion of recombinant tissue-type plasminogen activator and urokinase in patients with acute myocardial infarction. *Circulation* 1988;77:1100–1107.

Topol E J, Morris D C, Smalling R W, et al.: A multicenter, randomized, placebo-controlled trial of a new form of intravenous recombinant tissue-type plasminogen activator (activase) in acute myocardial infarction. *J Am Coll Cardiol* 1987;9:1205–1213.

Vaughan D E, Mendelsohn M E, Declerck P J, Van Houtte E, Collen D, Loscalzo J: Characterization of the binding of human tissue-type plasminogen activator to platelets. *J Biol Chem* 1989;264:15869–15874.

Vaughan D E, Van Houtte E, Collen D C: Urokinase binds to platelets through a specific saturable, low affinity mechanism. *Fibrinolysis* 1990;4:141–146.

Vaughan D E, Van Houtte E, Declerck P J, Collen D: Streptokinase-induced platelet aggregation: prevalence and mechanism. *Circulation* 1991;84: 84–91.

Weiss H J, Hawiger J, Ruggeri Z M, Turitto V T, Thiagarajan P, Hoffman T: Fibrinogen-independent platelet adhesion and thrombus formation on subendothelium mediated by glocoprotein IIb-IIIa complex at high shear rate. J Clin Invest 1989;83:288–297.

Weiss H J, Meyer D, Rabinowitz R, et al.: Pseudo-von Willebrand's disease. An intrinsic platelet defect with aggregation by unmodified human factor VIII/von Willebrand factor and enhanced adsorption of its high-molecular-weight multimers. *N Engl J Med* 1982;306:326–333.

Willerson J T, Golino P, McNatt J, Eidt J, Yao S-K, Buja L M: Role of new antiplatelet agents as adjunctive therapies in thrombolysis. *Am J Cardiol* 1991;67:12A–18A.

Winters K J, Eisenberg P R, Jaffe A S, Santoro S A: Dependence of plasmin-mediated degradation of platelet adhesive receptors on temperature and Ca^{2+}. *Blood* 1990;76:1546–1557.

Yasada T, Gold H K, Fallon J T, et al.: Monoclonal antibody against the platelet glycoprotein (GP) IIb/IIIa receptor prevents coronary artery reocclusion after reperfusion with recombinant tissue-type plasminogen activator in dogs. *J Clin Invest* 1988;81:1284–1291.

Yasuda T, Gold H K, Leinbach R C, et al.: Lysis of plasminogen activator-resistant platelet-rich coronary artery thrombus with combined bolus injection of recombinant tissue-type plasminogen activator and antiplatelet GPIIb/IIIa antibody. *J Am Coll Cardiol* 1990;16:1728–1735.

Yasuda T, Gold H K, Yaoita H, et al.: Comparative effects of aspirin, a synthetic thrombin inhibitor and a monoclonal antiplatelet glycoprotein IIb/IIIa antibody on coronary artery reperfusion, reocclusion and bleeding with recombinant tissue-type plasminogen activator in a canine preparation. *J Am Coll Cardiol* 1990;16:714–722.

8

Relationships Between Suppression of Coagulation and Prevention of Reocclusion

Dana R. Abendschein
Washington University School of Medicine
St. Louis, Missouri

I. INTRODUCTION

Early reocclusion occurs in up to 20% of patients with coronary arteries initially recanalized by fibrinolytic agents and is associated with a high incidence of in-hospital mortality compared with that in patients exhibiting sustained coronary patency. Recognition that reocclusion is caused by a shift in the balance between clot lysis and thrombosis favoring rethrombosis has led to research to define the factors involved and to develop agents that when given together with fibrinolytic agents (i.e., conjunctive agents) might potentiate thrombolysis and inhibit subsequent reocclusion. This chapter discusses the role of thrombin in the pathogenesis of coronary reocclusion and the potential use of direct-acting inhibitors of thrombin and newly developed inhibitors of prothrombin activation as conjunctive agents.

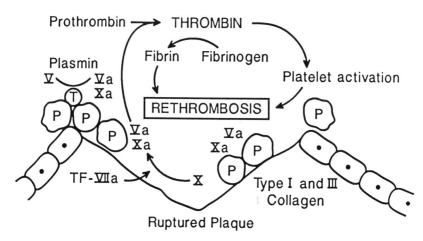

Figure 1   Diagram showing some of the factors contributing to re-occlusion after thrombolysis in an artery with initial thrombosis induced by plaque rupture. Plasmin and thrombin (T) bound to fibrin both activate factor V to Va, which leads to activation of more prothrombin via the prothrombinase complex formed with factor Xa on platelets (P). Factor X is activated by the complex of tissue factor and factor VIIa (TF-VIIa) exposed at the site of plaque rupture as are platelets by exposed collagen. Thrombin activates platelets and converts fibrinogen to fibrin, leading to accumulation of more thrombus.

A.   Factors Contributing to Reocclusion After Thrombolysis

Several factors appear to be active in shifting the balance during pharmacological thrombolysis toward rethrombosis (Figure 1), as listed below.

Fibrinolytic Agents

All fibrinolytic agents used clinically have procoagulant effects because they convert some plasminogen in the fluid phase surrounding thrombi to plasmin. This "free" plasmin converts prothrombin to thrombin directly and can activate factor X to Xa and factor V to Va, which together induce activation of prothrombin to thrombin. The thrombin thus formed degrades fibrinogen to fibrin and activates platelets causing accumulation of additional thrombus. Thrombin also markedly amplifies activation of prothrombin by activation of factors V, VIII, XI, and XIII.

Increased thrombin activity following administration of fibrinolytic agents is reflected by immediate increases in plasma levels of fibrinopeptide A, a 16-amino-acid polypeptide cleaved from fibrinogen by thrombin. Importantly, levels of fibrinopeptide A appear to increase more and remain higher in patients exhibiting failed thrombolysis and early reocclusion despite administration of heparin, indicating a close relationship between persistent thrombin activity and reocclusion.

Residual Thrombus

Fibrinolysis exposes enzymatically active thrombin and other procoagulant molecules to coagulation factors in the flowing blood. Although thrombin bound to fibrin has been thought to account for the majority of the procoagulant activity of thrombi, we have shown recently (Eisenberg et al.) that arterial thrombi exhibit relatively modest thrombin activity but marked factor Xa activity. Thrombus-associated factor Xa might represent that in complex with factor Va on the platelet membrane (the prothrombinase complex) or bound directly to fibrin. Nonetheless, factor Xa may be even more important than thrombin in accounting for the procoagulant activity of residual thrombus. Consistent with this hypothesis is the observation in patients given tissue-type plasminogen activator (t-PA) of increased plasma concentrations of prothrombin fragment 1.2, generated when prothrombin is activated to thrombin. Persistent activation of prothrombin by thrombus-associated factor Xa might also account for the rebound of thrombosis and reccurence of ischemia observed after the withdrawal of heparin.

Residual thrombus confers an additional risk for reocclusion by contributing to the severity of stenosis. High shear forces induced by the high velocity of blood flow through the stenosis can activate platelets directly or potentiate platelet adhesion mediated by interactions of platelet receptors for von Willebrand factor with von Willebrand factor in the wall of the vessel.

Exposed Vessel Injury

Fibrinolysis can reexpose blood to prothrombotic molecules including type I and type III collagen and tissue factor in the wall of the vessel at the site of plaque rupture. Tissue factor, which likely initiates thrombosis in response to vessel injury, is augmented in atherosclerotic plaque and forms a complex with factor VIIa to markedly accelerate factor VIIa–mediated activation of factor X. Plasminogen activator inhibitor type 1 is also increased in atheroma and upon reexposure might compromise the efficacy of fibrinolysis.

Thus, simultaneous, competing thrombosis during fibrinolysis is induced by procoagulant effects of fibrinolytic agents coupled with persistent thrombin activity and prothrombin activation in the thrombus and at the site of vessel injury. Platelet activation and aggregation induced by thrombin and by local shear forces also contribute. Accordingly, conjunctive therapy targeted at thrombin, its progenitors, or both appears essential to attenuate rethrombosis leading to vessel reocclusion with possibly some benefit derived from direct inhibition of platelets as well. Importantly, because procoagulant activity is greatly accelerated by fibrinolytic agents, sufficiently high plasma levels of anticoagulant agents must be achieved at or before the start of the infusion of lytic agents to attenuate reocclusion optimally.

II. RATIONALE FOR USE OF DIRECT INHIBITORS OF THROMBIN AS CONJUNCTIVE AGENTS

A. Limitations of Heparin

The underlying role of thrombin in reocclusion was doubted initially because heparin was only moderately effective for maintaining vessel patency in several thrombolysis studies. In some studies this might reflect inadequate doses and modes of administration or inappropriate timing of anticoagulation compared to the onset of the procoagulant activity associated with administration of fibrinolytic agents because others have reported better efficacy when heparin was administered intravenously with fibrinolytic agents. In addition to the dependence on dose and administration, however, heparin is also limited as an inhibitor of thrombin or factor Xa bound to fibrin in the milieu of the thrombus. Heparin must form an inhibitory complex with antithrombin III, which is bulky because of the relatively large size of antithrombin III (molecular weight 58,000) and thereby hindered from entry and association with thrombin and factor Xa bound to the thrombus. In addition, fibrin II monomer and platelet-derived proteins including platelet factor 4 and thrombospondin inhibit the formation of heparin-antithrombin III. Thus, low-molecular-weight, direct (i.e., antithrombin III–independent) inhibitors that easily penetrate the interstices of thrombi and are not deactivated by circulating factors have emerged as an important advance for the inhibition of bound thrombin.

B. Experimental Direct Inhibitors of Thrombin

Several direct inhibitors have been developed that exhibit diverse affinities for thrombin (Table 1). The most potent and specific known inhibitor of thrombin, and also the most extensively studied, is hirudin, a 65-amino-acid protein from the saliva of the medicinal leech, *Hirudo medicinalis*. Hirudin binds thrombin with 1:1 stoichiometry and with extraordinarily high affinity (K_D 2 $\times$ 10^{-14} M). It also exhibits high affinity for platelet thrombin receptors (10–100-fold higher than thrombin) and can displace thrombin bound to its platelet receptor. A recombinant form of hirudin is now available that differs from the native protein only in the absence of a sulfate group on tyrosine 63, but has nearly the same affinity for thrombin. Hirugen is a dodecapeptide modeled from the C-terminus of hirudin (N-acetyl-Hir53-64, sulfated Tyr63), which inhibits thrombin by binding to its anion-binding exosite. Hirugen's affinity for thrombin (K_D 1.5 $\times$ 10^{-7} M) is considerably lower than that of hirudin. Hirulogs are bifunctional oligopeptides

Table 1   Affinity of Inhibitors of Thrombin

Inhibitor	Molecular weight (Daltons)	K_D[a] of thrombin-inhibitor complex (M)
Heparin-antithrombin III	73,000	1.0×10^{-6} [b]
Recombinant desulfatohirudin	7,000	2.3×10^{-14}
DuP 714[c]	1,200	4.1×10^{-11}
Hirulog-1	8,000	2.3×10^{-9}
PPACK[d]	1,200	3.7×10^{-8} [b]
Argatroban[e]	526	3.9×10^{-8}
Hirugen	4,000	1.5×10^{-7}

[a]Dissociation constant.
[b]K_D for the initial reversible complex, which is followed by formation of an irreversible covalent bond.
[c]Ac-(D)-Phe-Pro-Boroarginine (Du Pont).
[d]D-Phe-L-Pro-L-Arg-chloromethyl ketone.
[e](2R,4R)-4-methyl-1-[N²-(3-methyl-1,2,3,4-tetrahydro-8-quinolinesulfonyl)-L-arginyl]-2-piperidinecarboxylic acid monohydrate (MCI-9038).

with both a C-terminal domain resembling hirudins and a synthetic N-terminal tripeptide domain that inhibits the amidolytic center of thrombin. The bifunctional interaction with thrombin increases hirulog's affinity for thrombin compared with hirugen. Among the smaller peptide inhibitors, the boroarginine tripeptide, DuP 714 (Du Pont), exhibits the highest affinity for thrombin compared with hirudin and has the potential for oral administration.

III.   RESULTS FROM STUDIES OF THROMBIN INHIBITORS IN VIVO

A.   Considerations Related to Animal Preparations of Thrombosis

Results of studies in experimental animals must be considered relative to the methods employed to induce recurrent thrombosis and their ability to simulate the anatomical and pathophysiological correlates of coronary thrombolysis in humans. Several diverse thrombosis preparations have been developed, including placement of a coil of thrombogenic copper wire within the artery, induction of deep vessel injury by application of electrical current to an indwelling transluminal electrode, surgical excision and eversion of a segment of artery followed by reattachment of the everted segment to the native vessel, and instillation of blood containing thrombin into a clamp-injured segment of artery to form a clot.

Copper-Coil Method

The copper-coil method has been used extensively to test the efficacy of fibrinolytic agents. It involves placement of a 3–4-mm coil of copper bell wire into the lumen of a coronary artery, usually over a guide wire introduced via a peripheral artery and advanced with the aide of a fluoroscope. Thrombotic occlusion typically occurs within 5 to 10 minutes. However, the thrombus evolved is composed predominantly of fibrin, which differs from the platelet-rich thrombus typically observed in the coronary arteries of patients. Furthermore, this technique is generally associated with minimal vascular injury, which differs from the trauma often seen clinically at the site of thrombosis that exposes highly thrombogenic matrix proteins to blood.

Electrical Injury Method

The most frequently used method for induction of coronary thrombosis in experimental animals involves electrical stimulation of the intima through an indwelling electrode. First reported by Romson and Lucchesi in 1980, the technique entails penetration of the vessel with an electrode consisting of the tip of a 23-gauge needle crimped on silver-coated copper wire and connected to the anode (positive terminal) of a 9-volt battery. Application of 250 μA of current results in disruption of the intima with exposure of the highly thrombogenic subendothelial matrix to blood. The occlusive thrombus that develops over 2 to 3 hours is composed primarily of platelets near the electrode tip surrounded by heterogeneous areas

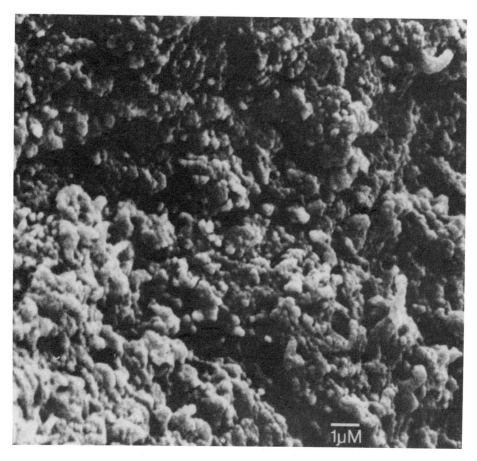

(a)

Figure 2   Scanning electron micrographs of the reoccluding coronary thrombus formed after initially successful thrombolysis in a dog with thrombosis induced by previous electrical vascular injury. The region adjacent to the electrode at the site of intimal injury is composed mainly of platelets (a). Regions rich in fibrin and erythrocytes as well as scattered platelets are evident both proximal and distal to the site of injury (b). (From Haskel, Prager, et al., with permission of the American Heart Association, Inc.)

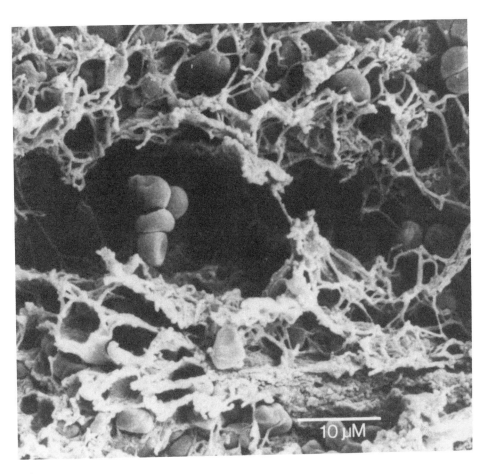

(b)

containing a mixture of fibrin, platelets, and red blood cells analogous to thrombi observed clinically (Figure 2). Reocclusion occurs virtually universally after fibrinolysis yielding the same platelet-rich thrombus, facilitating use of the preparation for studies of the effects of conjunctive agents. High-grade residual stenosis has been superimposed in some studies by mechanical obstruction of the artery just distal to the site of electrical stimulation to further mimic conditions in human arteries.

Arterial Eversion Method

A method involving surgical removal of a segment of the coronary artery, which is turned inside out and reattached end-to-end to the native artery, has been described. Although tedious, this technique exposes the adventitia—the primary location of tissue factor in normal vessels—to the flowing blood, making it analogous to the exposure of tissue factor in a ruptured atherosclerotic plaque. The resulting platelet-rich thrombus is highly resistant to fibrinolysis with t-PA, perhaps because of the intensity of the thrombogenic stimulus and the trauma to the vessel induced by surgery.

Clamp Injury and Thrombin Injection Method

Another surgical procedure for induction of thrombosis involves clamping the artery with hemostatic forceps to remove the endothelium and then injecting, usually through a sidebranch, a mixture of thrombin and blood into a segment of artery isolated with ligatures. After a clot forms, the ligatures are released. Although the initial clot is fibrin-rich, the reocclusive thrombus after fibrinolysis is typically platelet-enriched, depending on the extent of underlying vessel injury.

Among the various methods developed to simulate the conditions of thrombosis observed in human coronary arteries, the electrical injury and arterial eversion techniques might mimic the features of vessel injury and platelet-rich thrombosis most closely. With any method, however, extrapolations to humans based on results obtained in animals must be undertaken with caution because of differences in the hemostatic and coagulation systems and because the vessel in most animal experiments has not been modified by atherosclerosis.

B. Results from Studies of Thrombin Inhibitors in Experimental Animals

The pivotal role of thrombin in the pathogenesis of coronary reocclusion after thrombolysis was first demonstrated in experimental animals given direct inhibitors of thrombin conjunctively with fibrinolytic agents. Thus, in dogs with thrombosis induced in the left coronary artery by electrical vascular injury, coadministration of recombinant desulfatohirudin (1.5 mg/kg bolus followed by 1.5 mg/kg/h), a dose that increased the aPTT 1.5- to 2-fold baseline, and recombinant tissue-type plasminogen activator (rt-PA), 1 mg/kg, was shown to accelerate thrombolysis and universally prevent early thrombotic reocclusion (Figure 3). An infusion of heparin that prolonged the aPTT comparably was much less effective, as was aspirin and an antagonist of platelet glycoprotein IIb/IIIa receptors (Figure 3). Similarly, Markwardt has shown in dogs with thrombosis induced electrically in the right coronary artery, infusions of hirudin (1 mg/kg/h) after recanalization induced with streptokinase prevented reocclusion within 4 hours compared to an 80% reocclusion rate in control animals. In contrast to the results with hirudin, others have observed that argatroban, which exhibits moderate affinity for thrombin compared with hirudin (Table 1), did not completely prevent coronary reocclusion in the electrical vascular injury preparation even when given in doses that prolonged the aPTT more than threefold. Accordingly, results in vivo have appeared consistent with the expected differences attributable to the affinity of the inhibitors for thrombin.

Results in animals have also been consistent, with expected differences attributable to the type of thrombus evolved and the extent of stenosis in the coronary artery. Thus, argatroban was effective for preventing reocclusion after fibrinolysis when fibrin-rich thrombosis was induced with a copper coil. Conversely, we (Prager et al.) and others (Yasuda et al.) have shown that inhibition of thrombin alone does not appear sufficient to prevent reocclusion after fibrinolysis in the electrical injury preparation in the presence of severe residual coronary stenosis that induces high shear and thrombin-independent platelet activation (Figure 4). Thus, under these circumstances, both inhibition of thrombin and inhibition of platelets are required.

It is not clear from available data how long after the ad-

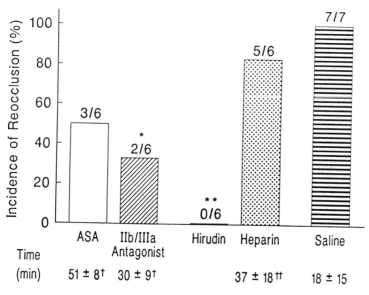

Figure 3   Effects of conjunctive antithrombotic agents on the incidence and time of reocclusion, if it occurred, after the end of an infusion of rt-PA that induced coronary recanalization in dogs with
thrombosis induced by previous electrical vascular injury. ASA =
5 mg/kg body weight of lysine acetylsalicylic acid, a water-soluble
analog of aspirin; IIb/IIIa antagonist = 0.5 mg/kg/min infusion for
10 min, then 0.2 mg/kg/min of a peptide mimetic of Arg-Gly-Asp
(SC 47643, Monsanto/Searle) that inhibits binding of fibrinogen to
platelet glycoprotein IIb/IIIa receptors. Heparin was given as 150 U/
kg, then 50 U/kg/hr. *$p < 0.02$ vs. saline, **$p < 0.001$ vs. saline,
†$p < 0.01$ by survival analysis vs. saline, ††$p < 0.05$ by survival analysis vs. saline. (From Haskel, Prager, et al., with permission of the
American Heart Association, Inc.)

ministration of fibrinolytic agents thrombin must be inhibited
to prevent reocclusion. However, conjunctive administration of
both aspirin and an infusion of either hirudin or argatroban for
1 to 2 hours after the end of administration of rt-PA has been
shown to prevent coronary reocclusion for up to 24 hours, suggesting that the interval may be brief.

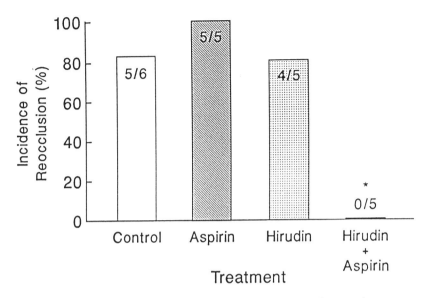

Figure 4   Effects of conjunctive agents on the incidence of coronary
.reocclusion in dogs with thrombosis induced by electrical vascular injury and with high-grade stenosis (85% area reduction of lumen) superimposed distally. Aspirin = 5 mg/kg of lysine acetylsalicylic acid;
hirudin = 1.5 mg/kg bolus followed by 1.5 mg/kg/hr of recombinant
desulfatohirudin; control = saline. *$p < 0.05$ compared with controls. (From Prager et al., *J Am Coll Cardiol* 1993;22, with permission of
the American College of Cardiology.)

C.   Results in Patients

Recently, preliminary results were reported (Cannon et al.) for
conjunctive administration of a direct antithrombin during fibrinolysis for prevention of reocclusion. Patients with acute
myocardial infarction enrolled in the Thrombolysis in Myocardial Infarction (TIMI 5) trial were given either recombinant
desulfatohirudin (ascending doses ranging from 0.15 mg/kg
bolus and 0.05 mg/kg/h infusion to 0.6 mg/kg bolus and 0.2 mg/
kg/h infusion) or heparin (5000 U bolus and 1000 U/h infusion)
together with a front-loaded regimen of t-PA (Activase) and

aspirin. Continuous infusion of hirudin for 5 days was associated with a 1% incidence of reocclusion ($n = 134$) assessed angiographically at 18 to 36 hours after the onset of therapy and did not potentiate spontaneous hemorrhage compared with a 7% incidence of reocclusion ($n = 80$; $p < 0.05$) and a 3% incidence of hemorrhage in heparin-treated patients. Studies to determine the efficacy of recombinant desulfatohirudin given together with streptokinase are in progress. Clinical studies with other direct antithrombins such as argatroban have shown them to be safe, but their efficacy for preventing reocclusion has not been proven.

IV. NOVEL ANTICOAGULANTS AS CONJUNCTIVE AGENTS

A. Rationale for Use of Inhibitors of Prothrombin Activation

Although initial results with high-affinity inhibitors of thrombin used as conjunctive agents are quite promising, there are several reasons why specific inhibition of prothrombin activation may be important in place of, or in addition to, conjunctive inhibition of thrombin during fibrinolytic therapy. One reason is that limiting thrombin formation may be more efficient than direct inhibition of thrombin already generated. Thrombin amplifies its own formation by activating factors VIII and V, which markedly increases the catalytic activity of factor IXa/VIIIa and factor Xa/Va complexes toward factor X and prothrombin. Thus, any thrombin that is allowed to escape inhibition, even transiently, could greatly accelerate coagulation. Furthermore, administration of antithrombin agents alone, although possibly effective in the short term, will not inhibit the activity of factors in the thrombus and vessel wall that promote prothrombin activation. Persistence of prothrombin activation could lead to recurrent increases in thrombin activity once administration of the thrombin inhibitor is discontinued. Another reason to consider conjunctive inhibition of prothrombin activation is that the effects of inhibitors might be more localized to constituents

of the thrombus, thereby contributing to less systemic anticoagulation and a lower risk of bleeding complications.

B. Experimental Inhibitors of Prothrombin Activation

Pharmacological approaches developed for attenuating activation of prothrombin have been based on the physiological regulation of coagulation mediated either through tissue factor or
by direct inhibition of selected factors including factor IXa and
Xa. Most of the inhibitors have been studied in experimental
animals, but have yet to be tested in patients.

Inhibitors of Tissue Factor/VIIa Complexes

As noted earlier, fibrinolysis may reexpose tissue factor in
the subendothelium or ruptured plaque to circulating factor
VII or VIIa with consequent activation of factors IX and X by
the complex. Agents to inhibit the activity of the tissue factor/
VIIa complex have been investigated, including the circulating
physiological inhibitor, tissue factor pathway inhibitor (TFPI,
previously known as lipoprotein-associated coagulation inhibitor and extrinsic pathway inhibitor), and monoclonal antibodies that inhibit the activity of either tissue factor or factor VII.
Among these, TFPI has been characterized most extensively
and produced by recombinant DNA technology in sufficient
quantities for use as an anticoagulant in vivo. TFPI is a multi-
variate, Kunitz-type, protease inhibitor that directly binds and
inactivates factor Xa and, in a factor Xa–dependent fashion,
produces feedback inhibition of the tissue factor/VIIa catalytic
complex. TFPI resides primarily on endothelium, where it is
likely synthesized and bound to heparan sulfate or other glu-
cosaminoglycans. Some TFPI also circulates bound to high-
density lipoprotein particles and in platelets. In studies to
determine whether pharmacological concentrations of TFPI
might inhibit reocclusion after thrombolysis, thrombi were induced in contralateral femoral arteries of dogs by electrical vascular injury invoking a platelet-rich thrombus in one and by
placement of a copper coil eliciting minimal vessel trauma and

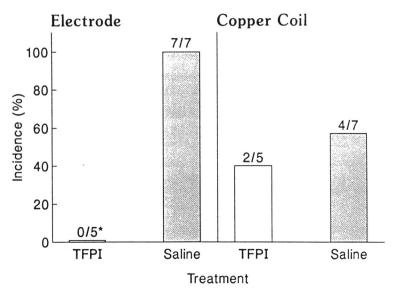

Figure 5   Effects of recombinant tissue factor pathway inhibitor (TFPI, Monsanto) (225 μg/kg followed by 4 μg/kg/min) or saline infused after the end of the infusion of rt-PA (1 mg/kg) on reocclusion after thrombolysis in femoral arteries in which thrombosis was induced by electrical injury (left panel) or with an implanted copper coil (right panel). *$p < 0.001$ vs. saline. (From Haskel, Torr, et al., with permission of the American Heart Association, Inc.)

a fibrin-rich thrombus in the other. Administration of recombinant TFPI after recanalization of both arteries induced by infusion of rt-PA prevented reocclusion in arteries with extensive injury but was less effective in arteries that contained copper wire and had minimal injury (Figure 5). These results are consistent with tissue factor present in the subendothelium and reexposed during fibrinolysis playing a role in reocclusion. Whether the benefit observed with TFPI is due primarily to inhibition of the activity of tissue factor/VIIa complex or might result from direct inhibitory effects on factor Xa as well remains to be elucidated. Nevertheless, the combined inhibitory properties of TFPI are unique compared to those of other available agents.

Monoclonal antibodies have also been developed against tissue factor and factor VIIa, and these might be useful in inhibiting the procoagulant activity of the complex. Experience with these antibodies as anticoagulants in vivo is limited, but Jang et al. have reported that brief infusion of an antibody against tissue factor prevented thrombosis over 2 hours in everted segments of the femoral artery in four of five rabbits compared to occlusion in five of six control animals, suggesting that this approach may have utility to attenuate reocclusion after fibrinolysis.

Inhibitors of Factor Xa/Va and Factor IXa/VIIIa Complexes

Another approach to limit the activation of prothrombin is with direct inhibitors of membrane-bound activation complexes. One such inhibitor is a highly selective and potent 60-amino-acid inhibitor of factor Xa derived from extracts of the soft tick, *Ornithodoros moubata*, and termed tick anticoagulant peptide. Coadministration of recombinant DNA produced tick anticoagulant peptide (100 μg/kg/min) and rt-PA in dogs with coronary thrombosis induced by electrical vascular injury and with superimposed critical coronary stenosis was observed to accelerate fibrinolysis and to prevent acute reocclusion in five of eight dogs (Sitko et al.). In the same study, a constant infusion of hirudin delayed reocclusion, but reocclusion ensued in six of eight animals after the end of the infusion. These results are consistent with persistent activation of prothrombin providing a major stimulus for reocclusion and show that inhibition of prothrombin activation may have more prolonged effects than inhibition of thrombin alone. Analogous results to those with the tick anticoagulant peptide have been obtained with low-molecular-weight heparin, which also inhibits factor Xa.

Inhibition of the factor IXa/VIIIa complex may provide an alternative strategy to limit procoagulant activity. Intravenous bolus injection of an active site-blocked factor IXa (glutamyl-glycyl-arginyl-factor IXa) in dogs with coronary injury induced electrically was shown to prevent complete thrombotic occlusion (Benedict et al.). In contrast, heparin given in concentrations analogous to those used clinically was much less effective. Although studies incorporating fibrinolysis are needed, the results suggest that factor IXa/VIIIa complexes are an important component of the procoagulant response to vessel injury and should be considered a target for conjunctive therapy.

Thus, results of studies in experimental animals showing marked attenuation of thrombosis achieved with selective inhibitors and antibodies directed toward factors eliciting activation of prothrombin emphasize the importance of de novo thrombin generation to the occurrence of reocclusion after fibrinolysis. They also imply that inhibition of prothrombin activation might complement direct inhibition of thrombin to achieve more prolonged efficacy.

V. CONCLUSIONS

Thrombin activity evolved by the action of fibrinolytic agents and by the persistent activity of procoagulant molecules in the residual thrombus and the wall of the injured vessel is primarily responsible for rethrombosis leading to reocclusion after initially successful thrombolysis. Although it is clear that anticoagulation with sufficiently high doses of intravenous heparin at the time of administration of fibrinolytic agents can attenuate reocclusion, preliminary results of recent studies suggest that direct inhibition of thrombin activity with agents such as recombinant desulfatohirudin may be even more efficient and reduce the risk of bleeding complications. However, the solution to the problem of reocclusion is more complex than utilization of direct and more potent antithrombins alone. Judging from the results in experimental animals, de novo generation of thrombin accounts for the majority of the procoagulant activity induced by fibrinolysis. Thus, inhibition of thrombin alone will be limited because the underlying stimuli for prothrombin activation persist, a hypothesis that is supported by clinical studies showing the rebound of coagulation after discontinuation of heparin. Persistent procoagulant activity might be suppressed by anticoagulants targeted to key moieties including factor Xa and the tissue factor/VIIa complex. Accordingly, a combination of direct inhibitors of thrombin, necessary to inhibit preformed thrombin, and selected inhibitors of the activation of prothrombin administered conjointly with fibrinolytic agents, and for an as yet undefined interval needed to achieve passivation of the recanalized vessel, may suppress procoagulant activity optimally. In addition, because high-grade residual stenosis appears to produce some thrombin-independent platelet activation, inhibition of platelets will be required as well for optimal maintenance of patency after thrombolysis. Potential advantages of this "cocktail" approach are greater efficiency for maintenance of vessel patency and the ability to lower doses of individual agents that may potentiate bleeding risk.

PERTINENT REFERENCES

Benedict C R, Ryan J, Wolitzky B, Ramos R, Gerlach M, Tijburg P, Stern D: Active site-blocked factor IXa prevents intravascular thrombus formation in the coronary vasculature without inhibiting extravascular coagulation in a canine thrombosis model. *J Clin Invest* 1991;88:1760–1765.

Cannon C P, McCabe C H, Henry T D, Rogers W J, Schweiger M, Gibson R S, Anderson J L, Williams D O, Braunwald E for the TIMI 5 Investigators: Hirudin reduces reocclusion compared to heparin following thrombolysis in acute myocardial infarction: Results of the TIMI 5 trial. *J Am Coll Cardiol* 1993;21:136A.

Haskel E J, Prager N A, Sobel B E, Abendschein D R: Relative efficacy of antithrombin compared with antiplatelet agents in accelerating coronary thrombolysis and preventing early reocclusion. *Circulation* 1991;83: 1048–1056.

Haskel E J, Torr S R, Day K C, Palmier M O, Wun T-C, Sobel B E, Abendschein D R: Prevention of arterial reocclusion after thrombolysis with recombinant lipoprotein-associated coagulation inhibitor. *Circulation* 1991; 84:821–827.

Jang I-K, Gold H K, Leinbach R C, Fallon J T, Collen D, Wilcox J N: Antithrombotic effect of a monoclonal antibody against tissue factor in a rabbit model of platelet-mediated arterial thrombosis. *Arteriosclerosis Thrombosis* 1992;12:948–954.

Markwardt F: Development of hirudin as an antithrombotic agent. *Sem Thromb Hemost* 1989;15:269–282.

Prager N A, Torr-Brown S R, Sobel B E, Abendschein D R: Maintenance of patency after thrombolysis in stenotic coronary arteries requires combined inhibition of thrombin and platelets. *J Am Coll Cardiol* 1993; 22:85–92.

Sitko G R, Ramjit D R, Stabilito I I, Lehman D, Lynch J J, Vlasuk G P: Conjunctive enhancement of enzymatic thrombolysis and prevention of thrombotic reocclusion with the selective factor Xa inhibitor, tick anticoagulant peptide. *Circulation* 1992;85:805–815.

Yasuda T, Gold H K, Yaoita H, Leinbach R C, Guerrero J L, Jang I-K, Holt R, Fallon J T, Collen D: Comparative effects of aspirin, a synthetic thrombin inhibitor and a monoclonal antiplatelet glycoprotein IIb/IIIa antibody on coronary artery reperfusion, reocclusion and bleeding with recombinant tissue-type plasminogen activator in a canine preparation. *J Am Coll Cardiol* 1990;16:714–722.

9

Strengths and Limitations of Specific Antithrombotic Regimens and Agents

Jack Hirsh
Hamilton Civic Hospitals Research Centre and McMaster University
Hamilton, Ontario, Canada

I. INTRODUCTION

The rationale for using antithrombotic therapy as a conjunct to thrombolytic therapy in patients with acute myocardial infarction is based on the premise that rapid coronary thrombolysis is important and that the beneficial effects of rapid coronary thrombolysis is reversed by early reocclusion. There is biochemical evidence that the induction of coronary thrombolysis is accompanied by new fibrin formation and platelet activation and that thrombosis occurs during and after successful thrombolysis. Thus, more than 10% of patients develop reocclusion and up to 20% develop recurrent ischemic events despite the concomitant use of aspirin and heparin.

Coronary thrombolysis produces conditions in the newly opened coronary artery that favors rethrombosis, since blood perfusing the newly reopened artery is exposed to thrombin, which is adsorbed onto fibrin on the surface of the lysing coronary thrombus, onto the surface of the ruptured atherosclerosis plaque, which is also rich in tissue factor, and onto soluble fibrin fragments that are generated during thrombolysis. The surface-bound thrombin is enzymatically active and promotes rethrombosis. More importantly, the fibrin-bound thrombin in the vicinity of the lysing thrombus amplifies its own production many thousand-fold by activating factors V and VIII, so producing an explosive burst of thrombin activity through an autocatalytic process. In addition, plasmin released from the lysing clot has the potential to activate blood coagulation and so lead to more thrombin generation.

Thrombin is fundamental to the process of reocclusion and contributes to this complication by converting fibrinogen into fibrin; activating factors V and VIII, which in turn amplifies thrombin generation; activating factor XIII, a process that renders the fibrin more resistant to lysis; and activating platelets to produce platelet aggregation. Thrombin binds to receptors on the platelet surface, where it activates platelets and stimulates the release of adenosine diphosphate (ADP) and the synthesis and release of thromboxane $A_2(TXA_2)$. These three platelet agonists (thrombin, ADP, and TXA_2) bind to their specific receptors on the platelet surface and trigger a series of intracellular biochemical events, which culminate in the exposure of a fibrinogen glycoprotein receptor [glycoprotein IIb/IIIa (GPIIb/IIIa)] on the platelet surface. Plasma fibrinogen, a bivalent ligand, binds to its receptors on the surface of adjacent platelets and links them together to form platelet aggregates.

Two approaches are used currently to reduce the thrombogenic tendency during and after thrombolysis. The first is to inhibit thrombin formation and thrombin activity with heparin, and the second is to inhibit platelet activation with aspirin. Both of these antithrombotic agents have been shown to be effective clinically, but both have limitations which provide opportunities for a number of the new classes of antithrombotic agents.

Heparin suppresses the burst of thrombin activity that accompanies coronary thrombolysis, improves patency after recombinant tissue plasminogen activator (rt-PA)-induced coronary thrombolysis, and reduces myocardial ischemia, and even in subtherapeutic doses has a small effect on reducing re-infarction and mortality after coronary thrombolysis. Sub-group analysis of two prospective studies indicates that heparin's effectiveness in improving coronary patency and re-ducing recurrent ischemia is critically dependent on obtaining an adequate anticoagulant effect, as reflected by the activated partial thromboplastin time (APTT). However, the potential benefits of achieving a "therapeutic" anticoagulant effect might be offset to some degree by an increase in major bleeding.

Although heparin is an effective inhibitor of free throm-bin, it does not inhibit fibrin-bound thrombin when used in pharmacological concentrations. In contrast, the direct throm-bin inhibitors including hirudin and its derivatives, the chlor-methylketones and related small peptides, are able to inhibit fibrin-bound thrombin and soluble thrombin equally well. Ac-tivated protein C (APC), a natural anticoagulant that has now been produced by recombinant DNA technology, inactivates activated factors V and VIII and is an effective inhibitor of thrombin-induced autocatalysis. Novel direct factor Xa inhibi-tors derived from Tick and Leech and tissue factor pathway in-hibitor (TPI) have also been produced by recombinant DNA technology. These new anticoagulants have been shown to be more effective than heparin in accelerating lysis and/or pre-venting rethrombosis in experimental models of thrombolysis.

Aspirin inhibits TXA_2 synthesis but does not interfere with the other two pathways of thrombin-induced platelet ag-gregation. There is good evidence that aspirin is effective clin-ically in reducing mortality and reinfarction after thrombolytic therapy. The new antiplatelet agents, particularly the platelet GPIIb/IIIa-receptor antagonists, have the potential to be more effective than aspirin because they block all three mechanisms of platelet aggregation. In some but not all experimental mod-els, the GPIIb/IIIa-receptor inhibitors have been shown to be more effective than either aspirin or heparin in preventing re-occlusion in experimental models of arterial thrombolysis.

In this chapter, we will review (1) the mechanism of action and relevant pharmacokinetics of heparin and of aspirin, (2) the results of clinical studies evaluating the efficacy and safety of heparin and aspirin as adjuncts to thrombolytic therapy in myocardial infarction, and (3) the mechanism of action of the new anticoagulants and antiplatelet agents and the results of studies evaluating these new agents in animal models of thrombolysis.

II. HEPARIN

Heparin has the potential to prevent reocclusion by inactivating free thrombin formed in the vicinity of the lysing thrombus, but it is ineffective as an inhibitor of fibrin-bound thrombin and so has limitations as an adjunctive agent. These potential limitations have been borne out in studies in which heparin was shown to be less effective than antithrombin III (ATIII)–independent thrombin inhibitors and than new platelet aggregation inhibitors in accelerating lysis and preventing reocclusion of experimental arterial thrombi in animals.

A.   Structure and Mechanism of Action

Heparin is a glucosaminoglycan (GAG) which exerts its major anticoagulant effect through a unique pentasaccharide with a high affinity binding sequence to ATIII. The unique sequence is present in only one third of heparin molecules, which bind through the pentasaccharide to ATIII and produce a conformational change that markedly accelerates the ability of ATIII to inactivate the coagulation enzymes thrombin (factor IIa), factor Xa, and factor IXa. Of these three enzymes, thrombin is the most sensitive to inhibition by heparin-ATIII.

Heparin catalyzes the inactivation of thrombin by ATIII by acting as a template to which both the enzyme and inhibitor bind to form a ternary complex. In contrast, the inactivation of factor Xa by heparin-ATIII complex is achieved by binding of the enzyme to ATIII only and does not require ternary complex formation.

Heparin is heterogeneous with respect to molecular size, anticoagulant activity, and pharmacokinetic properties. The molecular weight of heparin ranges from 3000 to 30,000 with a mean molecular weight of 15,000 (approximately 50 monosaccharide chains). The anticoagulant activity of heparin is heterogeneous because (1) only one third of the heparin molecules administered to patients have an anticoagulant function, and (2) the anticoagulant profile and the clearance of heparin is influenced by the chain length of the molecules, with the higher molecular weight species being cleared from the circulation more rapidly than the lower molecular weight species. This differential clearance phenomenon results in an accumulation, in vivo, of the lower molecular weight species, which have a reduced ratio of antithrombin to anti–factor Xa activity. This effect is responsible for the differences observed when the relationship between the heparin level and the APTT is assessed in vivo and in vitro, since the lower molecular weight species retained in vivo are measured in the anti–factor Xa heparin assay but have minimal effects on the APTT. It is also responsible for the slower clearance of the low-molecular-weight heparins (LMWH).

B.   Administration, Pharmacokinetics, and Pharmacodynamics

The two preferred routes of administration of heparin are by continuous intravenous infusion and subcutaneous injection. If the subcutaneous route is selected, the initial dose must be sufficiently high to counteract the reduced bioavailability, which occurs when heparin is administered by the subcutaneous route. If an immediate anticoagulant effect is required and heparin is administered by subcutaneous injection, the initial dose should be accompanied by an intravenous bolus injection because an anticoagulant effect from subcutaneous heparin is delayed for 1–2 hours.

Following its passage into the blood stream, heparin binds to a number of plasma proteins, a phenomenon that contributes to its reduced plasma recovery (bioavailability) at low concentrations, to the variability of the anticoagulant response to fixed doses of heparin in patients with thromboembolic disorders, and to the laboratory phenomenon of heparin resistance. Binding of heparin to von Willebrand's factor (vWF) also results in the inhibition of vWF-dependent platelet function.

Heparin also binds to endothelial cells and macrophages, a property that contributes to its complicated pharmacokinetics. Heparin is cleared through a combination of a rapid saturable and a much slower first-order mechanism of clearance. The saturable phase of heparin clearance is thought to be due to heparin binding to receptors on endothelial cells and macrophages, where it is internalized and depolymerized. Clearance through the slower nonsaturable mechanism is largely renal. At therapeutic doses, a considerable proportion of the administered heparin is cleared through the rapid saturable, dose-dependent mechanism of clearance. Because of these kinetics, the anticoagulant response to heparin at therapeutic doses is not linear but increases disproportionally both in its intensity and duration with increasing dose. Thus, the apparent biological half-life of heparin increases from approximately 30 minutes with an intravenous bolus of 25 U/kg to 60 minutes with an intravenous bolus of 100 U/kg and to 150 minutes with a bolus of 400 U/kg.

The plasma recovery of heparin is reduced when the drug is administered by subcutaneous injection in low doses (e.g., 5000 U 12 hourly) or moderate doses of 12,500 U 12 hourly or 15,000 U 12 hourly. However, at high therapeutic doses of heparin (>35,000 U/24 h), the plasma recovery is almost complete. The difference between the bioavailability of heparin when administered by subcutaneous or intravenous injection was demonstrated strikingly in a study of patients with venous thrombosis. The patients were randomized to receive either 15,000 U of heparin 12 hourly by subcutaneous injection or 30,000 U of heparin by continuous intravenous infusion; both regimens were preceded by an intravenous bolus dose of 5000 U. Therapeutic heparin levels and APTT ratios were achieved at 24 hours in only 37% of patients randomized to receive subcutaneous heparin, while therapeutic heparin levels and APTT ratios were achieved at 24 hours in 71% given an identical dose of heparin by continuous intravenous infusion. These observations are relevant to the interpretation of the results of the GISSI-2 and ISIS-3 studies in which heparin was given in a fixed dose of 12,500 U subcutaneously twice daily commencing either 12 or 4 hours after thrombolytic therapy. Thus, an adequate anticoagulant effect would not have been achieved in a timely manner in either study.

C. Laboratory Monitoring and Dose-Response Relationships

The anticoagulant effects of heparin are usually monitored by the APTT, a test that is sensitive to the inhibitory effects of heparin on thrombin, factor Xa and factor IXa. When heparin is administered in fixed doses, the anticoagulant response to heparin varies among patients with acute venous thromboembolism and with myocardial ischemia. This variability is contributed to by differences between patients in their plasma concentrations of heparin-neutralizing plasma proteins and in their rates of heparin clearance. There is evidence from subgroup analysis of cohort studies that a relationship exists between ex vivo effect of heparin on the APTT and its clinical effectiveness for the prevention of recurrent thrombosis in patients with proximal vein thrombosis, prevention of mural thrombosis in patients with acute myocardial infarction, prevention of recurrent ischemia in patients following streptokinase therapy for acute myocardial infarction, and in the prevention of coronary artery reocclusion after thrombolytic therapy with tissue plasminogen activator (t-PA) (Table 1). For this reason, the dose of heparin administered to patients should be monitored by laboratory testing and adjusted to achieve a therapeutic level; this anticoagulant effect is referred to as the "therapeutic range."

Unfortunately, the different commercial APTT reagents vary in their responsiveness to heparin. For many APTT reagents, a therapeutic effect is achieved with an APTT ratio of 1.5–2.5 (measured by dividing the observed APTT by the mean

Table 1   Relationship Between Failure to Reach Lower Limit of Therapeutic Range and Thromboembolic Events from Subgroup Analysis of Prospective Studies

Type of patients	Outcome	Relative risk	Ref.
Deep vein thrombosis	Recurrent venous thromboembolism	15.0	Hull et al., 1986
Deep vein thrombosis	Recurrent venous thromboembolism	10.7	Basu et al., 1972
Acute myocardial infarction	Left ventricular mural thrombosis	22.2	Turpie et al., 1989
Acute myocardial infarction	Recurrent MI/AP	6.0	Kaplan et al., 1987
Acute myocardial infarction	Recurrent MI/AP	13.3	Camilleri et al., 1988
Acute myocardial infarction	Coronary artery patency	8.5	Arnout et al., 1992

MI/AP = Myocardial Infarction/Angina Pectoris.

of the laboratory control APTT). With very sensitive APTT reagents the therapeutic range is higher than a ratio of 1.5–2.5, while for insensitive reagents the therapeutic range is lower. Standardization of APTT reagents can be achieved by calibrating them against the heparin level (therapeutic range 0.2–0.4 U/ml by protamine titration or 0.3–0.7 U/ml by anti–factor Xa chromogenic assay) in a plasma system.

The risk of heparin-associated bleeding is increased with increasing heparin dose—which in turn is related to the anticoagulant response—the concomitant use of thrombolytic therapy, recent surgery, trauma, invasive procedures, or a generalized hemostatic abnormality.

A rapid therapeutic heparin effect is achieved by commencing with a loading dose of 5000 U as an intravenous bolus followed by 32,000 U/24 h by continuous infusion. A lower dose of 24,000 U/24 h is often used immediately after thrombolytic therapy because the plasma lytic state produces a variable anticoagulant effect, which prolongs the APTT in its own right. The APTT should be performed approximately 6 hours after the bolus and the heparin dose adjusted according to the result obtained. A heparin dose adjustment nomogram has been developed for APTT reagents for which the therapeutic range is 1.9–2.7 times control [based on a heparin level of 0.2–0.4 U/ml (Table 2)]. This nomogram is not applicable to all APTT reagents and should be adapted to the responsiveness of the local thromboplastin to heparin.

It is also possible to achieve therapeutic heparin levels with subcutaneous injection. The anticoagulant effects of subcutaneous heparin are delayed for approximately 1 hour and peak levels occur at approximately 3 hours. A high initial dose should be used (35,000 U/24 h in two divided doses) to overcome the poor bioavailability of moderate doses. Monitoring is performed 6 hours after injection with the aim of maintaining the APTT in the therapeutic range at this time.

III. ASPIRIN

Aspirin inhibits platelet aggregation by irreversibly inhibiting the enzyme cyclooxygenase. Cyclooxygenase is responsible for

Table 2   Heparin Dose Adjustment Protocol

Patients APTT[a]	Dosing Instructions			
	Repeat bolus dose	Stop infusion (min)	Change rate (dose) of infusion, ml/H[b] (U/24 h)	Timing of next APTT
<50	5000 U	0	+3 (+2880)	6 h
50–59	0	0	+3 (+2880)	6 h
60–85[c]	0	0	0	Next morning
86–95	0	0	−2 (−1920)	Next morning
96–120	0	30	−2 (−1920)	6 h
>120	0	60	−4 (−3840)	6 h

Starting dose of 5000 U intravenous bolus followed by 31,000 U/24 h as a continuous infusion. First APTT performed 6 h after the bolus injection, dosage adjustments made according to protocol, and the APTT repeated as indicated in the right-hand column.

[a]Normal range for APTT with Dade Actin FS reagent is 27–35 s.

[b]40 U/ml.

[c]Therapeutic range of 60–85 s equivalent to a heparin level of 0.2–0.4 U/ml by protamine titration or 0.35–0.7 U/ml as an anti–factor Xa level. The therapeutic range will vary with the responsiveness of the APTT reagent to heparin.

the conversion of arachidonic acid to TXA_2 in the platelet and in vascular wall cells is responsible for the conversion of arachidonic acid to prostaglandin I_2 (PGI_2). TXA_2 induces platelet aggregation and vasoconstriction, whereas PGI_2 inhibits platelet aggregation and induces vasodilation. Thus, aspirin has the potential to be both antithrombotic and thrombogenic.

Aspirin is rapidly absorbed in the stomach and upper intestine. Peak plasma levels occur 15–20 minutes after aspirin ingestion, and inhibition of platelet function is evident by 1 hour. The plasma concentration of aspirin decays with a half-life of 15–20 minutes. Despite the rapid clearance of aspirin from the circulation, the platelet-inhibitory effect lasts for the life span of the platelet because it irreversibly inactivates platelet cyclooxygenase. Aspirin also acetylates cyclooxygenase in megakaryocytes before new platelets are released into the circulation. The mean lifespan of the human platelet is approximately 10 days. Therefore, approximately 10% of circulating platelets are replaced every 24 hours. However, virtually complete inhibition of platelet TXA_2 synthesis persists for approximately 48 hours after a single dose of 300 mg aspirin, because the newly released platelets have had their prostaglandin synthetic mechanism inactivated before they are released from megakaryocytes.

Aspirin is effective in reducing the incidence of thrombotic complications of atherosclerosis. It has been shown to reduce the incidence of myocardial infarction and/or death in the following groups: patients with silent myocardial ischemia, with stable angina, with unstable angina and non–Q wave infarction, in which it appeared to be more effective than a short course of intravenous heparin; with acute myocardial infarction, 30-day incidence, and long-term incidence; and in patients with cerebrovascular disease. There is also evidence that aspirin prevents myocardial infarction in asymptomatic males and females over the age of 50, although the relative risks and benefits in asymptomatic individuals is less clear than in those with overt evidence of atherosclerotic vascular disease.

Aspirin is generally well tolerated, but some patients suffer gastrointestinal side effects that are dose related and reduced by using low doses (325 mg/day or less) and by using enteric-coated aspirin. If a rapid effect of aspirin is desired, then 325 mg of non–enteric-coated aspirin should be used, or, if enteric-coated aspirin is taken, it should be chewed and swallowed. The gastric side effects of aspirin can be reduced also by treatment with cimetidine, by antacids, and by the use of highly buffered aspirin. Aspirin is contraindicated in individuals with peptic ulcer disease, aspirin-induced asthma, and severe gastrointestinal side effects. Some of these patients should be considered for treatment with warfarin or with ticlopidine, a new antiplatelet agent.

IV. CLINICAL TRIALS IN CORONARY THROMBOLYSIS EVALUATING CONJUNCTIVE TREATMENT

Both heparin and aspirin have been evaluated as conjunctive antithrombotic agents in clinical trials of thrombolytic therapy in patients with acute myocardial infarction. Two types of outcome measures have been used: the angiographic endpoint of coronary artery patency and the clinical endpoints of reinfarction and death. Heparin has been shown to improve patency, but its overall benefit in reducing mortality and major morbidity is more controversial. Aspirin has been shown to reduce reinfarction and death, but is less effective than heparin in maintaining patency.

Controversy over a potential role for heparin as conjunctive treatment has intensified following the publication of the GISSI-2 and ISIS-3 studies in which one arm in each study was randomized to receive heparin administered in a dose of 12,500 U 12 hourly by subcutaneous injection 12 hours and 4 hours, respectively, after thrombolytic therapy. There was a marginal benefit from heparin, which was counteracted by a small increase in bleeding (see below).

The question of need or lack of need for heparin cannot be separated from the fundamental questions of dose of heparin, intensity of anticoagulant effect, and timing and route of heparin administration. It has been argued that the timing, dosage, and route of heparin administration in both the GISSI-2 study and the ISIS-3 study were suboptimal. Furthermore, it has been argued that the failure to use an optimal heparin regimen may have disadvantaged patients randomized to receive rt-PA more than those randomized to receive streptokinase since rt-PA produces less of a systemic anticoagulant effect than streptokinase.

V. PATENCY

There is good evidence that adjuvant treatment with intravenous heparin improves coronary artery patency in patients with myocardial infarction who are treated with rt-PA. Thus, subgroup analysis of two randomized studies revealed that patients whose APTT ratio was above 2.0 had a significantly higher patency rate than those whose APTT ratio was below 2.0. These findings suggest that the effectiveness of heparin in maintaining patency is critically dependent on maintaining an APTT in the therapeutic range.

VI. MORTALITY

The effectiveness of aspirin as adjunctive treatment to SK was clearly shown in the ISIS-2 study. The use of heparin after thrombolytic therapy for acute myocardial infarction has been evaluated in a number of randomized studies but the evidence supporting its effectiveness is more controversial. In the ISIS-2 study, heparin treatment was associated with a nonsignificant decrease in infarction. In the SCATI study, the mortality was reduced significantly in patients randomized to receive heparin (2000 U intravenous bolus followed by 12,500 U subcutaneous 12 hourly) after thrombolytic therapy for acute myocardial infarction. A small trend for efficacy of heparin was seen with streptokinase but not with tPA on subgroup analysis of the GISSI-2/International Study. In the ISIS-3 study, the addition of heparin (12,500 U subcutaneous 12 hourly starting 4 hours after commencing thrombolytic therapy) to aspirin and thrombolytic therapy resulted in a nonsignificant reduction of reinfarction of 3.1 events per thousand treated ($p < 0.09$) and a reduction in 35-day mortality of 3 events/1000 treated (NS).

VII. BLEEDING

The results of the GISSI-2 study and the ISIS-3 study show that the addition of heparin therapy to thrombolytic treatment increases the risk of bleeding. In the GISSI-2 study, the reported incidence of minor bleeds was 594/6195 (9.6%) among patients who received heparin and 328/6206 (5.3%) among those who did not (RR 1.88, $p < 0.001$), of major bleeds was 103/10361 (1%) in the heparin group and 57/10407 (0.5%) in the nonheparin group (RR 1.79, $p < 0.01$). The ISIS-3 study produced a small excess of major noncerebral bleeds (1.0% compared to 0.8% $p < 0.01$) and of cerebral bleeds (0.56% to 0.40%; $p < 0.05$). Thus, the addition of heparin, resulted in an excess of 3.6/1000 serious bleeding events.

Based on the combined findings of the patency and mortality studies, it is possible that patients might benefit from high-dose intravenous heparin monitored to maintain the APTT above 1.5 times control. It is possible also, however, that any potential benefits of high-dose intravenous heparin (in terms of reduction in mortality and reinfarction) will be offset, at least in part, by an increase in the incidence of cerebral hemorrhage.

VIII. PRACTICAL DOSING REGIMENS

Until more information becomes available from the GUSTO study (see Epilogue), the following would be a reasonable approach to the use of heparin and aspirin in patients with acute myocardial infarction.

All patients should receive non–enteric-coated aspirin, 325 mg. If rt-PA is used, heparin should be administered, 5000 U, intravenous bolus followed by 1000 U per hour by continuous infusion and the APTT maintained at 1.5–2.0 control. If streptokinase is used, the bolus of heparin can be omitted and the heparin given as a continuous infusion, 1000 U per hour, at 1–3 hours after start of streptokinase infusion to maintain the APTT at 1.5–2.0 control.

If thrombolytic therapy is not used in patients with anterior wall Q-wave infarcts, heparin should be administered in high doses to prevent mural thrombosis and systemic embolism, 5000 U intravenous bolus, followed by 32,000 U/24 h by continuous infusion or 17,500 U subcutaneous 12 hourly. The APTT should be adjusted at 1.5–2.0 control.

IX. NEW ANTITHROMBOTIC AGENTS AND THEIR POTENTIAL AS ADJUVANT ANTITHROMBOTIC AGENTS

The benefits and limitations of heparin and aspirin as conjunctive agents to thrombolysis have stimulated the development of new antithrombotic compounds. The most promising of these are the ATIII-independent thrombin inhibitors, LMWHs, APC, factor Xa inhibitors, TPI, platelet fibrinogen receptor inhibitors, and inhibitors of TXA_2.

A. Limitations of Heparin and Potential Opportunities for New Anticoagulants

The limitations of heparin are its highly variable anticoagulant response in sick patients, its poor bioavailability at low doses, its complicated dose-dependent clearance, its narrow benefit (antithrombotic) to risk (bleeding) ratio, and the interference of its anticoagulant effect by platelets, fibrin, and vascular surfaces. Some of these limitations can be overcome by three new classes of anticoagulants, the LMWHs, the ATIII-independent thrombin inhibitors, and the ATIII-independent factor Xa inhibitors. LMWHs have a more predictable anticoagulant response to fixed doses, a better bioavailability at low doses, a mechanism of clearance that is dose independent, and a broader benefit-to-risk ratio. The ATIII-independent thrombin inhibitors are equally effective against free and fibrin-bound thrombin and are not inhibited by platelets. The ATIII-independent factor Xa inhibitors are able to inhibit factor Xa in the prothrombinase complex and, therefore, have potential advantages over heparin and LMWHs. These properties might explain why heparin is less effective than the direct thrombin inhibitors and the direct factor Xa inhibitors at preventing arterial and venous thrombosis in experimental animals, and why the ATIII-independent inhibitors are more effective than heparin in preventing reocclusion after experimental coronary thrombolysis.

B. Low-Molecular-Weight Heparin

LMWHs are fragments of standard heparin produced by either chemical or enzymatic depolymerization. They are approximately one third the size of heparin and have a mean molecular weight of 4000–5000. Depolymerization of heparin results in a change in its anticoagulant profile, in its bioavailability and pharmacokinetics, and in its effects on platelet function and experimental bleeding.

Like heparin, LMWHs produce their major anticoagulant effect by binding to ATIII through an unique pentasaccharide sequence, which is present on less than one third of LMWH molecules. A minimum chain length of 18 saccharides is required for heparin to inactivate thrombin, because to be effective it must be large enough to bind to both thrombin and ATIII. In contrast, inactivation of factor Xa by ATIII does not require binding of the heparin molecules to the clotting enzyme and is, therefore, achieved by small molecular weight heparin fragments, provided that they contain the high-affinity pentasaccharide. Therefore, compared with heparin, LMWHs have a reduced anti-Xa–to–anti-IIa ratio.

LMWHs have superior bioavailability at low doses and a more predictable anticoagulant response than heparin because they do not bind to heparin-binding proteins. LMWHs also do not bind to endothelial cells in culture, a property that could account for their longer plasma half-life compared to heparin.

LMWHs produce less bleeding than heparin for equivalent antithrombotic effects in experimental animals, a property that has been attributed to their different effects on platelet function, reduced binding to vWF, and reduced vascular permeability. LMWHs have been investigated in humans and have been shown to be very effective in the prevention and treatment of venous thrombosis. Their potential role in the treatment of arterial thrombosis and as a conjunct to thrombolytic therapy is unknown.

C. ATIII-Independent Inhibitors

Several ATIII-independent inhibitors are now available. These include hirudin, hirudin fragments, argatroban, and the peptide chloromethyl ketone inhibitor, D-Phe-Pro-Arg-CH$_2$Cl (PPACK) and its derivatives. Although all of these inhibitors bind directly to thrombin, they have different mechanisms of action. The potential advantage of the ATIII-independent inhibitors is that, unlike heparin, these agents can access and inactivate thrombin that is bound to fibrin. Possibly because of this property, these inhibitors have proven to be more effective than heparin in experimental animal models of venous and arterial thrombosis and as conjuncts to t-PA–induced thrombolysis using a variety of model systems.

Hirudin and Derivatives

Hirudin is a 65-amino-acid-residue protein isolated from the salivary glands of the medicinal leech. It is a potent and specific thrombin inhibitor, which is now available through recombinant DNA technology. It forms an essentially irreversible, stoichiometric complex with thrombin. Analysis of the crystal structure of the thrombin-hirudin complex illustrates the extensive contact that hirudin makes with thrombin as it binds to both the active center and the substrate recognition site of the enzyme.

Synthetic C-terminal peptide fragments of hirudin have been developed and provide a novel class of bivalent thrombin inhibitors. The first of these fragments is hirugen, a synthetic dodecapeptide, which binds to the substrate recognition site of thrombin, thereby blocking its interaction with its substrates. By adding D-phe-pro-arg-pro-(gly)$_4$ to the amino-terminal region, hirugen has been converted from a weak competitive inhibitor to a potent bivalent inhibitor known as hirulog. Like hirudin, this inhibitor blocks both the active center and the substrate recognition site. However, active site inhibition is transient, because once complexed, thrombin can slowly cleave the pro-arg bond on the amino terminal extension, thereby converting hirulog to a hirugenlike species.

Argatroban

This synthetic arginine derivative is a relatively weak competitive inhibitor of the enzyme. Argatroban interacts with the active site of thrombin and has a half-life of only a few minutes.

PPACK and Derivatives

The tripeptide chloromethyl ketone, PPACK, irreversibly inhibits thrombin by alkylating the active center histidine. Since thrombin binds to fibrin through a site distinct from its catalytic center, PPACK readily inhibits clot-bound thrombin. Recently, a PPACK derivative, D-phe-pro-arg-borate, has been developed which is a more specific inhibitor of thrombin than the parent molecule.

D. Experimental Animal Studies with ATIII-Independent Inhibitors

A number of studies have been performed in animal models comparing the relative efficacy of the direct thrombin inhibitors with heparin or aspirin or platelet GPIIb/IIIa receptor antagonists in accelerating t-PA–induced thrombolysis or preventing reocclusion (see below). In most studies, the direct thrombin inhibitors proved to be more effective than the other antithrombotic agents. In a coronary thrombosis model in dogs, hirudin was more effective than heparin, aspirin, or a platelet GPIIb/IIIa fibrinogen receptor antagonist in accelerating t-PA–induced thrombolysis. Hirudin was also shown to be much more effective than high-dose heparin and aspirin in reducing platelet deposition and thrombosis after angioplasty in pigs. Other studies in a rat aortic thrombosis model compared the effects of heparin, hirudin, the synthetic hirudin-derived peptide hirulog, and PPACK in accelerating thrombolysis and preventing reocclusion following t-PA–induced thrombolysis. Compared to saline control, heparin had no significant effect on time to reperfusion or reocclusion. All three direct thrombin inhibitors tested decreased the number of reocclusions. Hirulog and PPACK accelerated thrombolysis. The superiority of hirudin over heparin in preventing thrombosis during and after thrombolysis and in permanently inactivating clot-bound thrombin has also been demonstrated in experimental venous thrombosis.

E. Activated Protein C

Natural and recombinant forms of APC have been developed and studied in experimental models of thrombosis and hemostasis. APC inhibits coagulation and prolongs the APTT by inactivating activated factors V and VIII (factor Va and factor VIIIa) on endothelial and platelet surfaces. By so doing, APC inhibits thrombin generation induced by thrombin and factor Xa. APC has been shown to inhibit platelet deposition in a baboon model of acute arterial thrombosis, to prevent experimental venous thrombosis, and to prevent rethrombosis after experimental thrombolysis.

F. Direct Factor Xa Inhibitors

Two ATIII-independent factor Xa inhibitors have been developed: the tick anticoagulant peptide (TAP) and the leech anticoagulant peptide (antistasin). TAP is a 60-amino-acid polypeptide, which is now produced as a recombinant tick anticoagulant peptide (rTAP) in yeast. It is a potent and selective inhibitor of factor Xa, which, unlike heparin, can access and inhibit factor Xa in the prothrombinase complex. rTAP has been shown to effectively prevent venous thrombus formation in rabbits, to suppress systemic elevations in FPA induced by intravenous administration of thromboplastin in conscious Rhesus monkeys, and to inhibit thrombosis in a silastic femoral arteriovenous shunt in baboons, a model used extensively to simulate arterial thrombosis produced under conditions of high shear.

The relative effects of TAP, rHirudin (rHIR), and heparin have also been compared in a model of rt-PA–mediated thrombolysis and subsequent acute reocclusion in a canine model of platelet-dependent coronary artery thrombosis. Both rTAP and rHIR, but not heparin, significantly accelerated rt-PA–mediated thrombolysis and prevented acute reocclusion. Heparin had a modest effect on enhancing thrombolytic reperfusion but failed to prevent or significantly delay reocclusion even in doses that elevated the APTT approximately eightfold over baseline values. This finding suggests that de novo thrombin formation mediated by factor Xa in the prothrombinase complex (where it is inaccessible to heparin) is an important source of thrombin in this occlusive experimental arterial thrombosis model.

Like TAP, recombinant antistasin (rATS) is a potent and selective inhibitor of factor Xa. Antistasin was originally isolated from the Mexican leech. rATS has a molecular weight of 13,341 and produces potent anticoagulant properties for a period of more than 30 hours following a single subcutaneous administration. The in vivo antithrombotic effects of rATS following continuous intravenous infusion have been demonstrated in a rabbit model of venous thrombosis and a rhesus monkey model of mild DIC.

G. Tissue Factor Pathway Inhibitor

One of the potential mechanisms of reocclusion following successful thrombolysis is through exposure of tissue factor in the depths of the lipid-rich atherosclerotic plaque. TPI forms a complex with activated factor X, which binds to and inhibits tissue factor/activated factor VII complex, and so inhibits thrombin generation. TPI has been cloned, and limited studies with recombinant TPI have been performed in a canine femoral artery model in which TPI infusion prevented reocclusion following t-PA–induced lysis.

H. New Antiplatelet Agents

There is evidence that platelets are activated during thrombolysis and that the formation of new platelet aggregates at the site of the lysing thrombus both delays thrombolysis and leads to reocclusion. Therefore, agents that inhibit platelet function have the potential to both accelerate thrombolysis and prevent reocclusion.

Platelet aggregation is mediated through the platelet glycoprotein receptor GPIIb/IIIa, which only becomes functional after the platelet surface has been activated by exposure to platelet agonists, such as ADP, epinephrine, collagen, or thrombin. TXA_2 can also activate platelets and expose the GPIIb/IIIa complex. The exposed GPIIb/IIIa receptors bind the large adhesive glycoproteins, fibrinogen, vWF, fibronectin, and vitronectin, which promote platelet aggregation. Of these, fibrinogen is present in the blood in the highest concentration and is, therefore, the most important mediator of platelet aggregation.

Three broad classes of fibrinogen receptor blocking agents have been developed-(1) Fab fragments of monoclonal antibodies to the platelet fibrinogen receptor GP, (2) nonenzymatic snake venom proteins, which have high affinity for the platelet GPIIb/IIIa receptor by virtue of containing the arginine-glycine-aspartate (RGD) binding recognition sequence, and (3) synthetic RDG-containing peptides, which compete with fibrinogen for binding to the platelet GPIIb/IIIa receptor. These antagonists of platelet GPIIb/IIIa receptor binding are much more potent as inhibitors of platelet aggregation than aspirin since they inhibit platelet aggregation by all of the biologically important agonists (thrombin, ADP, TXA_2, and collagen). On the other hand, these GPIIb/IIIa receptor antagonists do not inhibit the platelet release reaction or platelet thromboxane synthesis.

The murine monoclonal antibodies (7E3-F[ab']$_2$ and 10E5-F[ab']$_2$) have been shown in experimental models to prevent platelet thrombus formation after vascular injury and to significantly shorten the time to reperfusion and prevent reocclusion after thrombotic coronary occlusion in studies in dogs with experimental coronary thrombosis. The efficacy of 7E3 in combination with t-PA is currently being tested in patients with acute myocardial infarction.

Limited experience has been obtained with the synthetic peptides that mimic the RGD-containing sequence on fibrinogen and other adhesive proteins. In vitro they have similar activity to the monoclonal antibodies: they inhibit platelet aggregation in humans in a dose-related manner and prevent reocclusion after successful t-PA–induced thrombolysis in the femoral and coronary arteries of dogs. The peptide bistatin has also been shown to augment the effect of heparin in accelerating thrombolysis and preventing reocclusion following t-PA–induced thrombolysis in a canine model of coronary thrombolysis. Studies performed with a cyclic heptapeptide antagonist of GPIIb/IIIa binding indicate that this is also a potent antithrombotic compound in experimental models of arterial thrombosis.

I. Thromboxane A$_2$ Synthetase Inhibitors

There is experimental evidence that inhibition of both TXA_2 synthetase and thrombin activity may be more effective than inhibition of either one alone in shortening the time to reperfusion and preventing reocclusion. Thus Ridogrel, a combined TXA_2 synthetase inhibitor and receptor antagonist, when added to hirulog, reduced the frequency of reocclusion after t-PA–induced lysis of coronary arteries of experimental thrombi in dogs more effectively than hirulog and t-PA. These findings suggest that both TXA_2 and thrombin contribute to the process of reocclusion.

PERTINENT REFERENCES

Arnout J, Simoons M, de Bono D, Rapold H J, Collen D, Verstraete M: Correlation between level of heparinization and patency of the infarct-related coronary artery after treatment of acute myocardial infarction with alteplase (rt-PA). *JACC* 1992;20:513–519.

Basu D, Gallus A, Hirsh J, Cade J: A prospective study of the value of monitoring heparin treatment with the activated partial thromboplastin time. *N Engl J Med* 1972; 287:324–327.

Camilleri J F, Bonnet J L, Bouvier J L, Levy G, Djiane P, Bory M, Serradimigni A: Intravenous thrombolysis in myocardial infarction. Influence of the quality of the anticoagulation on the early recurrence rate of angina or infarction. *Arch Mal Coeur Vaiss* 1988;81:1037–1041.

Coller B S: Platelets and thrombolytic therapy. *N Engl J Med* 1990;322:33–42.

de Swart C A M, Nijmeyer B, Roelofs J M M, Sixma J J: Kinetics of intravenously administered heparin in normal humans. *Blood* 1982;60: 1251–1258.

Eisenberg P R, Miletich J P: Induction of marked thrombin activity by pharmacologic concentrations of plasminogen activators in nonanticoagulated whole blood. *Thromb Res* 1989;55:635–643.

Fitzgerald D J, Catella F, Roy L, Fitzgerald G A: Marked platelet activation in vivo after intravenous streptokinase in patients with acute myocardial infarction. *Circulation* 1988;77:142–150.

Fitzgerald D J, Fitzgerald G A: Role of thrombin and thromboxane A_2 in reocclusion following coronary thrombolysis with tissue-type plasminogen activator. *Proc Natl Acad Sci USA* 1989;86:7585–7589.

Haskel E J, Prager N A, Sobel B E, Abendschein D R: Relative efficacy of antithrombin compared with antiplatelet agents in accelerating coronary thrombolysis and preventing early reocclusion. *Circulation* 1991;83: 1048–1056.

Haskel E J, Torr S R, Day K C, Palmier M O, Wun T-C, Sobel B E, Abendschein D R: Prevention of arterial reocclusion after thrombolysis with recombinant lipoprotein associated coagulation inhibitor (LACI). *Circulation* 1991;84:821–827.

Heras M, Chesebro J H, Penny W J, Bailey K R, Badimon L, Fuster V: Effects of thrombin inhibition on the development of acute platelet-thrombus deposition during angioplasty in pigs: heparin versus recombinant hirudin, a specific thrombin inhibitor. *Circulation* 1980;79:657–665.

Hirsh J: Heparin. *N Engl J Med* 1991;324:1565–1574.

Hirsh J, Levine M N: Low molecular weight heparin. *Blood* 1992;79(1):1–17.

Hull R D, Raskob G E, Hirsh J, Jay R M, Leclerc, J R, Geerts W H, Rosenbloom D, Sackett D L, Anderson C, Harrison L, Gent M: Continuous intravenous heparin compared with intermittent subcutaneous heparin in the initial treatment of proximal-vein thrombosis. *N Engl J Med* 1986;315: 1109–1114.

Kaplan K, Davison R, Parker M, Mayberry B, Feiereisel P, Salinger M: Role of heparin after intravenous thrombolytic therapy for acute myocardial infarction. *Am J Cardiol* 1987;59:241–244.

Mickelson J K, Simpson P J, Cronin M, Homeister J W, Laywell E, Kitzen J, Lucchesi B R: Antiplatelet antibody [7E3 F(ab′)₂] prevents rethrombosis after recombinant tissue-type plasminogen activator-induced coronary artery thrombolysis in a canine model. *Circulation* 1990;81:617–627.

Prins M H, Hirsh J: Heparin as an adjunctive treatment after thrombolytic therapy for acute myocardial infarction. *Am J Cardiol* 1991;67:3A–11A.

Rapold H J: Promotion of thrombin activity by thrombolytic therapy without simultaneous anticoagulation. *Lancet* 1990;335:481–482.

Shebuski R J, Stabilito I J, Sitko G R, Polokoff M H: Acceleration of recombinant tissue-type plasminogen activator-induced thrombolysis and prevention of reocclusion by the combination of heparin and the Arg-Gly-Asp-containing peptide bitistatin in a canine model of coronary thrombosis. *Circulation* 1990;82:169–177.

Turpie A G G, Robinson J G, Doyle D J, Mulji A S, Mishkel G J, Sealy B J, Cairns J A, Skingley L, Hirsh J, Gent M: Comparison of high dose with low dose subcutaneous heparin to prevent left ventricular mural thrombosis in patients with acute transmural anterior myocardial infarction. *N Engl J Med* 1989;320:352–357.

Vlasuk G P, Ramjit D, Fujita T, Dunwiddie C T, Nutt E M, Smith D E, Shebuski R J: Comparison of the in vivo anticoagulant properties of standard heparin and the highly selective factor Xa inhibitors antistasin and tick anticoagulant peptide (TAP) in a rabbit model of venous thrombosis. *Thromb Haemost* 1991;65:257–262.

Weitz J I, Hudoba M, Massel D, Maraganore J, Hirsh J: Clot-bound thrombin is protected from inhibition by heparin-antithrombin III but is susceptible to inactivation by antithrombin III-independent inhibitors. *J Clin Invest* 1990;86:385–391.

Willerson J T, Golino P, McNatt J, Eidt J, Yao S K, Buja L M: Role of new antiplatelet agents as adjunctive therapies in thrombolysis. *Am J Cardiol* 1991;67:12A–18A.

10

Discrepancies Between End-Point Results in Clinical Trials of Thrombolytic Therapy
The Salvage Paradigm Revisited

Frans Van de Werf
University of Leuven and University Hospital Gasthuisberg
Leuven, Belgium

The rationale for thrombolytic therapy of acute myocardial infarction was initially based on the concept that salvage of acutely ischemic, but viable, myocardial tissue (=infarct size reduction) and preservation of left ventricular contractile function are the mechanisms responsible for improved early and late survival. And indeed, reductions in infarct size (both enzymatic and scintigraphic), preserved left ventricular contractile function, and improved survival have been demonstrated in placebo-controlled studies of thrombolytic therapy. After a few years it was shown, however, that successful coronary reperfusion could attenuate infarct expansion and subsequent remodeling and dilatation of the left ventricle, even when early salvage was not possible. In several studies, patients given thrombolytic agents had smaller left ventricular volumes compared with control patients. It was postulated that these effects on left ventricular volumes and shape also contribute to the improved survival. Additional clinical observations suggest that the relationships between coronary reperfusion, infarct size reduction, and preservation of left ventricular function on the one hand and early and late survival on the other hand are complex.

I. DISCREPANCIES BETWEEN THE EFFECTS OF THROMBOLYSIS ON LEFT VENTRICULAR FUNCTION AND SURVIVAL

A number of clinical results suggest that improved early and late survival after thrombolysis cannot be attributed solely to preservation of left ventricular function.

All placebo-controlled trials (Table 1) with intravenously administered thrombolytic agents in which more than 100 patients were randomized failed to show a statistically significant improvement in both survival and global ejection fraction for the total population studied. In some trials there was a striking beneficial effect on ejection fraction with a minimal or even an adverse effect on hospital mortality, while in other trials the opposite was observed. If one plots the absolute gains in ejection fraction against the absolute reductions in hospital mortality, reported in the 11 largest placebo-controlled trials of intravenous thrombolytic therapy (Table 1), a significant linear correlation ($r = 0.62$, $p = 0.04$) is obtained, but not in the direction one would expect: the greater the gain in ejection fraction the smaller the benefit in survival!

In the West-Washington trial with intracoronary streptokinase and in the TIMI phase I trial, improved long-term survival in the thrombolysis group was observed without a significant effect on left ventricular ejection fraction. Patency of the infarct-related coronary artery was the most important predictor for long-term clinical benefit in both studies.

In two directly comparative trials with left ventricular function as primary end point, a similar angiographic ejection fraction was found in patients allocated to alteplase or streptokinase. However, hospital mortality rates were lower in alteplase-treated patients as compared to those treated with streptokinase: 3.7 vs. 7.4% and 4.7 vs. 8.2%.

Table 1 Early Mortality and Global Left Ventricular Ejection Fraction in Placebo-Controlled Trials of Intravenous Thrombolytic Therapy with >100 Patients Randomized

n	Ejection fraction (%)			Early mortality (%)			Ref.
	Placebo	Thrombolysis		Placebo	Thrombolysis		
1741	53.9	56.8	+2.9*	7.1	6.3	−0.8	ISAM, 1986
721	48.5	50.7	+2.2*	5.7	2.8	−2.7†	Van de Werf and Arnold, 1988
368	50.7	54.3	+3.6‡	9.6	6.3	−3.3	Kennedy et al., 1988
313	54	53	−1.0	12.6	5.6	−7*	Meinertz et al., 1988
231	47	53	+6.0*	5.0	6.2	+1.2	Bassand et al., 1989
219	50.7	54.0	+3.3	12.5	3.7	−8.8*	White et al., 1987
147	54	61	+7.0*	5.6	5.4	−0.2	O'Rourke et al., 1988
145	51.7	57.7	+6.0*	4.2	9.6	+5	National Heart Foundation of Australia, 1988
138	46.4	53.2	+6.8*	7.6	5.6	−2	Guerci et al., 1987
115	47.8	53.6	+5.8*	8.9	5.1	−3.8	Armstrong et al., 1989
107	44	45	+1.0	12.7	7.7	−5	Bassand et al., 1987

*Statistically significantly different from placebo.
†$p = 0.056$.
‡$p = 0.053$.

169

All placebo-controlled trials of intravenous thrombolytic therapy have shown that the survival benefit, observed during the hospital phase, is maintained for at least 1 year. If preservation of left ventricular contractile function and shape is the only responsible mechanism for clinical benefit, one would expect divergent survival curves in hospital survivors of placebo-controlled trials of thrombolytic therapy. This, however, is not observed. In all trials, the survival curves run perfectly parallel for 1–2 years, even in patients who were treated within 1 hour after the onset of symptoms, as was shown in GISSI-1. In the latter group one would expect substantial salvage of ischemic myocardium and improved left ventricular contractile function and, therefore, an extra survival benefit after hospital discharge. A recent meta-analysis of the long-term benefit of intravenous thrombolytic therapy in more than 40,000 patients participating in placebo-controlled trials (Fibrinolytic Therapy Trialists' Collaboration, Oxford, UK, September 1992, publication in preparation) has clearly shown that the risk of death after 1 month is equal in survivors of an acute myocardial infarction whether or not thrombolytic therapy was given on admission and, importantly, also irrespective of the time this treatment was started (e.g., within or after 3 hours following the onset of infarction).

Important mortality reductions were observed in patients treated 6–12 hours after the onset of symptoms in the EMERAS and LATE trials, and also 12–24 hours in ISIS-2. These time windows are much too large to allow for substantial salvage of ischemic myocardial tissue. Yet clinical benefit was consistently observed.

II. IS EARLY CORONARY REPERFUSION A PREREQUISITE FOR CLINICAL BENEFIT?

Although preservation of left ventricular function may contribute to improved survival, it may not be a necessary condition for improved survival. Some authors have therefore challenged the concept that improved survival is causally dependent on early reperfusion. In two large comparative trials of thrombolytic agents, GISSI-2 with its international extension and ISIS-3, no difference in mortality was found between the different treatments (alteplase and streptokinase in GISSI-2/International and duteplase, streptokinase, and anistreplase in ISIS-3) in spite of demonstrated differences in efficacy for early reperfusion in other studies when these drugs were compared in a setting in which vigorous anticoagulation was employed. If differences in early reperfusion were actually present in the ISIS-3 and GISSI-2/International trials and if the paradigm that early reperfusion → infarct size reduction → preservation of left ventricular function → improved early and late survival is correct, one would expect to have seen lower mortality rates after tissue plasminogen activator than after streptokinase or anistreplase, since higher early reperfusion rates have been demonstrated with tissue plasminogen activator.

III. POSSIBLE EXPLANATIONS AND NEW INSIGHTS

There are at least three sets of explanation for the diversity in end point results observed in clinical trials of thrombolysis.

A. The Illusion of Salvage

The first and probably most important explanation can be described as the "illusion of salvage": substantial salvage of ischemic myocardium occurs presently in only a minority of patients with an acute myocardial infarction because (1) reperfusion therapy is often started too late and (2) optimal reperfusion of tissue is presently obtained infrequently.

In their pioneering experimental work in dogs, Jennings and Reimer have shown that if reperfusion is obtained after 3 hours of occlusion, only 20% of the ischemic myocardium can be salvaged. In order to recanalize an infarct-related artery within 3 hours after occlusion (and thus reduce infarct size by more than 20%) and assuming that the experimental conditions of the work of Jennings and Reimer are applicable to patients with an acute myocardial infarction, the time delay between the onset of symptoms and arrival at the emergency room must be less than 2 hours. Presently, at least 30 minutes more are often lost in the emergency department before administration of a thrombolytic agent is initiated ("door-to-needle" time), and a minimum of 30–40 minutes of continuous infusion are required on average to obtain recanalization if treatment is successful. Presently, only a few patients arrive at the hospital less than 2 hours after onset of infarction.

Recently the TEAM investigators have asserted that a TIMI perfusion grade 2 (so-called "partial reperfusion") should be considered as a mostly occluded artery. If only a TIMI grade 3 represents optimal reperfusion, the percentage of successful recanalization that can be obtained with the present thrombolytic regimens (including front-loaded alteplase) is disappointingly low: in a recent survey by Appel and coworkers in Germany, the incidence of a TIMI grade 3 flow at 60 minutes without subsequent reocclusion was only 46% (293 out of 644 patients studied).

The above-mentioned percentages are flow grades in the epicardial coronary arteries as judged from standard coronary angiograms. Recanalization of an epicardial coronary artery is not the final aim of thrombolytic therapy. What is important is restoration of capillary flow in the jeopardized, ischemic myocardium. In recent work, Ito and co-workers, using contrast echocardiography, showed that 23% of the patients with TIMI flow 3 after thrombolysis had inadequate tissue reperfusion. The presence of residual contrast defects after intracoronary injection of sonicated contrast (thus the demonstration of "no reflow") in spite of TIMI flow 3 in the infarct-related coronary artery at angiography was a predictor of poor functional recovery.

In summary, adequate tissue reperfusion within 1–3 hours after the onset of an infarction is obtainable presently in only a minority of patients with an acute myocardial infarction. Clearly, this conclusion is an oversimplification of the time dependency of myocardial salvage. The presence of collateral flow may extend the time window before necrosis occurs. Furthermore, thrombotic occlusion of a coronary artery is a dynamic event due to the interplay of procoagulant and thrombolytic processes. Intermittent opening and closure of the vessel have been observed and may explain why some patients presenting after a certain time may actually have had a shorter period of occlusion. It may also be responsible for "preconditioning" of the myocardium to withstand longer periods of ischemia. To which extent and in which percentage of patients these mechanisms play a significant part and thus contribute to the extension of the time window for myocardial salvage are largely unknown.

B. Other Mechanisms of Action

Though the conditions for timely reperfusion and salvage of ischemic myocardium may not be fulfilled in many patients, important reductions in mortality have been observed in all large placebo-controlled trials of thrombolytic therapy, suggesting that other mechanisms may contribute to improved early and late survival. Such mechanisms include increased electrical stability, reduced risk of cardiac rupture, attenuation of infarction expansion and left ventricular remodeling/dilatation, and provision of collaterals to another myocardial region in the event of occlusion of another coronary vessel. Smaller left ventricular volumes and lower incidences of cardiac rupture (or electromechanical dissociation), ventricular fibrillation, and "late potentials" (late potentials on the signal-averaged surface electrocardiogram have been associated with an increased risk of ventricular arrhythmias and sudden death early and late after an acute myocardial infarction) have been observed after thrombolysis. Infarct size reduction by provision of collateral flow in the event of a new occlusion in another coronary vessel has not been demonstrated in patients to date.

C. Time-to-Treatment Paradox

A third explanation for the observed discrepancies in clinical end points is the so-called time-to-treatment paradox. A post hoc analysis of the results of the ECSG-4 trial showed that in patients treated with alteplase within 3 hours after the onset of symptoms, the reduction in mortality at 14 days was 82% (1.1% vs. 6.3% in controls), whereas global ejection fraction at 10–22 days was not different from that observed in placebo-treated patients (Table 2). By contrast, in patients who received alteplase between 3 and 5 hours after onset of infarction, 14-day mortality was only slightly lower than in controls, while global ejection fraction was significantly higher (4 absolute % points) (Table 2). Similar findings were reported in the Western Washington trial with intravenous streptokinase: a 54% reduction in mortality at 14 days (from 11.3% to 5.2%) was observed in patients treated within 3 hours with an improvement in ejection fraction of only 2% in surviving patients; no difference in mortality, however, was observed in those treated after 3 hours in spite of a 5% higher global ejection fraction in the streptokinase group as compared with controls (Table 2). In the ISAM trial the reductions in early mortality were very similar in patients treated within and after 3 hours. Accordingly, the absolute differences in global ejection fraction between controls and streptokinase were also very similar for the two time windows (Table 2). Thus, based on these results from the three largest placebo-controlled left ventricular function trials with intravenous thrombolysis, it can be argued that when thrombolytic agents are given very early after the onset of an infarction, some patients with a very poor residual left ventricular function will be saved. These patients would have died if no thrombolytic agent had been given or if treatment had been started later (e.g., after 3 hours). The very low global ejection fractions of the patients in whom reperfusion is induced early will mask the gain in ejection fraction obtained in other reperfused patients and therefore distort the comparison of average values with those in surviving controls. The greater the reduction in early mortality obtained with a thrombolytic agent, the more prominent the paradox is likely to be. This may provide a partial explanation for the surprising, negative linear correlation

Table 2   Early Mortality and Global Left Ventricular Ejection Fraction According to Time-of-Treatment:Time-to-Treatment Paradox

	<3 hours		>3 hours	
	Controls	Alteplase or streptokinase	Controls	Alteplase or streptokinase
ECSG-4 (alteplase)				
Mortality at 14 days (%)	6.3	1.1	5.0	4.5
EF (%) at 10–22 days	50	51	47	51
WW (streptokinase)				
Mortality at 14 days (%)	11.3	5.2	7.5	7.5
EF (%) at 2 months	49	51	45	50
ISAM (streptokinase)				
Mortality at 21 days (%)	6.5	5.2	7.7	6.8
EF (%) at 3–4 weeks	54	57	54	57

WW: Western Washington trial with intravenous streptokinase; ECSG: European Co-operative Study Group, trial 4; EF: global ejection fraction; ISAM: Intravenous streptokinase in acute myocardial infarction trial.

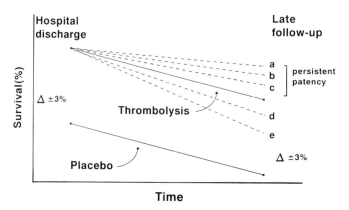

Figure 1   Schematic representation of mechanisms that could explain better or worse survival after hospital discharge in patients treated with thrombolytic agents as compared to control patients. (a) Infarct size reduction, (b) attenuation of LV dilatation, (c) electrical stability, (d) excess of reinfarction, (e) disappearance of short-term benefit. Data from more than 40,000 patients have shown that there is no added long-term survival benefit of thrombolytic therapy.

between survival benefit and gain in ejection fraction that has been observed above.

These observations may also explain the absence of an extra survival benefit after hospital discharge. Indeed, it can be assumed that survival after hospital discharge in a population treated with thrombolytic agents is the net result of different survival curves: on one hand, better survival than that in controls because of reduction in infarct size (myocardial salvage), attenuation of left ventricular dilatation (shape salvage), and greater electrical stability and, on the other hand, poorer survival than that in controls (Fig. 1). Poorer survival compared with the average survival rate in controls in patients successfully treated with thrombolytic agents might be due to a higher incidence of reinfarction (which has been observed consistently in the large placebo-controlled trials) and to a higher mortality in those patients with very poor left ventricular function who survived the acute phase because of early treatment.

The disappearance after hospital discharge of this short-term survival benefit because of very poor left ventricular function may partly neutralize the survival benefit observed in other treated patients and therefore explain the lack of an added long-term survival benefit in the total population studied.

IV. CONCLUSIONS

Intravenous administration of thrombolytic agents has dramatically improved the clinical outcome of patients with an acute myocardial infarction. Whatever the responsible mechanisms of action might be, the clinical benefit obtained is impressive. It is uncommon in the history of modern medicine to find a novel treatment for a common disease associated with mortality reductions of more than 25%. Nevertheless, results of clinical trials require refinement or reconsideration of well-accepted concepts thought to underlie benefits of thrombolysis. The original "salvage" paradigm can no longer be considered to be the only beneficial mechanism of action of thrombolytic therapy. Other mechanisms may contribute, as judged from analyses of the results of clinical trials. Although the importance of early reperfusion has recently been questioned because of the equal survival benefit obtained with different agents in spite of proven differences in efficacy for early recanalization, alternative explanations for the lack of thrombolytic drug–dependent differences may apply.

In view of the present confusion regarding mechanisms of action and (closely related to this) end points to be studied in future trials, the results of the GUSTO (Global Utilization of Streptokinase and t-PA for Occluded Coronary Arteries) trial are eagerly awaited. The angiographic and other substudies within GUSTO will give the GUSTO investigators the unique opportunity to correlate survival with early and late patency, left ventricular ejection fraction and volumes, enzymatic infarct size, electrical stability, etc. New developments in the field will undoubtedly be stimulated greatly by the outcomes in these GUSTO substudies.

PERTINENT REFERENCES

AIMS Trial Study Group: Long-term effect of intravenous anistreplase in acute myocardial infarction: final report of the AIMS study. *Lancet* 1990;335:427–431.

Appel K-F, Vogt A, von Essen R, et al.: Do we achieve optimal reperfusion in acute myocardial infarction by thrombolysis? *Eur Heart J* 1992;13 (Suppl):155 (abstract).

Armstrong P W, Baigrie R S, Daly P A, et al.: Tissue plasminogen activator Toronto (TPAT): Placebo-controlled randomized trial in acute myocardial infarction. *J Am Coll Cardiol* 1989;13:1469–1476.

Bassand J P, Faivre R, Becque O, et al.: Effects of early high dose streptokinase intravenously on left ventricular function in acute myocardial infarction. *Am J Cardiol* 1987;60:435–439.

Bassand J P, Machecourt J, Cassagnes J, et al.: Multicenter trial of intravenous anisoylated plasminogen streptokinase activator complex (APSAC) in acute myocardial infarction: effects on infarct size and left ventricular function. *J Am Coll Cardiol* 1989;13:988–997.

Braunwald E. Myocardial reperfusion, limitation of infarct size, reduction of left ventricular dysfunction, and improved survival—should the paradigm be expanded? *Circulation* 1989;79:441–444.

Califf R M, Harrelson-Woodlief L, Topol E J: Left ventricular ejection fraction may not be useful as an endpoint of thrombolytic therapy comparative trials. *Circulation* 1990;82:1847–1853.

Dalen J E, Gore J M, Braunwald E, et al.: Six- and twelve-month follow-up of the phase I thrombolysis in myocardial infarction (TIMI) trial. *Am J Cardiol* 1988;62:179–185.

EMERAS (Estudio Miocardio Estreptoquinasa Republic Americas Sud). Presented at the American College of Cardiology 46th Annual Scientific Session, Atlanta, March 1991.

Gang E, Lew A, Hong M, Wang F, Siebert C, Peter T: Decreased incidence of ventricular late potentials after successful thrombolytic therapy for acute myocardial infarction. *N Engl J Med* 1989;321:712–716.

Granger C B, Califf R M, Topol E J: Thrombolytic therapy for acute myocardial infarction. A review. *Drugs* 1992;44:293–325.

Gruppo Italiano per lo Studio della Sopravivenza nel'Infarto miocardico. GISSI-2: a factorial randomised trial of alteplase versus streptokinase and heparin versus no heparin among 12,490 patients with acute myocardial infarction. *Lancet* 1990;336:65–71.

Gruppo Italiano per lo Studio della Streptochinasi nell'Infarto Miocardico (GISSI): Effectiveness of intravenous thrombolytic treatment in acute myocardial infarction. *Lancet* 1986;i:397–402.

Gruppo Italiano per lo Studio della Streptochinasi nell'Infarto Miocardico: Long-term effects of intravenous thrombolysis in acute myocardial infarction: final report of the GISSI-study. *Lancet* 1987;2:871–874.

Gruppo Italiano per lo Studio della Streptochinasi: Global and regional left ventricular function and tomographic radionuclide perfusion: The Western Washington Intracoronary Streptokinase in Acute Myocardial Infarction Trial. *Circulation* 1984;70:867–875.

Guerci A D, Gerstenblith G, Brinker J A, et al.: A randomized trial of intravenous plasminogen activator for acute myocardial infarction with subsequent randomization to elective coronary angioplasty. *N Engl J Med* 1987;317:1613–1618.

Hochman J S, Choo H: Limitation of myocardial infarct expansion by reperfusion independent of myocardial salvage. *Circulation* 1987;75:299–306.

The International Study Group: In-hospital mortality and clinical course of 20,891 patients with suspected acute myocardial infarction randomised between alteplase and streptokinase with or without heparin. *Lancet* 1990;336:71–75.

ISAM Study Group: A prospective trial of intravenous streptokinase in acute myocardial infarction (ISAM). Mortality, morbidity and infarct size at 21 days. *N Engl J Med* 1986;314:1465–1471.

ISIS-2 Collaborative Group: Randomised trial of intravenous streptokinase, oral aspirin, both, or neither among 17,187 cases of suspected acute myocardial infarction: ISIS-2. *Lancet* 1988;2:349–360.

ISIS-3: A randomised comparison of streptokinase vs tissue plasminogen activator vs anistreplase and of aspirin plus heparin vs aspirin alone among 41,299 cases of suspected acute myocardial infarction. *Lancet* 1992;339:753–770.

Ito H, Tomooka T, Sakai N, Yu H, Higashino Y, Fujii K, Masuyama T, Kitabatake A, Minamino T: Lack of myocardial perfusion immediately after successful thrombolysis. *Circulation* 1992;85:1699–1705.

Jennings R B, Reimer K A: Factors involved in salvaging ischemic myocardium: effect of reperfusion of arterial blood. *Circulation* 1983;68 (Suppl):I25–I36.

Karagounis L, Sorenson S G, Menlove R L, Moreno F, Anderson J L for the TEAM-2 Investigators: Does thrombolysis in myocardial infarction

(TIMI) perfusion grade 2 represent a mostly patent artery or a mostly occluded artery? Enzymatic and electrocardiographic evidence from the TEAM-2 study. *J Am Coll Cardiol* 1992;19:1–10.

Kennedy J W, Martin G V, Davis K B, et al.: The Western Washington Intravenous Streptokinase in Acute Myocardial Infarction Randomized Trial. *Circulation* 1988;77:345–352.

Kennedy J W, Ritchie J L, Davis K B, Fritz J K: Western Washington randomized trial of intracoronary streptokinase in acute myocardial infarction. *N Engl J Med* 1983;309:1477–1482.

LATE (Late Assessment of Thrombolytic Efficacy). Presented at the XIVth congress of the European Society of Cardiology in Barcelona Spain, September 1992.

Magnani B for the PAIMS Investigators: Plasminogen Activator Italian Multicenter Study (PAIMS): Comparison of intravenous recombinant single-chain human tissue-type plasminogen activator (rt-PA) with intravenous streptokinase in acute myocardial infarction. *J Am Coll Cardiol* 1989; 13:19–26.

Marino P, Zanolla L, Golia G, Zardini P: Effects of intravenous streptokinase on left ventricular modeling after myocardial infarction: the GISSI-trial. *Circulation* 1988;78(Suppl. II):275.

Meinertz T, Kasper W, Schumacher M, Just H, for the APSAC Multicenter Trial Group: The German multicenter trial of anisoylated plasminogen streptokinase activator complex versus heparin for acute myocardial infarction. *Am J Cardiol* 1988;62:347–351.

National Heart Foundation of Australia Coronary Thrombolysis Group: Coronary thrombolysis and myocardial salvage by tissue plasminogen activator given up to 4 hours after onset of myocardial infarction. *Lancet* 1988;i:203–208.

O'Rourke M, Baron D, Keogh A, et al.: Limitation of myocardial infarction by early infusion of recombinant tissue-type plasminogen activator. *Circulation* 1988;77:1311–1315.

Ritchie J L, Cerqueira M, Maynard C, Davis K, Kennedy J W: Ventricular function and infarct size: the Western Washington Intravenous Streptokinase in myocardial infarction trial. *J Am Coll Cardiol* 1988;11:689–697.

Stadius M L, Davis K, Maynard C, Ritchie J L, Kennedy J W: Risk stratification for 1 year survival based on characteristics identified in the early hours of acute myocardial infarction. The Western Washington Intracoronary Streptokinase Trial. *Circulation* 1986;74:703–711.

Tranchesi B Jr, Verstraete M, Van de Werf F, et al.: Usefulness of high-frequency analysis of signal-averaged surface electrocardiograms in acute myocardial infarction before and after coronary thrombolysis for assessing coronary reperfusion. *Am J Cardiol* 1990;66:1196–1198.

Tiefenbrunn A J, Sobel B E: The impact of coronary thrombolysis on myocardial infarction. *Fibrinolysis* 1989;3:1–15.

Topol E J, Armstrong P, Van de Werf F, et al.: Confronting the issues of patient safety and investigator conflict of interest in an international clinical trial of myocardial reperfusion. *J Am Coll Cardiol* 1992;19:1123–1128.

Van de Werf F: Discrepancies between the effects of coronary reperfusion on survival and left ventricular function. *Lancet* 1989;i:1367–1369.

Van de Werf F, Arnold A E R: Intravenous tissue plasminogen activator and size of infarct, left ventricular function, and survival in acute myocardial infarction. *Br Med J* 1988;297:1374–1379.

White H D: Thrombolytic therapy for patients with myocardial infarction presenting after six hours. *Lancet* 1992;340:221–222.

White H D, Norris R M, Brown M A, Brandt P W T, Whitlock R M L, Wild C J: Left ventricular end-systolic volume as the major determinant of survival after recovery from myocardial infarction. *Circulation* 1987; 76:44–51.

White H D, Norris R M, Brown M A, et al.: Effect of intravenous streptokinase on left ventricular function and early survival after acute myocardial infarction. *N Engl J Med* 1987;317:850–855.

White H D, Rivers J T, Maslowski A H, et al.: Effect of intravenous streptokinase as compared with that of tissue plasminogen activator on left ventricular function after first myocardial infarction. *N Engl J Med* 1989; 320:817–821.

Wilcox R G, von der Lippe G, Olsson C G, et al.: Effects of alteplase in acute myocardial infarction: 6 month results from the ASSET study. *Lancet* 1990;335:1175–1178.

11

Coronary Artery Patency

Alan J. Tiefenbrunn
Washington University School of Medicine
St. Louis, Missouri

I. BACKGROUND/GENERAL CONSIDERATIONS

The goal of reperfusion therapy during evolving myocardial infarction, whether mechanical or pharmacological, is prompt and sustained restoration of nutritive myocardial blood flow. It is now well accepted that patency of the infarct-related artery is the prime correlate of myocardial salvage, clinical improvement, and decreased mortality rates. Since the potential benefits of reperfusion depend on the duration of occlusion, knowing when reperfusion occurs is of critical importance. It is also essential to identify the occurrence of reocclusion, or a high potential for reocclusion, since much of the benefit of early reperfusion is lost when reocclusion occurs. In assessing coronary artery patency, therefore, it is important to know not only that a vessel is open, but when patency was restored, the extent of improved flow and the probability that the vessel will remain patent.

Unfortunately, noninvasive assessment of reperfusion is notoriously unreliable. While complete resolution of chest discomfort in association with complete resolution of ST segment elevation is fairly specific, this occurrence is relatively unusual. Patients more often have ongoing or intermittent chest discomfort and fluctuating ST segment shift, making bedside documentation of reperfusion difficult. Computerized electrocardiographic monitoring and rapid turnover enzymatic estimates of reperfusion are still undergoing evaluation, but coronary arteriography remains the only definitive way of ascertaining coronary artery patency at this time.

II. ANGIOGRAPHIC ASSESSMENT

Angiography provides precise information not only about whether or not a vessel is patent, but also about the degree of flow, residual narrowing, residual macroscopic thrombus, extent of plaque, and presence of ulceration. "No reflow" may also be observed, in which there is no proximal focal obstruction to blood flow but runoff is impaired because of ischemia-induced myocardial and vascular endothelial cell damage and edema. In addition to detailed information about the infarct vessel, angiography also provides evaluation of the noninfarct vessels and may demonstrate the presence of collaterals that could influence the time window for myocardial salvage. Serial angiography over hours or days can provide invaluable information regarding the incidence of reocclusion and factors that might be predictive of increased tendency for reocclusion.

III. LIMITATIONS OF ANGIOGRAPHY

Emergency angiography, either before or immediately after initiation of activators of the lytic system, is not feasible for the majority of patients receiving lytic therapy, even in controlled trials. Medical risks are small, but there is increased bleeding at catheterization sites in association with thrombolytic and heparin therapy. Logistic constraints and inherent time delays, especially if a patient presents at a center without a cardiac catheterization laboratory and team experienced in emergency mobilization and procedures, limit applicability. The expense of angiography is warranted by the value of the information obtained, but expanding the number of facilities available solely for the purpose of improving access to emergency angiography is more difficult to justify. A major limitation of angiography is the inability to observe patients continuously over a prolonged period of time.

IV. DEFINING PATENCY

While it is convenient to think of vessels as open or closed, various degrees of flow may be observed in reviewing coronary angiograms. A flow grading scale initially developed at Washington University has become widely applied as the TIMI (Thrombolysis in Myocardial Infarction) grading scale since its use in the TIMI-I trial. Vessels with no antegrade flow are TIMI grade 0. Vessels with normal antegrade flow, with or without residual stenosis, are TIMI grade 3. Vessels thought to be functionally occluded but with limited antegrade penetration of contrast material are TIMI grade 1. Vessels that appear patent but with delayed antegrade visualization and/or delayed washout of contrast are TIMI grade 2.

The TIMI flow grades were developed as defined descriptors of the angiographic appearance of a vessel, and were not initially correlated with clinical outcome. Recently, Karl Neuhaus and others have pointed out that mortality rates in patients with 90-minute TIMI-2 flow are closer to the those of patients with TIMI-0 or 1 flow than to those with TIMI-3 flow, suggesting that patients with TIMI-2 flow should be considered as having occluded vessels, rather than patent as in most reports. However, in the European t-PA versus APSAC (Anisolated Plasminogen Streptokinase Activator Complex) Patency Study (TAPS), patients with TIMI grade 2 flow at 60 minutes had a significantly lower mortality of 3.4% compared to 11.5% for patients with TIMI grade 0 or 1 flow. Mortality was 1.1% for

patients with TIMI grade 3 flow at 60 minutes. Patients with
TIMI-2 flow probably represent a mixed group; some may still
be in the process of thrombolysis at the time of angiography
and subsequently develop TIMI-3 flow, some may never open
further or be in the process of reoccluding, while some may
have no focal epicardial limitation of flow but delayed runoff
because of the "no-reflow" phenomenon at the tissue level.
Approximately 20% of patients with "patent" vessels exhibit
TIMI-2 flow.

V. RECANALIZATION VERSUS PATENCY

Ideally, angiographic trials would all be recanalization studies
in which angiographic assessment is available prior to the start
of reperfusion therapy. This study design provides documentation of thrombotic occlusion and allows demonstration of collateral flow to distal vessels, if present. Without pretreatment
angiography, vessels will be included in the successful reperfusion group even if occlusion was never present (incorrect
clinical impression), if coronary artery spasm was primarily responsible for occlusion and subsequently resolved, or if spontaneous fibrinolysis occurred before the start of thrombolytic
therapy. Furthermore, the exact time of reperfusion can be documented in a recanalization study, relative to both symptom
onset and to the initiation of reperfusion therapy. Unfortunately, a recanalization trial is logistically cumbersome and results in unavoidable delay in starting therapy. The only major
reported recanalization trial is the TIMI-I study. Most trials are
"patency" studies, where intravenous thrombolytic therapy is
started prior to angiography.

VI. REOCCLUSION

The clinical importance of reocclusion of an infarct-related artery was well presented in the review of the first four TAMI
(Thrombolysis and Angioplasty in Myocardial Infarction) studies by Ohman et al., where an over 100% increase in mortality

was observed in the presence of reocclusion within the first week of myocardial infarction treated successfully with pharmacological and/or mechanical reperfusion therapy. This high mortality rate was observed in spite of emergency revascularization procedures in nearly half of those patients suffering reocclusion.

Reocclusion tends to occur because of the continued presence of the underlying unstable plaque that precipitated thrombosis in the first place, aggravated by the systemic procoagulant effect of plasminogen activation. Reocclusion may be minimized, though not completely prevented, by aggressive antithrombin and antiplatelet therapy, which is especially important in patients receiving a fibrin-specific agent with a short circulating half-life such as t-PA. Documenting reocclusion is difficult; it is clinically manifest in only approximately one half of patients. Angiographic documentation is more definitive but limited by the inability to monitor patients continuously. Even with angiography at 90 minutes, 24 hours, and 7 days, one cannot ascertain the complete picture of reperfusion and reocclusion in large groups of patients. Reported rates of reocclusion vary from approximately 2% to 50%! This wide variation is in part related to whether appropriate conjunctive therapy to prevent reocclusion is employed, but also relates to problems of documentation, including whether clinical or angiographic criteria, or both, are employed, and the time intervals and frequency of angiography.

Well-done angiographic studies, such as the TAMI series, suggest reocclusion rates on the order of 10–15% within one week after myocardial infarction, with about half of the reocclusions occurring within the first 24 hours. Patients who have clinically manifest reocclusion may benefit from repeat intervention to again achieve recanalization.

VII. TIME COURSE OF REPERFUSION

Thrombolysis resulting in reperfusion in a patient receiving an activator of the fibrinolytic system requires a finite period of time. Variables affecting time to reperfusion include the mass, age, and composition (fibrin versus platelet rich) of the clot; the ability of the lytic agent to reach the thrombus; the blood level of the lytic agent; the fibrin specificity of the lytic agent; the availability of plasminogen for activation to plasmin; the degree of systemic and local thrombin activation; and the nature of the underlying stenosis/plaque. Thus, a population receiving lytic therapy during myocardial infarction will exhibit reperfusion over a range of time intervals—while most occluded vessels may have patency restored between 30 and 90 minutes after initiation of therapy, some vessels may open more rapidly and some may not open for many hours. For example, in the European Cooperative Study Group trial of angioplasty following therapy with intravenous t-PA, patency was observed in 15 of 44 patients (34%) undergoing angiography within 30 minutes, 51 of 81 (63%) at 30–60 minutes, 25 of 37 (68%) at 60–90 minutes, and 14 of 14 (100%) at 90–120 minutes. In addition, initial reperfusion may be incomplete or intermittent, or fully patent vessels may subsequently reocclude. While angiography is precise in identifying patency, continuous monitoring is not feasible and we are thus limited to one or a few "snapshots" of the infarct vessel.

The snapshot at 90 minutes after the start of lytic therapy has become a standard of comparison for several reasons. In a recanalization trial, such as TIMI-I, 90 minutes approaches a reasonable limit for patient endurance in the catheterization laboratory. In a patency trial, 90 minutes is the approximate time interval until the first angiogram can consistently be performed after initiation of therapy. Ninety minutes is a long enough time interval to expect lytic therapy to work in the majority of patients who will respond, and short enough to anticipate significant myocardial salvage in those patients treated early after onset of occlusion.

Comparing angiographic patency rates for different lytic regimens at 90 minutes "favors" more rapidly acting agents such as t-PA, which is relatively fibrin specific, with patency rates up to twofold higher than those observed for non–fibrin specific agents at this point in time. Even more rapid reperfusion has been observed in patients receiving "front-loaded" regimens of t-PA, in which up to two thirds of a 100-mg dose is given in the first 30 minutes, with 90-minute patency rates of 85–90% reported. Patients treated with non–fibrin specific agents, such as streptokinase or APSAC, eventually catch up in terms of patency, however, such that 24-hour patency rates among all agents are similar (Fig. 1).

Whether the more rapid response to therapy with a fibrin-selective plasminogen activator results in a significant improvement in clinical outcome has been intensely debated. Shorter occlusion intervals are associated with improved myocardial salvage in experimental studies, and more rapid treat-

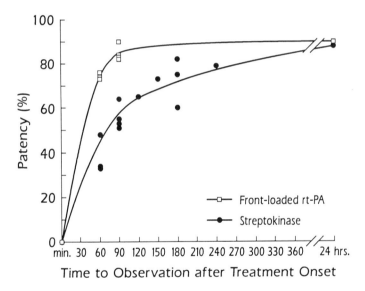

Figure 1   Extrapolated profiles of coronary artery patency rate relative to time after initiation of therapy with intravenous streptokinase or front-loaded recombinant tissue-type plasminogen activator (rt-PA). (Figure concept and streptokinase data from Sherry and Marder, 1991; front-loaded rt-PA data from Neuhaus, 1989; RAAMI, 1992; TAPS, 1992; and TAMI-7, 1992.)

ment relative to symptom onset is associated with improved mortality rates in clinical trials. However, time to clot lysis from start of therapy is one of several component intervals that compose the total time from occlusion to reperfusion. These include the time required for the patient to seek medical assistance, emergency medical service response and transportation times, time for clinical assessment and deciding to institute lytic therapy, and actually starting the thrombolytic agent (Fig. 2). Whether a more rapidly acting agent will provide additional benefit in a given patient will depend on the other components of delay, the time window for myocardial salvage in that particular patient, and whether a plateau of potential benefit has already been reached.

Neither the international t-PA/streptokinase mortality trial nor the more recent ISIS-3 (International Study of Infarct Survival) trial demonstrated a mortality difference among pa-

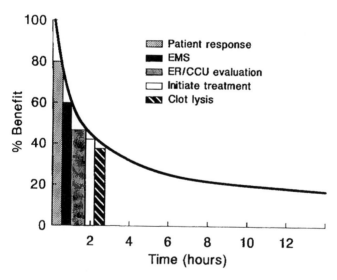

Figure 2 Curve depicting decreasing benefit of recanalization relative to duration of occlusion with superimposed potential delays in achieving coronary patency. (Curve modified from Tiefenbrunn and Sobel, 1992. EMS = emergency medical service; ER = emergency room; CCU = Coronary Care Unit.)

tients receiving different lytic regimens (streptokinase, alteplase, duteplase, or APSAC). However, patients in both of these studies received either no antithrombin therapy or a suboptimal heparin regimen, which likely mitigated the advantage of earlier reperfusion by allowing high and differential rates of reocclusion. The primary goal of the ongoing GUSTO (Global Utilization of Streptokinase and t-PA for Occluded Coronary Arteries) trial is to determine whether treatment with lytic regimens known to differ in time to lysis leads to a measurable difference in mortality in large groups of patients who also receive appropriate therapy to minimize the impact of reocclusion.

PERTINENT REFERENCES

Abendschein D R, Avery K E, Eisenberg P R, Klocke F J, Sobel B E, Jaffe A S: Prompt detection of coronary recanalization by analysis of rates of change of concentrations of macromolecular markers in plasma. *Coronary Artery Dis* 1991;2:201–212.

Califf R M, O'Neill W, Stack R S, Aronson L, Mark D B, Mantell S, George B S, Candela R J, Kereiakes D J, Abbottsmith C, Topol E J, and the TAMI Study Group: Failure of simple clinical measurements to predict perfusion status after intravenous thrombolysis. *Ann Intern Med* 1988; 108:658–662.

Chesebro J H, Knatterud G, Roberts R, Borer J, Cohen L S, Dalen J, Dodge H T, Francis C K, Hillis D, Ludbrook P, et al.: Thrombolysis in myocardial infarction (TIMI) trial, phase I: a comparison between intravenous tissue plasminogen activator and intravenous streptokinase. Clinical findings through hospital discharge. *Circulation* 1987;76:142–154.

Collen D. Coronary thrombolysis: streptokinase or recombinant tissue-type plasminogen activator? *Ann Intern Med* 1990;113:171.

Krucoff M W, Wagner N B, Pope J E, Mortara D M, Jackson Y R., Bottner R K, Wagner G S, Kent K M: The portable programmable microprocessor-driven real-time 12-lead electrocardiographic monitor: a preliminary report of a new device for the noninvasive detection of successful reperfusion or silent coronary reocclusion. *Am J Cardiol* 1990;65:143–148.

Neuhaus K L, Feuerer W, Jeep-Tebbe S, Neiderer W, Vogt A, Tebbe U: Improved thrombolysis with a modified dose regimen of recombinant tissue-type plasminogen activator. *J Am Coll Cardiol* 1989;14:1566–1569.

Neuhaus K, Von Essen R, Tebbe U, Vogt A, Roth M, Riess M, Niederer W, Forycki F, Wirtzfeld A, Maeurer W, Limbourg P, Merx W, Haerten K: Improved thrombolysis in acute myocardial infarction with front-loaded administration of Alteplase: results of the rt-PA–APSAC patency study (TAPS). *J Am Coll Cardiol* 1992;19:885–891.

Ohman E M, Califf R M, Topol E J, Candela R, Abbottsmith C, Ellis S, Sigmon K N, Kereiakes D, George B, Stack R, and the TAMI study group: Consequences of reocclusion after successful reperfusion therapy in acute myocardial infarction. *Circulation* 1990;82:781–791.

Carney J, Murphy G A, Brandt T R, Daley P J, Pickering E, White H J, McDonough T J, Vermilya S K, Teichman S L, for the RAAMI study investigators: Randomized angiographic trial of recombinant tissue-type plasminogen activator (alteplase) in myocardial infarction. *J Am Coll Cardiol* 1992;20:17–23.

Sherry S, Marder VJ: Streptokinase and recombinant tissue plasminogen activator (rt-PA) are equally effective in treating acute myocardial infarction. *Ann Intern Med* 1991;114;417–423.

Sobel B E, Hirsh J: Principles and practice of coronary thrombolysis and conjunctive treatment. *Am J Cardiol* 1991;68:382–388.

Tiefenbrunn A J, Sobel B E. Thrombolysis and myocardial infarction. *Fibrinolysis* 1991;5:1–15.

Tiefenbrunn A J, Sobel B E: Timing of coronary recanalization: paradigms, paradoxes, and pertinence. *Circulation* 1992;85:2311–2315.

Wall T C, Califf R M, George B S, Ellis S G, Samaha J K, Kereiakes D J,. Worley S J, Sigmon K, Topol E J, for the TAMI-7 study group: Accelerated plasminogen activator dose regimens for coronary thrombolysis. *J Am Coll Cardiol* 1992;19:482–489.

12

Mortality as an End Point in Studies of Coronary Thrombolysis

Burton E. Sobel
Washington University School of Medicine and Barnes Hospital
St. Louis, Missouri

I. GENERAL CONSIDERATIONS

Mortality is a popular end point in studies of coronary thrombolysis, particularly for the media and lay press. Its appeal includes definitiveness, convenience of tabulation, ease of ascertainment, and the unequivocal importance of survival as a criterion of success. Unfortunately, however, mortality as an end point is limited by often unacknowledged intrinsic weaknesses. Low death rates require huge trials if differences in mortality attributable to specific therapeutic regimens are to be identifiable. Mortality studies often fail to identify mechanistic factors responsible for results and may obscure important differences or principles. For example, if one drug compared with another were more effective in inducing coronary thrombolysis but also elicited an increased rate of death from a complication such as hemorrhage, the two agents might result in comparable mortality. Should it be the case that the complication (in this case hemorrhage) occurred primarily or exclusively in a particular subset of patients (e.g., those with antecedent cerebrovascular disease) or that it could be obviated by more appropriate dosage of the treatment drug, potentially beneficial features of the drug could be obfuscated by the simplistic consideration of its impact on mortality under a given set of conditions as a sole end point and criterion of its utility.

Additional weaknesses of mortality as an end point are apparent upon even modest reflection. Coronary thrombolysis evolved from a well-supported conceptual framework that identified preservation of jeopardized ischemic myocardium, consequent maintenance of regional left ventricular function, and enhancement of the quality of life as primary objectives and consequences of early and sustained recanalization. Although mortality reduction is clearly an objective, the implication that regimens with equivalent impacts on mortality are necessarily equivalent in terms of overall clinical efficacy is certainly not valid. For example, one therapeutic regimen might preserve ventricular function, reduce late arrhythmogenicity, and improve quality of life by diminishing heart failure without necessarily changing short-term mortality. If this were the case, the regimen in question might well be a superior one.

We and others have noted that simplistic consideration of mortality as a sole end point can be quite misleading. For example, the lack of recognition of statistically significant differences in mortality between two regimens in some large-scale, multicenter, clinical trials has been used as a criterion of the lack of a difference in their efficacy. If, however, a flaw in the design of such studies were present such that the efficacy of one or both regimens was compromised, comparisons of mortality would no longer be valid. Fundamental design flaws such as the omission of heparin and the predisposition to early thrombotic reocclusion offsetting initially beneficial thrombolysis with clot-selective thrombolytic agents as an example may have obscured real differences between regimens evident in terms of more fundamental properties including the frequency and rapidity of induction in recanalization.

One additional limitation of mortality as an end point has to do with eligibility criteria in clinical trials and is applicable to some extent to all end points. Trials are designed to maximize potential event rates and assure homogeneity of populations studied and compared. Thus, many trials of coronary thrombolysis excluded patients 70 years of age or greater. If, however, the mortality difference conferred by one regimen compared with another were most evident when the event rate (mortality) was great, as in the elderly, the difference might be missed.

A. A Corollary Regarding Eligibility for Treatment

Unfortunately, factors driving the design of clinical trials are not the same as those that must be considered often in treatment of individual patients. Trials are designed to maximize potential differences. Thus, for example, a trial designed to demonstrate differences in ventricular function between two regimens (e.g., ACE inhibitors vs. placebo) might select patients according to criteria in which heart failure was profoundly advanced so that a potential treatment effect could be easily identified. Regrettably, when such trials have been implemented and results have been positive, pundits have claimed that the inverses of criteria for inclusion should be considered also to be criteria for exclusion for treatment. In this hypothetical case, they would argue that treatment with ACE inhibitors should not be used for a patient with failure that happened to be even slightly more mild than the inclusion criteria for the trial had defined. Thus they would discard the principle (that ACE inhibitors ameliorate failure) and focus instead on limiting treatment to those who fulfilled the arbitrary criteria used for the selection criteria in the trial. Such reasoning is patently spurious. If, for example, a trial were undertaken to compare two thrombolytic drug regimens with respect to mortality among patients with extensive infarction (with plasma CK values exceeding 5000 U/ml, for example) in subjects of less than 60 years of age with initial infarcts associated with hypercholesterolemia, the results of the trial, no matter how dramatic, should not be used to limit the population of pa-

tients (to those less than 60 years of age with hypercholesterolemia) who might benefit from treatment with the regimen
demonstrated to be more favorable. Nevertheless, because
most clinical trials of coronary thrombolysis have used cut-offs
for age, electrocardiographic criteria (e.g., ST segment elevation of a specified magnitude), or other inclusion criteria designed to assure a high event rate in the trial, many clinicians
have been led to believe that these same criteria must be met if
patients are to be treated with thrombolytic drugs.

In an "ideal world," we could have an infinite number of
clinical trials to test all potential inclusion criteria for treatment
with respect to all end points of potential interest. However,
this is neither feasible nor probably truly desirable. In fact, the
principle elucidated by results of a clinical trial is what is important. In the case of coronary thrombolysis, demonstration
of the salutary effect of early and sustained coronary recanalization is applicable for clinical consideration in patients with
thrombotic coronary occlusions without contraindications for
thrombolysis even if the patient's characteristics do not con-
form entirely to the arbitrary "eligibility" criteria used to define inclusion of patients in the trial itself.

An analogous conundrum exists in legal parlance. The
"best" law is, in one sense, the most specific law (e.g., a law
designating as a violation driving a motor vehicle at a specific
speed, [e.g., greater than 31.5 mph] past a specific intersection
[e.g., a specific corner when populated by two cars and three
pedestrians] under highly specific conditions). The determination of whether or not such a law is violated in a specific case
is relatively straightforward. However, it's applicability to the
general case is virtually nil. Alternatively, the "best" law can
be considered to be the one that defines speeding in general
terms as traveling in excess of a desirable rate of speed (e.g.,
more than prudent) under diverse circumstances (at virtually
all times unless specific exceptions had prevailed such as flee-
ing a fire). Such a law is more broadly applicable but more difficult to apply for the specific cases actually encountered.

Clinical trials seek to define principles by selecting homogeneous populations for study with rigorously defined inclusion criteria utilized, in part, to provide populations with high event rates. The principles discerned from such trials have, however, broader applicability. In the imperfect clinical world in which we must practice, it is inappropriate to exclude patients for treatment simply because their particular characteristics do not match the arbitrary, research-driven inclusion criteria of a trial undertaken to define principles when, in fact, the disease entity with which they are afflicted and the pathophysiological processes by which they are affected are likely to be amenable to favorable modification by the treatment regimen proven to have been effective in the more restrictive circumstances of the clinical trial.

B.   Evaluation of Risk

Interpretation of results of mortality trials has been beclouded by confusion regarding definitions of risk. Absolute risk, defined as the incidence of death within a specified time frame, may be low or high. If it is low, the impact of any putative therapeutic regimen can be only modest (in absolute terms). Thus, for example, if the death rate from acute myocardial infarction in a particular population were only 0.5%, the maximal benefit achieved by any therapeutic regimen in terms of mortality could be only 0.5%. What may be much more pertinent is relative risk—namely, the relationship between risk with and without therapy or with one therapy as opposed to another. If, for example, the mortality risk in a placebo-treated population were 1% and the risk of death in the treated population were 0.5%, the difference would, in fact, represent a relative risk reduction of 50%. Relative risk is often the critical criterion, particularly if the one considering the implications is the one at risk.

An analogous set of considerations pertains to the justification for universal use of polio vaccine to protect the population against paralytic poliomyelitis. Within our population, the incidence of poliomyelitis was quite high before the advent of vaccine. However, the incidence of paralytic polio, even among those infected with the virus, was quite low in absolute terms (approximately 25,000 cases/year in the United States at the peak of the epidemic). Nevertheless, the devastating impact of paralytic polio on any given individual cannot be overestimated. Accordingly, even though the absolute risk of paralysis might be low, the reduction of risk achieved with a vaccine is sufficient justification for utilization of the vaccine in the population as a whole.

With respect to the impact of specific thrombolytic regimens on mortality it is therefore necessary to consider not only absolute mortality but differences in mortality in patients treated with one compared with another regimen or with one regimen compared with placebo (relative mortality). So-called small differences in relative mortality (of the order of 25%) may be terribly important even though their impact in terms of reduction of absolute mortality might be modest (e.g., a 2% reduction with a reduction of absolute mortality from 8% to 6%).

The concept of attributable risk is of particular importance in this regard. Attributable risk in a given subset of the population is the product of the anticipated mortality in that subset multiplied by the fraction of the population comprising the subset (e.g., age greater than 75 years). Thus, if the anticipated mortality from acute myocardial infarction were to be high (as it is in the very elderly) and the anticipated reduction of mortality were to be of the order of 25% in the subset of the population (those aged greater than 75 years), the reduction in attributable risk might be profound (as it actually is) in a population dominated by that particular subset.

C. Factors Obfuscating Interpretation of Results of Trials in Which Mortality Is an End Point

All subjects die ultimately. Obviously then, the age of the patients studied, their anticipated life expectancy, and the number of years at risk will influence rates of death in any given study. For this reason, comparisons between trials must be based on appropriate selection of subsets of the populations studied so that comparability of age is assured or normalization for disparities in age is incorporated in the comparison. A given therapeutic intervention cannot be anticipated to exert consistent effects on mortality, in quantitative terms, over time. Thus, coronary artery bypass grafting may reduce mortality in the immediate postoperative period by obviating the likelihood of acute myocardial infarction. However, over time, the graft itself may become a nidus for thrombotic occlusion with consequent increases in mortality relatively late after surgery. Alternatively, and perhaps of even more importance, a patient who has been restored to health by an operation may be exposed to risks that do not apply to his more severely ill counterparts, such as driving or indulging in physically demanding recreational or occupational activity which may increase the risk of death directly or indirectly. The fact that ambulatory patients may be at higher risk of death secondary to traffic accidents should not be construed to be a damnation of the efficacy of coronary artery bypass grafting that enables the patient to pursue vigorous activities such as walking and driving in the first place. The practical implication of these considerations is that comparisons of mortality in diverse clinical trials can be made only under conditions in which comparable intervals of exposure to comparable conditions of risk are present in all groups compared.

A corollary of these considerations is that therapeutic interventions that set the stage for patients to be treated definitively for complications of coronary artery disease that would otherwise be disabling or lethal cannot be considered only in terms of a short-term, putative mortality benefits. Such interventions may, in fact, be beneficial in "buying time" so that patients can benefit from other procedures that may improve the quality of life or prolong it.

A subtle, potentially confounding aspect of mortality trials concerns the basis of comparison. If, for example, two regimens are being compared, a beneficial effect ascribed to one may not be truly beneficial compared with the natural history of the disorder being treated if mortality associated with the other regimen used in the comparison has been inflated. In some early studies of anticoagulants, for example, the "placebo" group was actually given a low dose of anticoagulant that may have modified mortality unfavorably such that differences between the treatment regimen that would have been seen with respect to a true placebo effect may have been obscured.

Fibrinolytic agents have been shown to exert prothrombotic effects. Accordingly, their favorable impact on mortality may be obscured compared with mortality in placebo-treated subjects when they are used in the absence of concomitant, vigorous anticoagulation. Under such circumstances, prothrombotic effects may actually precipitate recurrent infarction or sudden cardiac death leading to a higher mortality in the subset of patients treated without concomitant anticoagulants that may offset the lower mortality that would be evident in a subset treated either with another agent or with a regimen including vigorous anticoagulation.

D. Statistical Power

Because the absolute incidence of death is relatively low among patients hospitalized with acute myocardial infarction, the number of patients required for a study in which reduction of mortality is the primary end point is prodigious. It has been estimated, for example, that a mortality trial comparing two thrombolytic drugs would require a sample size of at least 10,000 patients in each arm. The astute clinician will recognize, however, that large numbers alone do not assure validity of conclusions of clinical trials. For example, if a study were to be performed in which the response of pneumococcal pneumonia to penicillin were being tested with mortality as an end point under conditions prevailing at the end of World War II, the maximal dose of penicillin that might have been used (because of limitations of availability of the drug at that time) might be as low as 1000 units per day if a decision had been made to treat a large number of patients (e.g., 50,000). Under such circumstances, the placebo-treated patients would fare no worse than those treated with the homeopathic dose of penicillin used, but the conclusion that penicillin was ineffective in the treatment of pneumococcal pneumonia would not be justified. Conversely, should such a study be undertaken today, under conditions in which massive amounts of penicillin are available at low cost, and if the decision were made to treat large numbers of patients with huge amounts of the drug to avoid the risk of undertreatment (e.g., 1,000,000 units of penicillin per day), the treatment group might fare no better than the placebo-treated group because of toxic effects of the excessive dose of penicillin (e.g., seizures with aspiration pneumonitis, secondary infections, anaphylaxis, and other untoward consequences). Again, the conclusion that treatment of pneumococcal pneumonia with penicillin was ineffective would not be justified despite the lack of an observed difference in mortality. Thus, large numbers do not obviate deficiencies in study design even when mortality is the end point.

What large numbers do provide is statistical power—by definition, a high likelihood that results will identify small but real differences. If, for example, one wished to know whether students in the third grade on the west coast of the United States differed in height compared with those in the third grade on the east coast of the United States, and if a real difference existed (because of increased exposure to sunlight on the west coast, for example), a large sample size (of the order of 100,000 students in each group) might be necessary to demonstrate a small, real statistically significant difference in height (of the order of 0.1 cm). Unfortunately, the lay press and media confuse statistical power (the capacity to detect small, real differences as a result of large sample size) with validity of conclusions that can be obviated by design flaws in studies despite large sample size.

II. MORTALITY RESULTS BEFORE ISIS-3
AND GISSI-2

A. The Impact of Coronary Thrombolysis
on Mortality

The landmark GISSI-1 trial demonstrated that patients treated within 1 hour after the onset of symptoms of infarction with streptokinase exhibited 50% lower relative mortality than that seen in patients treated with placebo. Confirmatory results were obtained in the ISIS-2 and European Cooperative Study Group trials. Salutary effects on mortality are particularly striking among patients treated very early after the onset of infarction. Thus, in the GISSI-1 trial, the reduction of mortality associated with treatment with intravenous streptokinase compared with placebo was 50% in patients treated within 1 hour after the onset of chest pain but negligible in those treated 4 or more hours after its onset. In addition, in the MITI trial of prehospital treatment, mortality in patients treated with t-PA and i.v. heparin within 90 minutes after seeking medical attention was only 1%. It was 10-fold greater in patients treated after an interval exceeding 90 minutes. Analogous, though quantitatively less dramatic differences were seen in the EMIP study.

In some studies, mortality has been remarkably low among patients treated with thrombolytic drugs. For example, in the TIMI-II trial, mortality in patients treated with t-PA was less than 5% despite a high index of severity of illness in the study population (with 60% of the patients categorized clinically as not being at low risk). These results are consistent with the low mortality in all patients treated with t-PA in the United States followed in the National Registry maintained by Genentech, Inc. (5.6% in more than 20,000 patients with no exclusion criterion based on age).

Improved survival appears to depend on early induction of patency of infarct-related arteries. Late thrombolysis may reduce mortality through diverse mechanisms as judged from results of the recent LATE study and from meta-analyses. Although direct, beneficial effects of exclusively late thrombol-

ysis have been postulated including facilitated healing of myocardium and ventricular remodeling, provision of conduits
favoring development of collaterals, reduction of late ventricular aneurysm formation and of late arrhythmogenicity, among
others, it is equally possible that late thrombolysis benefits
those patients in whom earlier spontaneous intermittent recanalization had occurred and in whom, accordingly, some
myocardium remained viable and hence salvageable by the late
intervention. Both interpretations are consistent with the observation that untreated patients who are discharged with a
patent infarct-related artery have a better outcome than those
discharged with an occluded artery.

An additional factor that may account for benefit in patients reported in trials of exclusively late thrombolysis is the
inclusion of some patients whose infarction actually began
many hours after the onset of chest pain (misclassification with
respect to time of onset) and inclusion of some patients in
whom spontaneous endogenous fibrinolysis may have occurred with intermittent reperfusion anteceding pharmacologically induced thrombolysis that simply consolidated the
benefits of the occult, early, spontaneous recanalization.

Improved survival after coronary thrombolysis appears
also to be dependent on induction of sustained recanalization.
Coronary thrombolysis can, of course, be compromised by
early thrombotic reocclusion as a result of the persistence of
the atherogenic lesion that served as the initial nidus of thrombosis, the induction of prothrombotic effects by fibrinolytic
drugs secondary to plasminemia, or both. The persistence of
patency, potentiated by vigorous anticoagulation with bolus
administration of heparin intravenously followed by a steady-
state infusion, appears to be pivotal (Tables 1 and 2). Pooled
data demonstrate a 69% increase in mortality (from 5.5% to
9.3%) in studies in which fibrinolytic agents were used without
conjunctive intravenous heparin compared with those in
which conjunctive intravenous heparin was utilized (Table 3).

In order to determine whether prevention of early reocclusion of an infarct-related artery was a critical determinant of

Table 1   Early Mortality (≤ 42 days) in Trials of Intravenous Thrombolytic Drugs without Heparin

Trial	Placebo group		Treatment group	
	n	% mortality (n)	n	% mortality (n)
GISSI-1				
Times to treatment				
≤ 12 h	5852	13.0 (761)	5860	10.7 (627)
≤ 1 h	642	15.4 (99)	635	8.2 (52)
≤ 3 h	3078	12.0 (369)	3016	9.2 (277)
3–6 h	1800	14.1 (254)	1849	11.7 (216)
6–9 h	659	14.1 (93)	693	12.6 (87)
GISSI-2/Int'l. t-PA/SK	N/A		10,364(t-PA)	8.9 (922)
			10,385(SK)	8.5 (883)
ISIS-2	4300	13.2 (568)	1463 (SK + ASA)	9.6 (140)
HART	N/A		99	3.0 (3)
SCATI	N/A		217	8.8 (19)
Total	16,331	13.1 (2144)	34,581	9.3 (3226)

GISSI = Gruppo Italiano per lo Studio della Stretochinasi nell'Infarto Miocardico; ISIS = International Study of Infarct Survival; HART = Heparin or Aspirin Reocclusion Trial; SCATI = Studio sulla Calciparini nell'Angina nella Trombosi Ventriculare nell'Infarto; t-PA = tissue-type plasminogen activator; SK = streptokinase; ASA = aspirin; N/A = not applicable.
Source: Tiefenbrunn and Sobel, 1991.

Table 2   Early Mortality ($\leq$ 42 days) in Trials of Intravenous Thrombolytic Drugs with Heparin

Trial	Placebo group		Treatment group	
	n	% mortality (n)	n	% mortality (n)
ASSET	2495	9.8 (245)	2516	7.2 (181)
ECSG-I	N/A		64(t-PA)	4.7 (3)
			65(SK)	4.6 (3)
ECSG-II	65	6.2 (4)	64(t-PA)	1.6 (1)
ECSG-III			123(t-PA)	4.9 (6)
ECSG-IV	N/A		367	5.0 (18)
ECSG-V	366	5.7 (21)	355	2.8 (10)
HART			106	2.0 (2)
ISIS-2 ("intention to treat" with intravenous heparin)			1024 (SK + ASA)	6.4 (66)
NHF Australia	71	2.8 (2)	73	9.6 (7)
New Zealand I	93	12.9 (12)	79	2.5 (2)
New Zealand II	N/A		135(t-PA)	3.7 (5)
			135(SK)	7.4 (10)
SCATI	N/A		218	4.5 (10)
TIMI-II pilot	N/A		317	4.4 (14)
TIMI-IIa			195(t-PA + 2-h PTCA)	5.2 (11)
			200(t-PA + 24-h PTCA)	7.4 (15)
TIMI-IIb	N/A		3262	4.9 (160)
Total	3090	9.2 (284)	9298	5.5 (514)

ECSG = European Cooperative Study Group; NHF = National Heart Foundation; ASSET = Anglo-Scandinavian Study of Early Thrombolysis; TIMI = Thrombolysis in Myocardial Infarction Trial; PTCA = percutaneous transluminal coronary angioplasty; other abbreviations are as in Table 1.
Source: Tiefenbrunn and Sobel, 1991.

Table 3   Pooled Data on Early Mortality ($\leq$ 42 days) in Trials of Intravenous Thrombolytic Drugs with and without Heparin

	Placebo group		Treatment group		% Reduction in mortality (treatment vs. placebo)
	n	% mortality (n)	n	% mortality (n)	
With intravenous heparin	3090	9.2 (284)	9298	5.5 (514)	39
Without intravenous heparin	16,331	13.1 (2144)	34,581	9.3 (3226)	29

Source: Tiefenbrunn and Sobel, 1991.

reduction of mortality in studies with fibrinolytic agents, we recently analyzed results from all available trials of fibrinolytic agents for patients less than 70 years of age in whom treatment was initiated within 6 hours after the onset of chest pain and in whom ST segment elevation was present, indicative of probable infarction. All studies in which aspirin was included in the protocol and in which a minimum of 150 patients were included in the treatment arm were considered. As can be seen in Table 4, the use of concomitant intravenous heparin was associated with reduction of mortality induced by clot-selective fibrinolytic drugs, presumably because their lack of induction of high concentrations of fibrinogen degradation products with intrinsic anticoagulant properties provides no protection against early thrombotic reocclusion in the absence of concomitant anticoagulation. A similar trend, though not statistically significant, was evident with respect to nonselective agents. Perhaps of more importance, the analysis showed that patients treated with clot-selective agents, capable of initiating coronary recanalization more rapidly and more frequently compared with nonselective drugs, plus conjunctive intravenous heparin exhibited the lowest mortality (3.6%), a mortality considerably lower than the 5.8% mortality seen in comparably treated patients who were not given conjunctive, intravenous heparin ($\chi^2 = 3.38$, $p = 0.06$).

B. Mortality in Small, Randomized Patient Assignment, In-Hospital Studies of Clot-Selective Compared with Non–Clot-Selective Fibrinolytic Agents

Several factors can compromise clinical benefit otherwise resulting from initially successful coronary recanalization with fibrinolytic agents. None is more likely to compromise the outcome than early reocclusion. In addition to the persistence of the atheromatous nidus of the precipitating thrombus, induction of a procoagulant state secondary to plasminemia, encountered with all fibrinolytic agents given intravenously, can contribute to early thrombotic reocclusion. In view of these

Table 4 Early Mortality in Aspirin-Treated Patients < 70 Years Old Treated Within 6 Hours and Exhibiting ST-Segment Elevation

	Intravenous heparin			
	Yes	No	Chi-square	p-value
SK	ISAM: 38/730 (5.2%)	ISIS-2: 51/872 (5.8%) Int'l: 432/8005 (5.4%) ISIS-3: 369/5855 (6.3%)		
	Total: 38/730 (5.2%)	Total: 852/14,732 (5.8%)	0.33	0.57
rt-PA	ECSG-V: 10/355 (2.8%) TIMI-II: 55/1398 (3.0%) ECSG-VI: 9/324 (2.8%)	Int'l: 469/7986 (5/8%) ECSG-VI: 11/320 (3.4%)		
	Total: 74/2077 (3.6%)	Total: 479/8306 (5.8%)	15.6	< 0.001
Chi-square	3.38	0.001		
p-value	0.06	0.98		

Chi-square and p-values on the right pertain to effect of i.v. heparin with SK or t-PA; those at the bottom pertain to the effect of SK vs. rt-PA with or without i.v. heparin.
ISAM = Intravenous Streptokinase in Acute Myocardial Infarction Study; ISIS = International Study of Infarct Survival; Int'l. = International Tissue-type Plasminogen Activator/Streptokinase Study Group; ECSG = European Cooperative Study Group; TIMI = Thrombolysis in Myocardial Infarction Trial.
Source: Sobel and Collen, 1992.

considerations, vigorous anticoagulation with intravenously administered heparin accompanied by administration of aspirin to inhibit platelet activation is essential. We have referred to measures designed to potentiate or sustain clot lysis in this fashion as conjunctive measures.

Under conditions in which vigorous anticoagulation is employed, angiographic studies have demonstrated that fibrin-selective agents such as t-PA induce coronary patency more rapidly and more frequently than nonselective agents. Accordingly, it had been anticipated that mortality would be more markedly decreased with such agents when vigorous anticoagulation was employed.

A recent analysis of several available small, randomized, patient assignment, in-hospital studies in which t-PA was compared with non–fibrin-specific agents demonstrated a striking difference in mortality. Thus, mortality in patients treated with a non–fibrin-selective fibrinolytic agent averaged 7.3% compared with the 4.4% mortality experienced by patients treated with fibrin-selective agents in the same trials (Table 5). Although the absolute morality rates in both groups of patients were low, the 66% greater relative mortality in patients treated with non–clot-selective agents was significant and impressive.

Analogous results have been reported in the recently completed TAPS investigation. An increased incidence of early patency was seen with t-PA administered with conjunctive heparin compared with anistreplase (84% vs. 70% patency evident from 90-minute angiograms). Furthermore, the difference in patency was associated with a highly favorable hospital mortality with t-PA compared with anistreplase (2.4% with front-loaded t-PA as opposed to 8.1% with anistreplase, $p < 0.01$).

III. RESULTS IN THE MEGA-TRIALS

In view of the observations noted above, it had been anticipated by many that analogous results would be seen in two recently completed mega-trials: the International t-PA/SK and

Table 5   In-Hospital Mortality in Randomized Assignment, Large-Scale Studies of rt-PA Versus Non–Fibrin-Specific Thrombolytic Agents Combined with Immediate Intravenous Heparin for at Least 48 Hours in Patients with Acute Myocardial Infarction

Study	rt-PA	Non–fibrin-specific agent
TIMI-I	12/157	14/159 (SK)
ECSG-I	3/64	3/65 (SK)
White et al.	5/135	10/135 (SK)
PAIMS	4/86	7/85 (SK)
TAMI-5	8/191	5/190 (UK)
GAUS	6/124	5/121 (UK)
TAPS	5/218	17/217 (ASPAC)
Total	43/975 (4.4%)	71/972 (all) (7.3%)

Homogeneity index: $\chi^2 = 4.76$, $p = 0.57$.
Odds ratio: 0.59 (95% CI: 0.41 − 0.87), $p = 0.0067$.
TIMI = Thrombolysis in Myocardial Infarction Trial; ECSG = European Cooperative Study Group; PAIMS = Plasminogen Activator Italian Multicenter Study; TAMI = Thrombolysis and Angioplasty in Myocardial Infarction Trial; GAUS = German Activator Urokinase Study; TAPS = rt-PA − APSAC Patency Study; SK = streptokinase; UK = urokinase; APSAC = anisoylated plasminogen streptokinase activator complex; rt-PA = t-PA produced by recombinant DNA technology.
Source: Sobel and Collen, 1992.

ISIS-3 studies. In both of these trials, a non–clot-selective fibrinolytic agent was compared with a clot-selective agent (t-PA) in the form of alteplase in the International t-PA/SK trial and in the form of duteplase in the ISIS-3 investigation). However, no thrombolytic drug-dependent differences in mortality were observed. Furthermore, both trials reported an overall mortality that appears to be high in comparison with that in numerous other studies. Thus, overall mortality in the International t-PA/SK trial was 8.7%. The corresponding figure in the ISIS-3 study was 10.5%.

Several explanations have been offered to account for the high mortality experienced in those two mega-trials. The possibilities that inclusion of elderly patients may have influenced the mortality results adversely and that a relatively late onset of treatment (the median time to treatment in the ISIS-3 investigation was 4.1 hours after the onset of chest pain) may have precluded optimal reduction of mortality have been considered. However, differences in the age distribution of patients in the mega-trials do not appear to account for the high mortality because comparable age distributions were present in studies such as the TIMI-II investigation, yet mortality was much lower (4.9%). Even when patients are age-matched for purposes of comparison in ISIS-3 and TIMI-II, the mortality in the TIMI study is 37% lower (4.9% vs. 7.8% in ISIS-3 for patients 75 years of age or less).

Severity of illness does not appear to account for the higher mortality seen in the two mega-trials compared with that in numerous other studies. For example, 95% of patients in the International Study Group population were classified as being Killip class 1 or 2 at the time of admission.

Although some delay in the onset of treatment in the mega-trials may have contributed to the apparently high mortality, it appears unlikely that this factor alone accounts for the disparity between results in the mega-trials and those in numerous other studies. Very early treatment does result in the most marked reduction of mortality, as is evident from the recent report from the MITI trial in which mortality was only 1% in patients treated with t-PA and intravenous heparin plus aspirin within 90 minutes after the onset of chest pain as opposed to 10% in those treated later. However, time to treatment in the TIMI-II trial was not strikingly dissimilar from that in ISIS-3.

A third possibility appears much more likely to account for both the high mortality and the lack of apparent thrombolytic drug-dependent differences in mortality seen in the two mega-trials—namely, the omission of intravenous heparin. In both mega-trials, heparin was administered subcutaneously at a dose of 12,500 units at 12-hour intervals (beginning with 4 hours in the ISIS-3 study and within 12 hours in the International t-PA/SK trial). This regimen is known to fail to induce therapeutically effective blood levels for 24 hours or more, in part because of the high avidity of heparin for endothelial cell–binding sites that must be saturated before heparin entering the blood stream will remain there and in part because of the slow absorption of subcutaneously administered heparin.

Angiographic studies have demonstrated unequivocally that the initially higher patency rates seen with clot-selective as opposed to non–clot-selective fibrinolytic agents (approximately 80% compared with 50% patency in 90 minutes) are compromised by early reocclusion when fibrin-selective agents are administered in the absence of conjunctive intravenous heparin. The omission of intravenous heparin may compromise benefit otherwise seen with fibrin-selective agents more markedly than with nonselective agents because of the relative lack of generation of fibrinogen degradation products by the fibrin-selective agents with consequently less nonspecific partial anticoagulation compared with that induced by nonselective agents. In view of the omission of intravenous heparin in the two mega-trials, it appears quite likely that results with all of the fibrinolytic agents used were compromised by slowed recanalization (reflecting unmitigated ongoing thrombosis), early thrombotic reocclusion, or both. Accordingly, it is not surprising that the mortality encountered with all thrombolytic agents used in the two mega-trials were somewhat higher than that seen in numerous other trials. The same phenomenon may account for the lack of apparent thrombolytic drug-dependent differences in outcome in the mega-trials, since early thrombotic reocclusion may well have adversely affected patients treated initially with a fibrin-selective agent compared with those treated with a nonselective agent because of the lack of partial protection against thrombolysis conferred by fibrinogen degradation products in the absence of intravenous heparin.

IV.   CONCLUSIONS REGARDING MORTALITY

It has been established unequivocally that fibrinolytic agents reduce mortality associated with acute myocardial infarction. Reductions as great as 50% can be anticipated in patients treated within the first hour after onset of symptoms as judged from the GISSI-1 results. Dramatically low mortality may be possible when treatment is implemented within the first 60–90 minutes with fibrin-selective agents administered with conjunctive intravenous heparin and aspirin as judged from the remarkably low mortality (1%) seen in the recently reported MITI study. Analysis of data pooled from head-to-head comparisons of fibrin-selective and non–fibrin-selective agents demonstrate more favorable reductions of mortality with fibrin-selective compared with non–fibrin-selective drugs. Results of two recent mega-trials are inconsistent with these observations, and with the mounting evidence that the more rapid and more frequent induction of patency known to occur with fibrin-selective compared with non–fibrin-selective agents gives rise to more favorable effects on the heart and the patient. The explanation for the disparity may well be the omission of conjunctive intravenous heparin in the mega-trials with consequent compromise of the potential benefit of each of the fibrinolytic agents used. The high mortality seen in both mega-trials with all fibrinolytic drugs used is consistent with this possibility. Ongoing studies including the GUSTO investigation have been designed to definitively determine the extent to which reduction of mortality depends on prompt and sustained recanalization of infarct-related arteries. Corollary conclusions regarding the relative efficacy of fibrin-selective compared with nonselective fibrinolytic agents under conditions in which anticoagulation is optimal should be forthcoming as well (see Epilogue).

Because the absolute mortality associated with aggressively treated acute myocardial infarction is so low (5.6% in the 20,158 patients treated with t-PA followed in the national registry of myocardial infarction being compiled by Genentech,

Inc.) and because the sample size needed for detection of relative mortality differences as large as 30% between regimens is so high (well in excess of 20,000 patients according to many calculations), many investigators have relied on meta-analysis of results of diverse studies to reach conclusions. Such analyses pool data from disparate studies judged to be comparable as verified by calculation of homogeneity indexes and compare mortalities associated with specific regimens in terms of a hypothetical estimates of mean mortality calculated from the mortality observed in each of the studies weighted with respect to the size of the study population. A standard error of the hypothetical mortality rate applicable to the entire population with components from all the pooled studies (i.e., an estimate of the standard deviation of its estimated value) is calculated. The standard error depends not only on the overall observed mortality but also on the overall size of the pooled population. Deviations from the hypothetical mortality in terms of standard error units deviation can be used to determine the probability that a difference in mortality in one or more components of the pooled population occurred by chance and, conversely, that the difference is indicative of a real difference with a defined level of significance.

Despite the elegance and internal mathematical and statistical consistency of this approach, which has its basis in the central limit theorem of statistics, meta-analyses suffer from several inherent deficiencies including publication and overview bias, resulting in selectivity that may be unrecognized in the results being analyzed. Furthermore, such analyses do not take into consideration mechanistic determinants of outcome. Accordingly, they are prone to error if diverse causes of a common end point are not recognized. Such "lumping" has occurred in analysis of trials of thrombolytic agents that concluded that fibrin-selective drugs may be associated with an increased incidence of cerebrovascular accidents attributable to their intrinsic properties.

In a meta-analysis, for example, based on results of the two recently completed mega-trials (the International t-PA/SK

trial and ISIS-3), there was no overall increase in the incidence
of hemorrhagic stroke with the fibrin-selective drug used in
the International trial (t-PA in the form of alteplase) in contrast
to the case in the ISIS-3 study in which t-PA in the form of
duteplase was associated with an increased incidence of hemorrhagic stroke (probably because the dose of duteplase was
equivalent to 160–200 mg of conventionally used t-PA [al-
teplase] in terms of plasmin-generating activity quantified with
a kinetic, chromogenic substrate assay). Because of the omission of protocol-mandated intravenous heparin in both mega-
trials, it is not surprising that the incidence of overall stroke
was greater with t-PA compared with streptokinase in the International t-PA/SK trial as a result of an excess of ischemic
strokes attributable to unopposed procoagulant effects of fibrinolytic agents given in the absence of intravenous heparin. After combining incidences of increases in stroke apparently
attributable to ischemia with increases apparently attributable
to hemorrhage, it was concluded from the meta-analysis that
fibrin-selective agents had deleterious, stroke-producing properties. However, the validity of this conclusion is highly ques-
tionable in view of the disparate causes of strokes in the two
studies from which results were combined (ischemia related to
inadequate heparinization in patients subjected to procoagulant effects of a fibrinolytic drug and hemorrhage attributable
to a dose regimen of duteplase in which the amount of t-PA activity administered was consistent with that shown previously
to incur an increased risk of hemorrhagic stroke).

Despite the appeal of meta-analysis as a mathematical and
biostatistical procedure designed to acquire insights from
pooled data from diverse trials, the risk of erroneous conclusions is real. Accordingly, ongoing investigations such as the
GUSTO trial have been implemented to compare mortality pro-
spectively in patients treated with diverse fibrinolytic agents
with and without intravenous heparin to clarify the extent to
which reduction of mortality is contingent upon early and sustained recanalization and accordingly on specific fibrinolytic
drug regimens. Pending these results (see Chapter 13), it

seems prudent to reduce mortality by prompt implementation of fibrinolysis as early as possible after the onset of infarction. This can be done with aggressive concomitant anticoagulation with conjunctive agents such as intravenous heparin and, in the near future, direct-acting antithrombins (e.g., hirudin, hirugen, hirulog, argatroban), suppression of platelet activation (with vigorous use of antithrombins, antiplatelet drugs, or both), and other measures designed to prevent early thrombotic reocclusion by inhibiting procoagulant rebound with the use of novel anticoagulants such as inhibitors of factors VII, Xa, and tissue factor.

PERTINENT REFERENCES

Gruppo Italiano Per Lo Studio Della Streptochinasi Nell'infarto Miocardico (GISSI): Effectiveness of intravenous thrombolytic treatment in acute myocardial infarction. *Lancet* 1986;1:397–401.

Bleich S D, Nichols T C, Schumacher R R, Cooke D H, Tate D A, Teichman S L: Effect of heparin on coronary arterial patency after thrombolysis with tissue plasminogen activator in acute myocardial infarction. *Am J Cardiol* 1990;66:1412–1417.

Boissel J -P: European Myocardial Infarction Project (EMIP): short-term mortality and nonfatal outcomes. Presented at the National Meeting of the American College of Cardiology, Dallas, April 15, 1992.

Chesebro J H, Knatterud G, Roberts R, Borer J, Cohen L S, Dalen J, Dodge H T, Francis C K, Hillis D, Ludbrook P A, Markis J E, Mueller H, Passamani E R, Powers E R, Rao A K, Robertson T, Ross A, Ryan T J, Sobel B E, Willerson J, Williams D O, Zaret B L, Braunwald E: Thrombolysis in myocardial infarction (TIMI) trial, phase I: a comparison between intravenous tissue plasminogen activator and intravenous streptokinase. *Circulation* 1987;76:142–154.

de Bono D P, Simoons M L. Tijssen J, Arnold A E, Betriu A, Burgersdijk C, Lopez Bescos L, Mueller E, Pfisterer M, van de Werf F: Effect of early intravenous heparin on coronary patency, infarct size, and bleeding complications after alteplase thrombolysis: results of a randomised double blind European Cooperative Study Group trial. *Br Heart J* 1992; 67:122–128.

Eisenberg P R, Miletich J P, Sobel B E: Factors responsible for differential procoagulant effects of diverse plasminogen inhibitors in plasma. *Fibrinolysis* 1991;5:217–224.

Eisenberg P R, Miletich J P, Sobel B E, Jaffe A S: Differential effects of activation of prothrombin by streptokinase compared with urokinase and
tissue-type plasminogen activator. *Thromb Res* 1988;50:707–717.

Eisenberg P R, Sherman L, Rich M, Schwartz D, Schechtman K, Geltman
E M, Sobel B E, Jaffe A S: Importance of continued activation of throm-
bin reflected by fibrinopeptide A to the efficacy of thrombolysis. *J Am
Coll Cardiol* 1986;7:1255–1262.

Eisenberg P R, Sobel B E, Jaffe A S: Activation of prothrombin accompanying
thrombolysis with recombinant tissue-type plasminogen activator. *J Am
Coll Cardiol* 1992;19:1065–1069.

Hsia J, Hamilton W P, Kleiman N, Roberts R, Chaitman B R, Ross A M,
Heparin-Aspirin Reperfusion Trial (HART) Investigators: A comparison
between heparin and low-dose aspirin as adjunctive therapy with tissue
plasminogen activator for acute myocardial infarction. *N Engl J Med*
1990;323:1433–1437.

International Study Group: In-hospital mortality and clinical course of 20,891
patients with suspected acute myocardial infarction randomised between alteplase and streptokinase with or without heparin. *Lancet* 1990;
336:71–75.

ISIS-2 Collaborative Group: Randomised trial of intravenous streptokinase,
oral aspirin, both, or neither among 17,187 cases of suspected acute myocardial infarction: ISIS-2. *Lancet* 1988;2:349–360.

ISIS-3: A randomized comparison of streptokinase vs tissue plasminogen activator vs anistreplase and of aspirin plus heparin vs aspirin alone
among 41,299 cases of suspected acute myocardial infarction. *Lancet*
1992;339:753–770.

Kahn H A, Sempos C T: *Statistical Methods in Epidemiology.* New York, Oxford
University Press, 1989.

Maroko P R, Kjekshus J K, Sobel B E, Watanabe T, Covell J W, Ross J, Jr.,
Braunwald E: Factors influencing infarctsize following experimental coronary artery occlusions. *Circulation* 1971;43:67–82.

Neuhaus K L, von Essen R, Tebbe U, Vogt A, Roth M, Riess M, Niederer W,
Forycki F, Wirtzfeld A, Maeurer W: Improved thrombolysis in acute
myocardial infarction with front-loaded administration of alteplase: results of the rt-PA-APSAC patency study (TAPS). *J Am Coll Cardiol* 1992;
19:885–891.

Ohman E M, Califf R M, Topol E J, Candela R, Abbottsmith C, Ellis S, Sigmon K N, Kereiakes D, George B, Stack R: Consequences of reocclusion
after successful reperfusion therapy in acute myocardial infarction.
TAMI Study Group. *Circulation* 1990;82:781–791.

Rogers W J: Update on recent clinical trials of thrombolytic therapy in myocardial infarction. *J Invasive Cardiol* 1991;3(suppl A):11A.

Sobel B E: Thrombolysis in the treatment of acute myocardial infarction, in Fuster V, Verstraete M (eds): *Thrombosis in Cardiovascular Disorders*. Philadelphia, W. B. Saunders, 1992, pp. 289–326.

Sobel B E, Collen D: After ISIS-3. *Lancet* 1992;339:1225–1226.

Sobel B E, Collen D: Questions unresolved by the Third International Study of Infarct Survival. *Am J Cardiol* 1992;70:385–389.

Sobel B E, Collen D: Strokes, statistics and sophistry in trials of thrombolysis for acute myocardial infarction. *Am J Cardiol* 1993;71:424–427.

Sobel B E, Hirsh J: Principles and practice of coronary thrombolysis and conjunctive treatment. *Am J Cardiol* 1991;68:382–388.

Tiefenbrunn A J, Sobel B E: The impact of coronary thrombolysis on myocardial infarction. *Fibrinolysis* 1989;3:1–15.

Tiefenbrunn A J, Sobel B E: Thrombolysis and myocardial infarction. *Fibrinolysis* 1991;5:1–15.

Tiefenbrunn A J, Sobel B E: Timing of coronary recanalization. Paradigms, paradoxes, and pertinence. *Circulation* 1992;85:2311–2315.

TIMI Study Group: Comparison of invasive and conservative strategies after treatment with intravenous tissue plasminogen activator in acute myocardial infarction: results of the Thrombolysis in Myocardial Infarction (TIMI) Phase II Trial. *N Engl Med* 1989;320:618–627.

Topol E J, Armstrong P, van de Werf F, Kleiman N, Lee K, Morris D, Simoons M, Barbash G, White H, Califf RM: Confronting issues of patient safety and investigator conflict of interest in an international clinical trial of myocardial reperfusion. *J Am Coll Cardiol* 1992;19:1123–1128.

Topol E J, George B S, Kereiakes D J, Stump D C, Candela R J, Abbotsmith C W, Aronson L, Pickel A, Boswick J M, Lee K L: A randomized controlled trial of intravenous tissue plasminogen activator and early intravenous heparin in acute myocardial infarction. *Circulation* 1989;79:281–286.

Torr S R, Eisenberg P R, Sobel B E: The dependence of activation of platelets by a plasminogen activator on the evolution of thrombin activity. *Thromb Res* 1991;64:435–444.

Turpie A G, Robinson J G, Doyle D J, Mulji A S, Mishkel G J, Sealey B J Cairns J A, Skingley L, Hirsh J, Gent M: Comparison of high-dose with low-dose subcutaneous heparin to prevent left ventricular mural thrombosis in patients with acute transmural anterior myocardial infarction. *N Engl J Med* 1989;320:352–357.

van de Werf F, Arnold A E, for the European Cooperative Study Group for Recombinant Tissue-type Plasminogen Activator: Intravenous tissue plasminogen activator and size of infarct, left ventricular function, and survival in acute myocardial infarction. *Br Med J* 1988;297:1374–1379.

Verstraete M, Bernard R, Bory M, Brower R W, Collen D: Randomised trial of intravenous recombinant tissue-type plasminogen activator versus intravenous streptokinase in acute myocardial infarction. Report from the European Cooperative Study Group for Recombinant Tissue-type Plasminogen Activator. *Lancet* 1985;i:842–847.

Verstraete M, Bleifield W, Brower R W, Charbonnier B, Collen D, DeBono D P, Dunning A J, Lennane R J, Lubsen J, Mathey D G, Michel P L, Raynaud P H, Schofer J, Vahanian A, Vanhaecke J, van de Kley G A, van de Werf F, von Essen R: Double-blind randomised trial of intravenous tissue-type plasminogen activator versus placebo in acute myocardial infarction. *Lancet* 1985;2:965–969.

Weaver W D: Myocardial Infarction Triage and Intervention (MITI) trial of pre-hospital initiated thrombolysis—results. Presented at the American College of Cardiology National Meeting, Dallas, April 14, 1992.

Weaver W D, for National Registry of Myocardial Infarction Investigators: Factors influencing the time to hospital administration of thrombolytic therapy: results from a large national registry. *Circulation* 1992;86 (suppl I):I–16 (Abstract).

Yusuf S, Collins R, Peto R, Furberg C, Stampfer M J, Goldhaber S Z, Henekens C H: Intravenous and intracoronary fibrinolytic therapy in acute myocardial infarction: overview of results on mortality, reinfarction and side effects from 33 randomized controlled trials. *Eur Heart J* 1985; 6:556–585.

13

Clinical Factors Militating Against Sustained Patency and Their Consequences

Stanley D. Bleich
Tulane University School of Medicine
Metairie, Louisiana

I. INTRODUCTION

The value of prompt reperfusion utilizing thrombolytic therapy in acute myocardial infarction has been well established. Data from a recently presented abstract by Appel et al. suggests that "optimal reperfusion" is not solely based on early patency. The role of complete and sustained reestablishment of coronary perfusion has been shown to be of equal importance. Although adjunctive and conjunctive therapy have not been proven to contribute significantly to early patency, they have demonstrated a vital function in reducing the incidence of coronary reocclusion. This, in turn, positively affects recurrent ischemia and reinfarction following thrombolysis in the clinical setting of acute myocardial infarction. In the absence of conjunctive and adjunctive therapy, as represented by adequate anticoagulation and antiplatelet therapy, rapid reperfusion generated by potent thrombolytic agents may not be sustained, thereby negating complete or partial clinical benefit.

Therapies commonly used in practice today that have been shown to exhibit a positive effect on clinical outcome as adjuncts to thrombolysis include beta-adrenoreceptor–blocking agents, nitrates, aspirin, and heparin. Although it has been demonstrated that beta blockers prevent recurrent ischemia and decrease the incidence of both reinfarction and serious ventricular arrhythmias, this does not appear to be secondary to the prevention of reocclusion. These agents acutely decrease heart rate, blood pressure, and tension-time index levels. This directly reduces myocardial oxygen consumption, which in turn manifests its positive effect on clinical outcome. Nitrates, however, contribute a favorable clinical response by decreasing preload, which in turn limits infarct size, conferring a beneficial effect on the development of congestive heart failure. The administration of beta blockers and nitrates is not considered an absolute necessity to the success of thrombolytic therapy, and they are therefore referred to as "adjunctive" agents. Aspirin and heparin, however, exhibit their positive clinical influence by aiding in the prevention of reocclusion and reinfarction. This potentiates a beneficial clinical impact on thrombolysis in the treatment of acute myocardial infarction. It is for this reason that aspirin and heparin are often referred to as "conjunctive" agents, as they are essential to the clinical success of thrombolytic therapy. This is in comparison to the term "adjunctive agents," which implies an additive influence that is not essential to a favorable clinical outcome. Commonly utilized and investigational conjunctive and adjunctive agents along with their doses and indications are summarized in Tables 1 and 2.

II. CLINICAL MANIFESTATIONS
OF REOCCLUSION

It has been well recognized that the propagation of a pathophysiologically procoagulant effect is elicited by fibrinolytic agents during thrombolysis. It has also been suggested that this clinically important effect is particularly evident with the

Table 1   Conjunctive Agents to Thrombolytic Therapy in AMI

Agent	Dosage	Indication	Clinical benefit
Heparin	5000 U i.v. bolus during initial infusion. 1000 U/h (1200 U/h for pts > 85 kg) titrating drip to aPTT of 2–2.5 x control	All	Prevent reocclusion reducing recurrent ischemia and reinfarction
Aspirin	160–324 mg (1/2–1 adult tab.) given acutely (chewed) and then daily (oral)	All (If truly allergic substitute dipyridamole.)	Prevent reocclusion reducing recurrent ischemia and reinfarction

Investigational agents include glycoprotein IIb-IIIa receptor blockers, ticlopidine, serotinin inhibitors, anti-vWF, disintegrins, prostacyclin, and prostaglandin E_1.

Table 2   Adjunctive Agents to Thrombolytic Therapy in AMI

Agent	Dosage	Indication	Clinical benefit
Beta blockers			
Atenolol	5 mg i.v. × 2 50 mg p.o. Q.D.	All patients without con- traindications: hypoten- sion, bradycardia, COPD/ asthma, CHF	Decreased heart rate, B.P. and O_2 consumption de- creasing reinfarction, recur- rent ischemia, ventricular arrhthymias, and intracere- bral hemorrhage
Metoprolol	5 mg i.v. × 3 50 mg p.o. b.i.d.		
Nitrates	Start i.v. infusion at 5 μg/ min; titrate to decrease systolic B.P. 10%	Patients with persistent ischemia and hypertension	Decreases preload, limiting infarct size and decreasing incidence of CHF

Investigational agents include angiotensin-converting enzymes, calcium-channel blockers, neutrophil inhibitors, and oxy-gen free radical scavengers.

fibrin-specific agents (i.e., alteplase) because of their almost nonexistent anticoagulant properties. This is in comparison to somewhat more potent anticoagulant characteristics associated with the non–fibrin-specific agents (streptokinase and anistreplase).

The procoagulant effect of thrombolysis is one arm of an intensely sensitive balance. The opposing arm consists of the timing, aggressiveness, and subsequent success of concomitant anticoagulation. Tipping of the balance in favor of the procoagulant effect can cause significant and serious clinical ramifications, as described by the data discussed below. The incidence of reocclusion associated with the fibrin-specific and non–fibrin-specific agents are reviewed in Tables 3 and 4.

The negative effect of reocclusion following successful thrombolysis was defined in an important study by Ohman et al. In this trial, 810 patients with an acute myocardial infarction who had received one of three thrombolytic agents were evaluated. Thrombolytic therapy included tissue-type plasminogen activator (t-PA) in 517, urokinase in 87, and a combination regimen of t-PA and urokinase in 129 patients. All patients received intravenous heparin along with aspirin, nitroglycerin, and diltiazem during the recovery phase. Seven hundred and thirty-three patients were found to have successfully reperfused, as assessed by 90-minute angiography. Repeat cardiac catherization in 88% of patients at a median of 7 days from onset of symptoms revealed reocclusion of the infarct-related artery in 91 patients (12.4%). Only 58% of reocclusions that were documented by angiography were symptomatic. Patients who suffered reocclusion had similar left ventricular ejection fractions but had worse infarct zone function than those who remained patent. Also interesting to note is that patients who suffered an angiographic reocclusion had a more complicated hospital course and a significantly higher in-hospital mortality rate (11% as compared to 4.5% for the group that maintained vessel patency). This data clearly supports the theory that patients whose infarct-related arteries remain patent, despite a significant risk of rethrombosis, have a better initial prognosis

Table 3   Incidence of Reocclusion Associated with Alteplase

Method	Incidence	Time	Ancillary Tx	Dose	Ref.
Clinical	17% (12/71)	24 h	H,A,D,P	100 mg/3 h	Mueller et al., 1987
Angio	24% (12/51)	7–10 days	H,P	1.25 mg/kg/3 h	Topol et al., 1987
Angio	14% (28/205)	7 days	H,A,D,C,P	150 mg/6 h	Topol et al., 1988
Angio	18% (30/167)	7 days	H,A,D,C,P	150 mg/8 h	Topol et al., 1988
Angio	8% (11/134)	Hosp.	H,A,C,B	1.5 mg/kg/4 h	Topol et al., 1989
Angio	4.1% (4/98)	7 days	H,A	100 mg/3 h	Carney, 1992
Angio	4.6% (5/108)	7 days	H,A	100 mg/90 min	Carney, 1992
Angio	2.6%	21 days	H,A	100 mg/90 min	Neuhaus, 1992

H: heparin; A: aspirin; D: dipyridamole; P: PTCA; B: beta blockers; C: Ca^+ channel blockers.

Table 4   Incidence of Reocclusion Associated with Non Fibrin-Specific Agents

Agent	Method	Incidence	Time	Ancillary Tx	Dose	Ref.
Streptokinase	Angio	7% (5/64)	hosp.	H,A	Adjusted	Merx et al., 1981
	Angio	18% (6/34)	2 h	H	2–6000 U[a]	Gold et al., 1983
	Angio	45% (5/11)	10–14 days	NTG	240,000 U	Leibof et al., 1984
	Angio	29% (7/24)	8–14 days	None	177,000 U	Harrison, 1984
	Angio	34% (7/21)	9–14 days	H	850,000–1.5 M	Spann et al., 1984
Anisoylated plasminogen streptokinase activator complex	Clinical	21% (11/51)	hosp	H	30 U	Bossaert, 1987
	Angio	7.5% (3/40)	24 h	H	30 U	Anderson, 1988

H: heparin; A: aspirin; NTG: nitroglycerin.
[a]Intracoronary administration.

and subsequent clinical course than those who reocclude following reperfusion. The study affirms the favorable impact of sustained vessel patency in this clinical situation.

The clinical effect exhibited by the prevention of reocclusion is of particular importance, as the negative clinical consequence associated with rethrombosis can often occur without any significant symptomatic markers. Patients who experienced silent reocclusion in this series had degrees of global left-ventricular dysfunction that were similar to the group with clinically symptomatic reocclusion. It has been documented that reocclusion manifesting as reinfarction following successful reperfusion in the setting of acute myocardial infarction is a common cause of death, second only to progressive congestive heart failure. Therefore, prevention of recurrence of occlusion of infarct-related vessels should be of paramount importance. Significant attention and effort must be placed on the proper administration of aspirin and heparin as conjuncts to successful thrombolysis.

III. CLINICAL FACTORS PREVENTING REOCCLUSION WITH ASPIRIN

The benefit of aspirin as a preventative agent for ischemic coronary disease has been well established by many randomized trials. However, it was not until the results of the ISIS-2 trial were presented that the vital importance of aspirin as a conjunctive agent to coronary thrombolysis was realized. In this trial, 17,187 patients presenting within 24 hours of the onset of the clinical findings associated with acute myocardial infarction were randomized to one of four treatment groups utilizing a 2 × 2 factorial design. These groups were comprised of patients treated with placebo, 1.5 million units of intravenous streptokinase administered over 60 minutes, 162 mg of aspirin alone for 30 days, or a combination therapy of aspirin and streptokinase. Mortality for the placebo and aspirin-streptokinase combination-treated patients was 13.2% and 8%, respectively. The groups randomized to aspirin or streptokinase

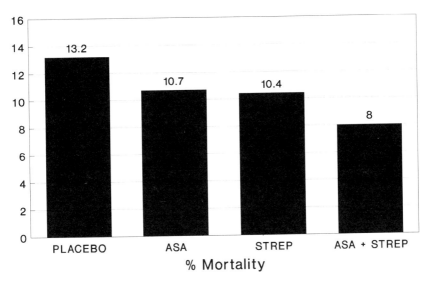

Figure 1   Results of the ISIS-2 trial.

as a sole therapy had 10.7% and 10.4% respective mortality. Deaths were reduced by 23% with the administration of aspirin ($p < 0.00001$). A similar reduction in mortality was seen in the group of patients treated with the thrombolytic agent alone. However, the most impressive reduction in mortality was demonstrated in those randomized to combination therapy. Close examination of these results provides the clinician with important therapeutic direction in the setting of acute myocardial infarction. As both platelet inhibition and thrombolysis play a crucial role in initial and sustained patency, they exhibit individual influences toward a single positive outcome. The most significant contribution that this trial makes towards directing clinical practice is not the fact that both platelet inhibition and thrombolysis exhibit a positive effect on mortality, but that together the beneficial outcome results in an additive effect. The results of the ISIS-2 trial are graphically depicted in Figure 1.

Further support for the utilization of aspirin in conjunction with thrombolytic therapy in acute myocardial infarction comes from a meta-analysis by Roux et al. incorporating 32 studies. The purpose of this analytical investigation was to evaluate whether platelet inhibition induced by aspirin plays a role in the prevention of coronary reocclusion and recurrent ischemia following thrombolysis. The reocclusion rate assessed by coronary angiography in 419 patients treated with aspirin was 11% as compared to 25% in 513 infarcts without aspirin ($p < 0.001$). Recurrent ischemic events were present in 25% of 2977 patients randomized to antiplatelet therapy and 41% of 721 patients ($p < 0.001$) who did not receive aspirin as a conjunct to their thrombolytic agent. Further subgroup evaluation revealed that the positive clinical benefit provided by the platelet inhibitory effect of aspirin was comparable to that of streptokinase or tissue-type plasminogen activator (rt-PA) utilized independently.

Recently presented results of the Apricot Trial compared the use of aspirin to coumadin and placebo-treated acute myocardial infarcts. Patients in this clinical study were treated with intravenous streptokinase and heparin. Angiography-proven infarct artery patency documented within 48 hours qualified them for study entry. Randomization of 300 patients was performed to result in equal adjunctive treatment groups of coumadin, aspirin, and placebo. To evaluate infarct artery patency and left ventricular ejection fraction, cardiac catherization was repeated at 3 months. Although there was no significant difference in infarct artery patency among the three groups, ejection fraction improvement was at least three times as great in those treated with aspirin compared to either the coumadin or placebo-randomized patients.

This study not only further supports the need for aspirin administration during acute myocardial infarction, but also shows its superiority as compared to the anticoagulant properties of coumadin. The distinction of the separate roles of platelet inhibition and anticoagulation is clarified by this important comparative trial.

The optimal dose of aspirin as a conjunctive agent to thrombolysis continues to be debated. Clinical trials have been conducted utilizing doses from as low as 75 mg to as high as 1500 mg. It is currently accepted that extremely low doses of aspirin (35 mg/day) can affect both platelet thromboxane A_2 and endothelial prostacyclin formation. However, the maximal clinical benefit is probably achieved when doses of at least 80 mg are administered during the acute ischemic event. Higher doses of aspirin (>324 mg) do not appear to be more efficacious, but can be associated with significantly increased gastrointestinal complications. Several of the thrombolytic trials conducted by the European Cooperative Study Group have utilized aspirin as an intravenous preparation (250 mg) during acute myocardial infarction. Although an intravenous route of administration would be better tolerated by patients, there is no evidence in the current literature of its clinical superiority over that achieved by chewing a dose of aspirin. Aspirin, in its nonenterically coated form, is rapidly absorbed from the stomach and upper small intestine. Appreciable plasma levels are achieved in 20 minutes, and platelet inhibition in approximately 1 hour. Absorption periods can be somewhat shortened when aspirin is chewed and not swallowed. Therefore, based on currently available data, patients undergoing thrombolytic therapy for acute myocardial infarction will obtain maximal clinical benefit and minimal complication risk when they are instructed to chew 80–324 mg of aspirin as early during the event as possible. It is the opinion of this author and many other clinical cardiologists that one adult aspirin (324 mg) is the easiest dose to administer and is not felt to be associated with a more significant side-effect profile. For the purpose of subsequent long-term administration of aspirin, this dose is relatively simple for the patient to remember, which translates into a higher compliance rate.

IV. CLINICAL FACTORS PREVENTING REOCCLUSION WITH HEPARIN

The utilization of heparin in acute myocardial infarction dates back many years. Clinical benefit in the prethrombolytic era was felt to be paramount as a prophylactic therapy to many of the frequently encountered complications of an acute coronary ischemic event. In fact, the incidence of these commonly presenting complicating events of myocardial infarction including left ventricular mural thrombus formation, deep vein thrombosis, and pulmonary embolization were significantly reduced with the introduction of intravenous heparin.

In the early years of administration of thrombolytic therapy for acute myocardial infarction, heparin therapy was often administered as a conjunctive agent in both clinical research and daily practice. It was not until some years later that the actual mechanism of clinical benefit and critical role of heparin therapy in the overall scheme of thrombolysis were realized. Although the importance of heparin as a conjunctive agent with thrombolytic therapy has been well established, the debate over the method of administration continues.

The rationale for intravenous heparin therapy, specifically in conjunction with fibrin-specific plasminogen activators (i.e., rt-PA), has been thoroughly documented. However, its role with non–fibrin-specific agents (i.e., streptokinase and anisoylated plasminogen streptokinase activator complex) has not been clearly defined. The prolonged half-life of these plasminogen activators and the generation of relatively high concentrations of fibrin degradation products is the theoretical reason for the less stringent anticoagulation requirement.

The pathophysiological rationale for the utilization of heparin is discussed in other chapters of this book in great detail. Researchers feel that the need for adequate heparinization in conjunction with the administration of fibrinolytic agents (especially fibrin-specific agents) is the direct result of events at the site of thrombolysis. When fibrinolysis occurs, there is reexposure of the original ruptured plaque that initiated the thrombotic process. In addition, constant release of thrombin and fibrin-bound thrombin as a result of clot dissolution occurs. Thrombin bound to fibrin fragments that are released during thrombolysis are more resistant to heparin inactivation, whereas thrombin produced through the catalytic effect of fibrin-bound thrombin is readily inactivated by the heparin–antithrombin-III complex. Therefore, the site at which thrombolysis occurs creates a perfect nidus for rethrombosis. Consequently, ongoing fibrinolysis is often an excellent setting for thrombogenesis and the initiation of reocclusion. The process of coronary reperfusion can be envisioned as a competitive event between thrombolytic activity and a constant threat of reocclusion. The ultimate fate of coronary flow is dependent on adequacy of anticoagulation and other factors described in previous chapters of this book.

Data from the ECSG-3 trial, published by Verstraete et al., reinforce the need for conjunctive heparin therapy for the prevention of reocclusion following alteplase-induced thrombolysis. In this interesting study, it was established that continued prolonged plasminogen activator infusion is not necessary to prevent rethrombosis and that heparin alone is sufficient.

A. Clinical Trials of Alteplase and Heparin

Substantial clinical information has been published in the recent literature supporting the critical role of conjunctive heparin administration for the prevention of coronary reocclusion following successful thrombolysis with alteplase in acute myocardial infarction. The characteristics of these trials are summarized in Table 5.

The first study to evaluate the necessity for heparin with alteplase was published in 1990 by Bleich et al. In this trial, 84 patients with an acute myocardial infarction were randomized to one of two treatment arms in conjunction with alteplase. Both groups received 100 mg of alteplase administered over 3 hours. The patients randomized to the anticoagulation treatment group were given 5000 U of an intravenous bolus of heparin followed by an initial infusion of 1000 U/h. Activated partial thromboplastin times (aPTT) were drawn at 12 hours following initiation of the heparin infusion. Subsequent blood sampling and rate of infusion were dependent on a standardized nomogram to maintain prolongation of the aPTT to 1.5–2 times control values. There was no aspirin administration required by the protocol.

Table 5   Study Design of Alteplase-Heparin Trials

Study	# pts.	Time of cath.	Heparin randomized group			
			Bolus	Initial infusion	Drip titration by aPTT	Aspirin
Bleich	84	48–72 h	5000 U	1000 U/h	Yes	No
HART	205	7–24 h	5000 U	1000 U/h	Yes	80 mg p.o. [a]
TOPOL	134	90 min	10,000 U	N/A	N/A	325 mg p.o.
ECSG-6	652	48–120 h	5000 U	1000 U/h	No	250 mg i.v.
Nat'l. Heart Foundation	241	7–10 days	5000 U	1000 U/h	Yes	325 mg [b]

[a] Control group.
[b] All patients received heparin for the first 24 hours, at which point half of the group had heparin drip stopped and replaced with 325 mg of aspirin and 300 mg of dipyridamole.

The primary end point of the trial was coronary angiography performed 48–72 hours (mean of 57 hours) from initiation of therapy. Patency rates were evaluated utilizing the thrombolysis in myocardial infarction (TIMI) flow grade criteria. Infarct arteries with TIMI flow grades 0 and 1 were classified as "occluded" and flow grades 2 and 3 as "patent."

Angiographic patency rates of 71% were reported in the anticoagulated patients and 43% in the control group at a mean of 57 hours following initiation of thrombolytic therapy. These results were found to be statistically significant with a p-value of 0.015. Among the patients deemed patent there was a significant inequality in favor of grade III flow. A clear clinical benefit has been recently reported with resultant TIMI grade III versus grade II coronary flow. The categorization of TIMI flow grading seen in this trial is depicted in Figure 2.

The secondary endpoint of this trial addressed an equally important question regarding bleeding complications suffered by the two treatment groups. Bleeding occurred in 64% of patients in the group receiving heparin (minor bleeding in 52%, moderate in 10%, and severe in 2%) and 36% of the control population. Although bleeding was more common in the heparinized patients, most of these events were classified as minor and were of no clinical significance. Bleeding complications are illustrated in Figure 12-3.

The HART trial further confirmed the need for heparinization as a conjunctive agent to alteplase. Two hundred and five patients suffering an acute myocardial infarction were administered 100 mg of alteplase over 6 hours and randomized to one of two conjunctive agent regimen. One hundred and six of the patients received an intravenous heparin bolus of 5000 U with a subsequent initial infusion of 1000 U/h. The control group (99 patients) received 80 mg of immediate and subsequent daily aspirin.

Angiographic evaluation of the infarct vessel was performed at 7–24 hours following initiation of the thrombolytic agent (average of 18 hours). Recocclusion of the patients with initial patency was assessed by repeat cardiac catherization on

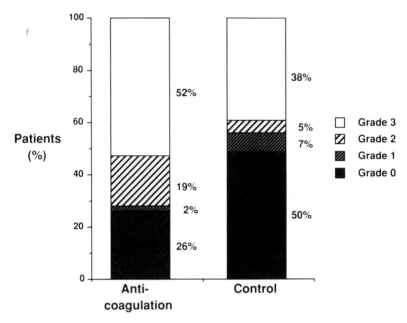

Figure 2   Percentage of patients demonstrating angiographic patency as graded by TIMI flow grades 0 to III. (From Bleich et al., 1990.)

day 7. Angiographic patency rates at 18 hours were 82% for the heparin-treated patients and 52% for the group randomized to aspirin with a statistical significance of $p < 0.0001$. Of the patients with initial coronary patency, 88% remained patent at 7 days from thrombolytic therapy. This was in comparison to 95% in the aspirin group ($p = $ NS). There was no statistical difference in hemorrhagic complications between the two treatment groups.

Review of the results of the above-cited trials contributed important information regarding clinical treatment directions in thrombolysis in acute myocardial infarction. However, an important piece of the puzzle was contributed by the results of the TAMI-3 trial. In this clinical investigative protocol, patients were randomized to receive either a 10,000 U bolus of heparin

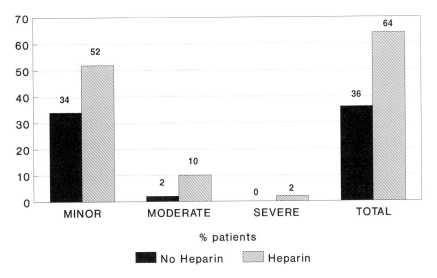

Figure 3   Bleeding complications. (From Bleich et al., 1990.)

during initial infusion of 100 mg of alteplase over a 4-hour period or no heparin at all. Angiography performed at 90 minutes from initiation of treatment revealed 79% patency in both
treatment groups. This data reinforces the theory that conjunctive therapy does not play a significant role in the actual
thrombolytic phenomenon. However, if data from the above-
mentioned trials are associated with the TAMI-3 results, a
meaningful concept is confirmed. Although conjunctive therapy plays essentially no proven role in lysis of clot, it serves an
important function in preventing rethrombosis and reocclusion resulting in positive prognostic implications.

The European Cooperative Study Group (ECSG-6) trial re-
affirmed the need for heparin following treatment with tissue
plasminogen activator (alteplase, 100 mg/3 h). Heparin was
administered to half of the randomized patients in this trial in
the form of a 5000 U bolus followed by an intravenous infusion of 1000 U/h. Patients who received heparin in conjunction
with alteplase had an angiographic patency rate of 83% at
81 hours as compared to 75% if they were randomized to the

no-heparin arm. The disparity of patent infarct arteries found in the two groups of this trial are statistically significant but show a smaller difference than previously demonstrated by the above-cited trials. The relative risk of an occluded vessel in the heparin-treated group was 0.66 (95% confidence interval 0.47–0.93). It has been postulated that the decreased disparity between the heparin- and non–heparin-treated patients was the result of administrative methods. Although aPTTs were drawn periodically, heparin drips were not titrated accordingly. This further dictates the importance of an adequate level of anticoagulation utilizing heparin drip titration.

A study from the National Heart Foundation (NHF) of Australia provides evidence that the continuation of heparin may not be necessary for longer than 24 hours if adequate antiplatelet therapy is instituted. Patients receiving 100 mg of alteplase were administered a bolus of heparin followed by an infusion of 1000 U/h. At 24 hours from initiation of thrombolytic therapy, patients were randomized to either continue the heparin infusion or to receive 325 mg of aspirin and 300 mg of dipyridamole. Coronary angiography revealed patency rates of 80% in both groups with no difference in reinfarction, recurrent ischemic events, or left ventricular function. Since angiography was not performed early, the exact time of reperfusion could not be evaluated. Therefore, there was no distinction between patients with continued perfusion versus late spontaneous reperfusion of previously reoccluded vessels. Secondary end point equality, as mentioned above, however, does support clinical relevance of this investigation.

The above-reviewed clinical data (summarized in Fig. 4) clearly supports the need for adequate anticoagulation with heparin in conjunction with alteplase therapy in acute myocardial infarction. Details regarding timing, route of administration, and dosing will be addressed later in this chapter.

B. Clinical Trials of Non–Fibrin-Specific Agents and Heparin

In contrast to the extensive investigation into the role of heparin in conjunction with the fibrin-specific plasminogen acti-

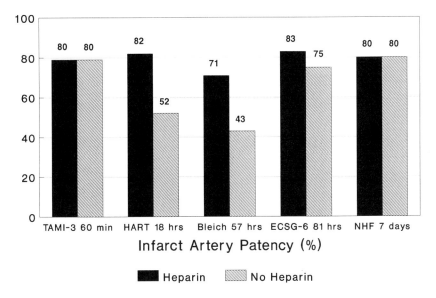

Figure 4   Summary of patency rates of clinical investigations of heparin as a conjunctive agent to alteplase in acute myocardial infarction.

vators, there is significantly less information present in the literature in response to the same question for the systemic plasminogen activators (streptokinase and anistreplase). This is somewhat surprising since the administration of early high-dose intravenous heparin was initiated due to frequent episodes of reocclusion following direct intracoronary infusion of streptokinase. As a result of this recognized phenomenon, anticoagulation with heparin as a conjunct to intracoronary streptokinase was considered the standard of care several years ago. Despite the lack of randomized studies utilizing angiographic patency as an end point in streptokinase-treated infarcts, the following clinical ischemia and mortality data exists and will be reviewed below.

In a study by Kaplan et al. in 1987, a significant correlation between the degree of prolongation of the aPTT produced as a result of heparin administration and the development of recurrent ischemia was established in patients receiving intravenous streptokinase for myocardial infarction. Clinical ischemic events were realized two to four times as often among those patients who did not achieve therapeutic levels of anticoagulation as determined by aPTT.

The Studio sulla Calciparina nell' Angina E Nella Trombosi Ventricolare nell' Infarto (SCATI) trial randomized 711 patients suffering an acute myocardial infarction. Patients received either calcium heparin administered as a bolus of 2000 U with a subsequent subcutaneous dose of 12,500 U every 12 hours (instituted 9 hours after the bolus) or no heparin at all. Patients presenting within 24 hours of symptom onset were considered for entry into the study. Four hundred and thirty-three of the infarcts admitted within 6 hours were treated with intravenous streptokinase. There was no aspirin administered in this study. The primary end point of the trial was in-hospital mortality with electrocardiographically documented ischemia as a secondary point of evaluation.

Of the group presenting late (nonlytic), heparin had no significant effect on mortality, recurrent ischemia, or reinfarction. Mortality in the patients presenting less than 6 hours from symptom onset (streptokinase-treated) was 4.5% for those randomized to heparin therapy in contrast to 8.8% in the no-heparin group ($p = 0.05$). Reinfarction and recurrent ischemia were reduced 28% and 15%, respectively. Statistical significance was not reached, however, due to the relatively small sample size.

The GISSI-2/International t-PA/SK Mortality Trial attempted to clarify the long-asked question of thrombolytic agent superiority randomizing more than 20,000 acute infarcts to receive either alteplase or streptokinase. A secondary randomization in this trial concerned anticoagulation. Half of the group received 12,500 units of subcutaneous heparin twice a day, which was introduced 12 hours after the initiation of thrombolytic therapy. The delay in heparin administration was apparently secondary to a fear of concomitant anticoagulation in the face of a lytic state possibly resulting in more significant bleeding.

Patients randomized to the alteplase-treatment group showed no benefit realized from the addition of adjunctive subcutaneous heparin. Mortality in the heparin-treated patients was 9.2% versus 8.7% among those without the addition of a conjunctive anticoagulant (p = NS). The streptokinase-treated patients, however, showed a mild reduction in mortality in the heparin group (7.9%) as compared to the nonheparin group (9.2%). The delay in heparin initiation along with the relatively slow rate of achieving therapeutic levels of anti-coagulation resulted in a serious lack of adequate anticoagulation when rethrombosis is most apt to occur, i.e., during thrombolysis.

It is, therefore, of interest to review the influence on mortality exhibited by patients who survived the first 12 hours of the GISSI-2/International t-PA/SK Trial and as a result became eligible for anticoagulant therapy. For those patients who had been treated with streptokinase and adjunctive heparin, a 5.0% mortality was realized as compared to 6.2% for those without heparin therapy (p < 0.01). The group randomized to alteplase and surviving the first 12 hours displayed a mortality of 5.9% regardless of their randomization to late subcutaneous heparin therapy or no heparin at all.

After reviewing the above-mentioned disparity in effect on mortality displayed by alteplase and streptokinase in the GISSI-2/International t-PA/SK Mortality Trial, an important hypothesis is realized regarding the delayed use of heparin. There is some positive effect on mortality seen in the group of patients treated with streptokinase and late low-dose subcutaneous heparin. However, there is no benefit to those randomized to alteplase and the anticoagulant. It can be inferred from the above findings that the disruption of coagulation factors associated with the use of streptokinase induces a state of anti-coagulation thereby reducing the requirements of heparin. This compares with a more timely and significantly greater degree of heparinization that is required as a conjunctive treatment with alteplase in the prevention of reocclusion following a previously successful reperfusion.

The ISIS-3 trial is the largest thrombolytic mortality trial to date comparing streptokinase, duteplase, and APSAC enrolling 41,299 patients. Heparin dosing and mode of delivery in this trial were similar to those utilized in the GISSI-2/International t-PA/SK Mortality Trial discussed above. Timing of the initiation of anticoagulation was the sole distinction between the two "mega" mortality trials. Both trials randomized patients to 12,500 U of subcutaneous heparin versus no heparin at all. In the GISSI-2/International t-PA/SK Mortality Trial heparin was delayed for 12 hours as compared to 4 hours of postponing anticoagulation in ISIS-3. The terms delayed and postponing are utilized above because of the relatively late initiation of anticoagulation based on the previously explained theory that the risk of thrombogenesis is extreme, especially with fibrin-specific agents, early during the thrombolytic process.

The resultant mortality in the ISIS-3 Trial was 10.3–10.6%. Regardless of thrombolytic agent randomization, no significant difference was realized. In fact, mortality was also not affected to a statistically significant degree when patients were subrandomized to receive heparin along with aspirin or aspirin alone.

The equalization in mortality among the three thrombolytic agents seen in this trial has been attributed to be a consequence of the relatively late, low-dose subcutaneous heparin administration. As discussed earlier and also later in this chapter, the benefit of relatively rapid reperfusion associated with fibrin-specific agents (i.e., alteplase and duteplase) is nullified by the late initiation and inadequate dosing of heparin utilized in ISIS-3. Overall stroke rates in the subcutaneous heparin and no-heparin arms were 1.28% and 1.18%, respectively (p = NS). A statistically significant difference was found in "probable" cerebral hemorrhage rates between the two groups (0.6% for the heparin/ASA versus 0.4% for ASA alone with a p value of <0.01). However, the increase in intracranial bleeding was offset by a decrease in mortality (0.5%) that was greater than the increase in stroke (0.2%) resulting in a positive net clinical benefit.

The Duke University Clinical Cardiology Studies (DUCCS-1) study looked at the need for conjunctive heparin with APSAC. In this trial, 250 patients with acute myocardial infarction were randomized to one of two anticoagulant regimen following 30 U of APSAC over 5 minutes within 12 hours from symptom onset. One hundred and twenty-two patients received no heparin therapy, while the remaining 128 received intravenous heparin at a dose of 150 U/kg/h beginning 4 hours after thrombolytic initiation. All patients received 325 mg of aspirin acutely and daily throughout the hospital course. Patients randomized to the heparin treatment group had drip adjustments to maintain aPTTs between 50 and 90 seconds. The primary end point of the trial was coronary angiography performed on day 5. Among the 231 patients who underwent cardiac catherization, patency of the infarct-related artery was seen in 80% of the heparin group as compared to 74% in the non–heparin-treated patients. Overall mortality of the trial was 8%, including 9% in the heparin group and 7% among the no-heparin patients. Data from this trial infers that heparin plays no significant clinical role as conjunctive therapy to APSAC. However, one must take into account the fact that angiography was performed 5 days following initial treatment, allowing for spontaneous reperfusion of vessels that may have remained occluded throughout the acute event. Although no statistical difference in patency was seen in this trial between the two treatment groups, heparin should continue to be used as a conjunctive agent with APSAC. However, the aggressiveness of therapy need not be as strict as that required for alteplase because of the significantly longer half-life, a less fibrin-specific mode of action, and a more systemic anticoagulant effect of APSAC.

To summarize this section, significant data exist to support aggressive heparinization with alteplase to obtain the maximal clinical benefit of the high rate of early patency associated with this agent. Although anticoagulation is also important with streptokinase and APSAC, a less aggressive approach might be adequate. Great care should be taken when interpreting the results of clinical trials that utilize relatively unaggressive, low-dose, nontitrated heparin regimens with fibrin-specific agents (i.e., alteplase and duteplase). A great disadvantage is placed on these agents if the procoagulant state that is generated by rapid reperfusion remains unprotected from rethrombosis. A heparin regimen that might be adequate for the non–fibrin-specific agents may prove to be insufficient for the fibrin-specific group.

V. MODE OF HEPARIN ADMINISTRATION

Much controversy continues to exist surrounding the correct mode of administration of heparin as a conjunctive agent for thrombolytic-treated acute myocardial infarction. Intravenous infusion is the most commonly utilized route of delivery of physicians in the United States, whereas subcutaneous treatment with heparin is often utilized in Europe. In addition to the ongoing clinical debate over the most efficacious and safest manner of heparin therapy, another equally important discussion continues: the ongoing question as to the therapeutic adequacy of subcutaneous heparin as conjuncts in large mortality trials. If these methods of administering heparin are adequate, then clinical comparisons can be fairly evaluated. However, if subcutaneous delivery is not satisfactory, especially as to the significant requirements of the fibrin-specific agents (i.e., alteplase), then mortality comparisons must be made with caution in trials utilizing what might be subtherapeutic heparin dosing.

An important trial that compared intravenous heparin administration versus intermittent subcutaneous therapy in the treatment of proximal vein thrombosis was published by Hull et al. in 1986. One hundred and fifteen patients with acute proximal deep vein thrombosis were treated with a 5000 U intravenous bolus of heparin followed by randomization to one of two maintenance regimen. Those assigned to the intravenous group were placed on continuous infusion of 20,000 U in 500 cc at 31 cc/h (24-hour dose of 29,760 U). The subcutaneous group received 15,000 U every 12 hours. Frequency of recurrent thromboemboli in the subcutaneous group was 19.3% as compared to 5.2% for the intravenous-treated patients ($p = 0.24$). The percentage of patients with an aPTT less than 1.5 times the control during the first 24 hours was 63.2% for the subcutaneous-treated and 29.3% for the intravenous patients ($p < 0.001$).

These data become a very interesting and pertinent addition to the thrombolytic literature in view of the fact that the subcutaneous dose administered in this trial was greater than that utilized in the GISSI-2 and ISIS-3 trials (12,500U twice daily). In addition, new data from the HART and ECSG-6 trials dictate that significantly increased patency rates are achieved postthrombolysis in those patients with aPTT prolongation of two times the control value. In the HART study, patients with aPTT values of less than 45 seconds had a patency rate of 45%. Those who displayed a greater prolongation of their aPTT achieved a more significant chance of coronary patency. Patients realizing aPTT values of greater than 45 and 60 seconds displayed angiographic patency rates of 88% and 95%, respectively. In the ECSG-6 study, similar findings were documented. Entries into the trial with aPTTs less than two times the control value achieved patency rates of 74.1% as compared to 95.6% for those with aPTT determinations of greater than two times control.

It was made clear in the trial by Hull et al. that, despite the addition of a bolus and a larger maintenance dose of heparin than utilized in the GISSI-2 and ISIS-3 trials, few patients will ever realize therapeutic coagulation with the administration of relatively low-dose subcutaneous heparin. It has been felt that the heparin dose used in GISSI-2 and ISIS-3 may have resulted in nontherapeutic anticoagulation, thereby adversely affecting mortality, particularly of the duteplase-treated patients.

Similarly, a trial published by Turpie et al. confirms a poor therapeutic response to subcutaneous heparinization. This double-blind study randomized 221 patients with acute anterior myocardial infarction to receive either low- or high-dose subcutaneous heparin therapy in the prevention of left ventricular mural thrombosis. The high-dose group received 12,500 U of heparin twice daily (the same dose utilized in the GISSI-2 and ISIS-3 trials) as compared to 5,000 U b.i.d. for those randomized to low-dose therapy. Activated partial thromboplastin times drawn from day 0 to day 10 provide interesting therapeutic response curves. Patients receiving the low-dose treatment never developed aPTTs greater than 30 seconds. Those treated with the higher dose only showed significant evidence of aPTT prolongation (greater than 50 seconds but never longer than 52 seconds) at day 2–3. However, at this relatively late point in time, a significant risk of rethrombosis has passed. Therefore, according to this data, utilization of the identical dose of heparin administered in the GISSI-2 and ISIS-3 trials results in very poor levels of therapeutic anticoagulation.

VI. DURATION OF HEPARIN THERAPY POSTTHROMBOLYTIC TREATMENT

The duration of heparin therapy following thrombolytic treatment remains an unanswered question. To date, one clinical trial has attempted to clarify this issue. The Australian National Heart Foundation study randomized 202 patients following treatment with alteplase and 24 hours of intravenous heparin therapy. At this juncture, half of the group continued to receive intravenous heparin for 6 days while the remaining patients were placed on a daily adult aspirin and 300 mg of dipyridamole. Angiography to determine infarct-artery patency was performed at 8 days from initial therapy. No statistical difference was seen between the two groups as both arms achieved 80% patency. This data is consistent with the previously cited hypothesis that thrombogenesis causing reocclusion exhibits the most significant threat during the early stages of thrombolysis. However, the ACC/AHA guidelines for the treatment of myocardial infarction recommend at least 48 hours of heparin therapy.

Until more data becomes available, it is recommended that all postthrombolytic anticoagulation (barring complications) should continue until angiography is performed (if indicated) or for at least 48 hours with continuation of adequate antiplatelet therapy.

VII. HEPARIN MONITORING AND TITRATION

The majority of physicians in the United States utilize intravenous heparin for their postthrombolytic patients. However, the most common technique for measuring anticoagulation and dictating drip titration is the activated partial thromboplastin, which may be inadequate and misleading. Heparin titration by aPTT was initially developed and utilized for the treatment of deep venous thrombosis. Heras et al. has presented significant data supporting the theory that the dose of heparin necessary for adequate anticoagulation in the setting of arterial injury is significantly greater than that required to treat venous thrombotic disease. Data from a recent study, along with a great degree of anecdotal personal communication, informs us that when patients return to the cardiac catherization laboratory while on heparin drips and have achieved therapeutic aPTTs, the measured activated clotting time (ACT) is often subtherapeutic. This phenomenon has also been frequently identified in patients presenting to the catherization laboratory for rescue angioplasty following coronary reocclusion.

A retrospective study by Bleich et al. looked at the comparison of ACT and aPTT as markers of adequate anticoagulation. Patients experiencing acute coronary syndromes undergoing continuous intravenous heparin therapy were identified. If found to have a therapeutic aPTT of 60–90 seconds, a bedside ACT was obtained within 4 hours prior to any changes in drug delivery rate. Of 57 eligible patients with therapeutic aPTTs, only 8.8% (5/57) of those exhibited an ACT that achieved the target range of 300 seconds or greater (level used for arterial intervention).

Attempts to maintain adequate anticoagulation are often difficult. A report by the GUSTO (Global Utilization of Streptokinase and t-PA for Occluded Coronary Arteries) pilot investigators suggests this in a recent report. In their pilot trial, 108 patients with acute myocardial infarction were treated with a combination of alteplase and streptokinase. Heparin was administered as a bolus of 5000 U at the onset of thrombolytic therapy followed by a drip of 1000 U/h for 48 hours or longer. Drips were titrated to attempt to maintain an aPTT of greater than 60 seconds. Despite what was previously felt to be aggressive heparinization, aPTTs at 24 hours were subtherapeutic in 55% of patients. It is based on this data that the therapeutic adequacy concerning the dose and manner in which heparin is currently titrated following thrombolysis is questioned.

The most significant obstacle associated with obtaining adequate anticoagulation is often a clinical problem and not a biochemical one. It is the delay of obtaining results and subsequent infusion adjustment based on a given aPTT value that leads to improper titration. This, in turn, often results in wide swings in levels of anticoagulation (the "roller coaster phenomenon"). It is therefore felt that the benefit of bedside ACT might prove to be clinically significant. A randomized trial is currently underway to evaluate the role of bedside ACT as compared to aPTT in the regulation of anticoagulation in post-thrombolytic patients.

VIII. CONCLUSION

With the availability of potent fibrinolytic agents and new dosage regimen providing increasingly improved patency rates, rapid reperfusion is commonly achieved. However, sustained patency has been shown to be as influential on long-term outcome as is early reperfusion. These important data along with the significant procoagulant effect produced by thrombolytic agents demonstrate the importance of vigorous well-controlled conjunctive therapy to thrombolysis. Evidence supporting the administration of aspirin in this clinical setting is well documented. A minimum of 160 mg of aspirin provides adequate alteration of platelet function without a significant increase in hemorrhagic risk. In view of the ease of administration of one adult aspirin (324 mg) with essentially no additional risk of bleeding, this regimen has been adopted by many centers as standard of care.

Much data support the important contribution made by heparin as a conjunct to thrombolysis if properly administered. The prevention of thrombogenesis and subsequent coronary reocclusion is the key role played by the anticoagulant. Significant data regarding the adverse role played by coronary reocclusion following a successful thrombolysis dictate the importance of careful utilization of conjunctive agents. Despite the fact that much evidence exists documenting the need for early, high-dose, intravenous heparin as a conjunct to thrombolytic therapy (especially fibrin-specific agents), the controversy surrounding this issue continues. Delayed subcutaneous administration of heparin, thought by some to be an adequate alternative to intravenous delivery, results in a less predictable, delayed, often subtherapeutic anticoagulative state. Therefore, the data obtained from thrombolytic trials that utilize inadequate anticoagulation should be carefully interpreted.

Ongoing clinical investigation continues to attempt to settle the controversy. The GUSTO trial has clarified the need for early and sustained patency supporting aggressive anticoagulation. It has also addressed the utilization of subcutaneous heparin with streptokinase. Other important research continues in search of the most reliable and efficacious mechanism of titration of heparin infusion. Despite the fact that heparin is known to be a potent anticoagulant, the utilization of the most reliable laboratory method for guiding therapy remains an important question. Promising clinical research continues to attempt to clarify these issues.

In summary, aspirin and heparin have been found to be imperative conjuncts to thrombolytic agents in the setting of acute myocardial infarction. Research into the development of new antiplatelet and antithrombin agents as well as new

innovative ways to deliver currently available agents continues
at a rapid pace. Until new developments emerge, aspirin
should be administered early, utilizing a dose of at least 160
mg. Heparin therapy should be initiated early with an adequate bolus of at least 5000 U followed by an initial minimal
infusion of 1000 U/h. Data from the GUSTO trial indicates that
patients weighing more than 85 kg should receive an initial infusion of 1200 U/h. Determination of aPTTs should be obtained
on a relatively frequent basis and drips adjusted to maintain
prolongation of 2–2.5 times the control value. However, infusion rates should not be adjusted downward during the first 12
hours to avoid sub- and supratherapeutic levels.

Careful monitoring of the literature regarding adjunctive
and conjunctive therapy in thrombolysis is recommended as
new data is constantly being generated regarding innovative
administrative strategies in addition to the advent of new
therapies.

ACKNOWLEDGMENTS

The development of this chapter was an extremely important
personal endeavor. It is therefore dedicated in memory of my
father, George Bleich, who suddenly passed away during its
writing. This manuscript is also dedicated in honor of my
mother, Yolanda Bleich, who loved him so dearly.

PERTINENT REFERENCES

Anderson J L, Rothbard R L, Hackworthy R A, et al. Multicenter reperfusion
    trial of intravenous anisoylated plasminogen streptokinase activator
    complex (APSAC) in acute myocardial infarction: controlled comparison
    with intracoronary streptokinase. *J Am Coll Cardiol* 1988;11:1153–1163.

Appel K F, Vogt A, von Essen R, Tebbe U, Feurerer W, Neuhaus K L: Do we
    achieve optimal reperfusion in acute myocardial infarction by thrombol-
    ysis?(abstr.) *European Heart J* 1992;13:155

Bleich S D, Ditta S, Mailander L, Leonhard R, Tilton G D, Rolston W A: A
    comparative analysis of activated clotting time (ACT) versus activated

partial thromboplastin time (aPTT) for heparin monitoring in acute coronary disease. 2nd International Symposium on Heart Failure-Mechanisms and Management, Palexpo, Geneva, Switzerland, May 16–20, 1993.

Bleich S D, Ditta S, Mailander L, Leonhard R, Tilton G D, Rolston W A: An analysis of activated clotting time (ACT) versus activated partial thromboplastin time (aPTT) for heparin monitoring in acute coronary disease. XIVth Congress of the International Society on Thrombosis and Haemostasis, New York, July 4–9, 1993.

Bleich S D, Nichols T C, Schumacher R R, Cooke D H, Tate D A, Teichman S L: Effect of heparin on coronary arterial patency after thrombolysis with tissue plasminogen activator in acute myocardial infarction. *Am J Cardiol* 1990;66:1412–1417.

Bleich S D, Rolston W A, Tilton G D, Mailander L: Adjunctive therapy in thrombolysis for acute myocardial infarction. *Z Kardiol* 1993;28:Suppl 1.

Bossaert L L. Safety and tolerance data from the Belgian multicentre study of anisoylated plasminogen streptokinase activator complex versus heparin in acute myocardial infarction. *Drugs* 1987;33(Suppl. 3):287–293.

Carney R J, Murphy G A, Brandt T R, Daley P J, Pickering E, White H, McDonough T J, Vermilya S K, Teichman S L: Randomized angiographic trial of recombinant tissue-type plasminogen activator in myocardial infarction. *J Am Coll Cardiol* 1992;20:17–23.

deBono D P, Simoons J T, Arnold A E R, et al.: Effect of early intravenous heparin on coronary patency, infarct size, and bleeding complications after alteplase thrombolysis: results of a randomized double blind European Cooperative Study Group Trial. *Br Heart J* 1992;67:122–8.

Gold H K, Leinbach R C, Palacios I F, et al.: Coronary reocclusion after selective administration of streptokinase. *Circulation* 1983;68(Suppl I):50.

Granger C B, Califf R M et al.: aPTT after thrombolysis and standard intravenous heparin are often low and correlate with weight, age and sex: experience from the GUSTO trial (abstr.). *Circulation* 1992;86:8–258.

Granger C, Kalbfeisch J, Califf R, et al.: The global utilization of streptokinase and tissue plasminogen activator for occluded coronary arteries (GUSTO) Pilot Study: Combines streptokinase and rt-PA (abstr.). *Circulation* 1991;84:573.

Gruppo Italiano Per Lo Studio Della Sopravivenza Nell-Infarto Miocardico: GISSI-2: a factorial randomized trial of alteplase versus streptokinase and heparin versus no heparin among 12,490 patients with acute myocardial infarction. *Lancet* 1990;336:65–71.

Gulba D C, Barthels M, Westhoff-Bleck M, et al.: Increased thrombin levels during thrombolytic therapy in acute myocardial infarction. Relavence for the success of therapy. *Circulation* 1991;83:937.

Heras M, Cheseboro J H, Penny W, Bailey K R, Badimon L, Fuster V: Effects of thrombin inhibition on the development of acute platelet-thrombus deposition during angioplasty in pigs. Heparin versus recombinant hirudin, a specific thrombin inhibitor. *Circulation* 1989;79:657–65.

Hsia J, Hamilton W P, Kleiman N, Roberts R, Chaitman B R, Ross A M: A comparison between heparin and low-dose aspirin as adjunctive therapy with tissue plasminogen activator for acute myocardial infarction. *N Engl J Med* 1990;323:1433–1437.

Hsia J, Kleiman N, Aguire F, Chaitman B R, Roberts R, Ross A M: Heparin induced prolongation of partial thromboplastin time after thrombolysis: Relation to coronary artery disease. *J Am Coll Cardiol* 1992;20:31–5.

Hull R D, Raskob G E, Hirsh J, et al.: Continuous intravenous heparin compared with intermittent sub-cutaneous heparin in the initial treatment of proximal-vein thrombosis. *N Engl J Med* 1986;315:1109–1114.

ISIS-2 (Second International Study of Infarct Survival) Collaborative Group: Randomized trial of intravenous streptokinase, oral aspirin, both or neither among 17,187 cases of suspected acute myocardial infarction: ISIS-2. *Lancet* 1988;2:349–360.

ISIS-3 (Third International Study of Infarct Survival) Collaborative Group: A randomised comparison of streptokinase vs. tissue plasminogen activator vs. anistreplase and of aspirin plus heparin vs. aspirin alone among 41,299 cases of suspected acute myocardial infarction. *Lancet* 1992; 339:753–770.

Johns J A, Gold H K, Leinbach R C, et al.: Prevention of coronary artery re-occlusion and reduction in late coronary artery stenosis after thrombolytic therapy in patients with acute myocardial infarction. *Circulation* 1989;79:546.

Kaplan K, Davison R, Parker M, et al.: Role of heparin after intravenous thrombolytic therapy for acute myocardial infarction. *Am J Cardiol* 1987; 59:241–244.

Leibof R H, Katz R J, Wasserman A G, et al.: A randomized, angiographically controlled trial of intracoronary streptokinase in acute myocardial infarction. *Am J Cardiol* 1984;53:404–407.

Meijer A, Werter C J, Verheugt F W A, et al.: The APRICOT Study: Aspirin versus coumadin in the prevention of recurrent ischemia and reocclusion after successful thrombolysis, a placebo-controlled angiographic follow-up study (abstr.). *J Am Coll Cardiol* 1992;19:91A.

Merx W, Dorr R, Rentrop P, et al.: Evaluation of the effectiveness of intra-coronary streptokinase infusion in acute myocardial infarction: procedural management and hospital course in 204 patients. *Am Heart J* 1981; 102:1181–1187.

Mueller H S, Rao A K, Forman S A, et al.: Thrombolysis in myocardial infarction (TIMI): comparative studies of coronary reperfusion and systemic fibrinogenolysis with two forms of recombinant tissue-type plasminogen activator. *J Am Coll Cardiol* 1987;10:479–490.

National Heart Foundation of Australia Coronary Thrombolysis Group: A randomized comparison of oral aspirin/dipyridamole versus intravenous heparin after rt-PA for acute myocardial infarction (abstr.). *Circulation* 1989;80(Suppl. II):114.

Neuhaus K -L, Feuerer W, Jeep-Tebbe S, et al.: Improved thrombolysis in acute myocardial infarction with front-loaded administration of alteplase: Results of the rt-PA APSAC patency study (TAPS). *J Am Coll Cardiol* 1992;19:885–891.

O'Connor C M, Meese R, Navetta F, et al.: A randomized trial of heparin in conjunction with anistreplase (APSAC) in acute myocardial infarction (abstr.). *Circulation* 1991;84(Suppl II):116.

Ohman E M, Califf R M, Topol E J, et al.: Consequences of reocclusion after successful therapy in acute myocardial infarction. *Circulation* 1990;82: 781–789.

Prins M H, Hirsh J: Heparin as an adjunctive treatment after thrombolytic therapy for acute myocardial infarction. *Am J Cardiol* 1991;67:3A–11A.

Roberts R, Rogers W J, Mueller H S, et al.: Immediate versus deferred beta-blockade following thrombolytic therapy in patients with acute myocardial infarction: results of the thrombolysis in myocardial infarction (TIMI) II B Study. *Circulation* 1991;83:422–437.

Roux S, Christeller, Ludin E: Effects of aspirin on coronary reocclusion and recurrent ischemia after thrombolysis: a meta analysis. *J Am Coll Cardiol* 1992;19:671–677.

The SCATI Studio Sulla Calciparina Nell'Angina E Nella Trombosi Ventricolare Nell'Infarto) Group: Randomized controlled trial of subcutaneous calcium-heparin in acute myocardial infarction. *Lancet* 1989;2:182–185.

Spann J F, Sherry S, Carabello B A, et al.: Coronary thrombolysis by intravenous streptokinase in acute myocardial infarction: acute and follow-up studies. *Am J Cardiol* 1984;53:655–661.

The TIMI Study Group: Comparison of invasive and conservative strategies after treatment with intravenous tissue plasminogen activator in acute myocardial infarction. Results of the thrombolysis in myocardial infarction (TIMI) phase II trial. *N Engl J Med* 1989;320:618.

Topol E J, George B S, Kereiakies D J, et al.: Comparison of two dose regimens of intravenous tissue plasminogen activator for acute myocardial infarction. *Am J Cardiol* 1988;61:723–728.

Topol E J, George B S, Kereiakes D J, et al.: A randomized controlled trial of intravenous tissue plasminogen activator and early intravenous heparin in acute myocardial infarction. *Circulation* 1989;79:281–286.

Topol E J, Morris D C, Smalling R W, et al.: A multicenter, randomized, placebo-controlled trial of a new form of intravenous tissue plasminogen activator (Activase) in acute myocardial infarction. *J Am Coll Cardiol* 1987; 9:1205–1213.

Turpie A G, Robinson T G, Doyle D J: Comparison of high-dose with low-dose sub-cutaneous heparin to prevent left ventricular mural thrombosis in patients with acute transmural anterior myocardial infarction. *N Engl J Med* 1989;320:352–357.

Verstraete M, Arnold A E R, Brower R W, et al.: Acute coronary thrombolysis with recombinant human tissue-type plasminogen activator: initial patency and influence of maintained infusion on reocclusion rate. *Am J Cardiol* 1987;60:231–237.

14

Efficacy of Currently Available Conjunctive Regimens

Uwe Zeymer and Karl-Ludwig Neuhaus
Medical Clinic II
Kassel, Germany

I. RATIONALE FOR THE USE OF CONJUNCTIVE THERAPY

Early intravenous thrombolytic therapy has proven to reduce mortality in patients with acute myocardial infarction. According to the open-artery hypothesis the aim of thrombolytic treatment is to achieve early, complete, and sustained patency of the infarct-related artery.

Various thrombolytic agents effect very early restoration of bloodflow in the infarct-related artery within 60 minutes in 50 to 75% of patients (Figure 1). Reocclusion rates vary between 8.0% (Streptokinase, APSAC) and 13.5% (rt-PA). The importance of optimal reperfusion has been shown in a retrospective analysis of four German multicenter trials, in which patients with a very early, complete, and sustained patency had a very low in-hospital mortality of about 1% (Figure 2). However, optimal thrombolysis was achieved in only 50% of patients. In the TAMI trials, patients with sustained

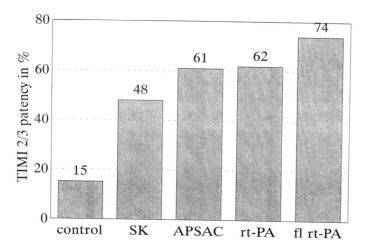

Figure 1   Standard (TIMI 2/3) patency 60 minutes after the initiation of thrombolytic therapy with different agents. Pooled meta-analysis of 13,728 angiographic observations. Control: patients without thrombolytic therapy; SK: streptokinase; APSAC: anistreplase; rt-PA: alteplase 100 mg/3 hours; fl rt-PA: front loaded rt-PA. (From Granger et al., 1992.)

reperfusion also showed a significantly lower mortality (4.5%) than did those with reocclusions (11.0%).

Thus, the potential of thrombolytic agents to create complete and sustained reperfusion in the infarct-related artery, even with the most efficacious regimen of front-loaded recombinant tissue-type plasminogen activator (rt-PA), is rather limited. New thrombolytics and/or combinations of fibrinolytic agents have not achieved better success rates. Therefore, in recent years, conjunctive treatment with thrombolysis has attracted more attention. Conjunctive treatment was defined initially by the editors of this monograph as therapy with anticoagulants and/or platelet inhibitors to enhance the efficacy of thrombolytic drugs, improve early and complete restoration of bloodflow in the infarct-related artery, and protect a successfully reopened artery from reocclusion.

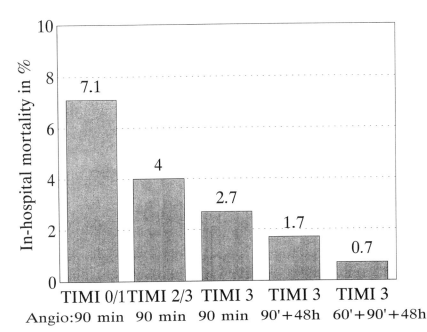

Figure 2   In-hospital mortality of patency of infarct-related artery. Meta-analysis of four multicenter trials with 907 patients. TIMI 0/1 = occluded vessel; TIMI 2/3 at 90 min = standard patency; TIMI 3 at 90 min = early and complete reperfusion; TIMI 3 at 90 min and 48 h = early, complete, and sustained reperfusion; TIMI 3 at 60 min, 90 min, and 48 h = very early, complete, and sustained perfusion. (From Vogt et al., in press.)

II. PRINCIPAL MECHANISMS OF CONJUNCTIVE THERAPY

Patients undergoing thrombolysis usually have residual fibrin-bound thrombin at the site of the arterial plaque rupture. The residual thrombin is highly prothrombogenic. In addition, paradoxically, thrombolysis itself can initiate activation of the coagulation system and platelets by generating plasmin. Platelet activation might reflect induction of thrombin activity secondary to procoagulant effects of plasminogen activators and to release of thrombin from clots undergoing lysis. The complex interactions between platelets and thrombolytic therapy have been reviewed in Chapters 6 and 7.

Therefore, the two most important mechanisms of conjunctive therapy are platelet and thrombin inhibition. This chapter focuses on the efficacy in patients of the antiplatelet and antithrombin agents that are currently available.

III. PLATELET INHIBITORS

A. Aspirin

Aspirin irreversibly blocks the enzyme cyclooxygenase and therefore inhibits prostaglandin biosynthesis. The dosage of aspirin that almost completely inhibits thromboxane A_2 synthesis is 20–40 mg. To date, no trials have directly compared the effect of aspirin versus placebo on early patency of infarct-related coronary arteries.

The clinical benefits of oral aspirin for patients with acute myocardial infarction have been impressively documented in the ISIS-2 trial. Patients on 160 mg aspirin daily had a reduction in hospital mortality of 23%, in the same range as with thrombolysis versus placebo. This benefit in survival was additive to that with streptokinase; the combination of aspirin and streptokinase reduced in-hospital mortality by as much as 42%. However, benefit with aspirin may have occurred largely in the subset of patients with unstable angina.

An unresolved problem is the dosage of aspirin. While antiplatelet properties have been well documented in doses lower than 100 mg, higher doses (>500 mg) seem to be necessary to induce suppression. After bypass surgery, shear-induced platelet thrombus formation, in which von Willebrand's factor plays a crucial role, was suppressed by high doses of aspirin (>300 mg per day) but not by low doses (75 mg per day), suggesting a mechanism other than interference with thromboxane formation. This antithrombotic effect of high-dose aspirin is possibly one reason for the low mortality in the ISAM trial, in which intravenous aspirin in a dose of 500 mg was given before thrombolysis.

B. Ticlopidine

Ticlopidine reduced the incidence of acute vessel closure and thrombosis after percutaneous transluminal coronary angioplasty (PTCA) and may be effective in the prevention of acute myocardial infarction in patients with unstable angina. Currently, data about ticlopidine as a conjunct to thrombolysis are not available, and the use may be limited in this setting by the 3-day delay in its optimal efficacy.

C. Ridogrel

Ridogrel is an inhibitor of thromboxane A_2 synthetase and antagonizes thromboxane A_2-prostaglandin endoperoxide receptors. In an uncontrolled pilot study of 50 patients treated with ridogrel in addition to rt-PA and heparin, a high early TIMI 2/3 patency of 86% after 90 minutes and 94% after 6–24 hours was observed, without excessive bleeding complications. In a randomized trial with 90 patients, ridogrel did not accelerate or increase early patency as a conjunct to rt-PA lysis when compared to aspirin. In 900 patients treated with streptokinase in the RAPT study, the angiographic patency rate after 7 to 14 days in the group allocated to aspirin (73.5%) did not differ from that with ridogrel (70.5%). Thus, ridogrel does not appear to increase early or late patency after thrombolysis.

D. Prostacyclin and Prostaglandin

Prostacyclin is the most potent endogenous platelet inhibitor known and is a relatively strong vasodilator. In experimental models, prostacyclin (PGI_2) was able to accelerate thrombolysis and reduce reocclusions and myocardial stunning. In patients with acute myocardial infarction, however, Iloprost, a stable analog of prostacyclin, did not improve immediate or follow-up coronary artery patency or left ventricular function recovery in combination with rt-PA compared with that achieved with rt-PA alone. Another prostacyclin analog, Taprostene, did not affect 90-minute patency when combined with saruplase, but seemed to reduce the rate of reocclusions at higher doses.

Prostaglandin E_1 in a small pilot trial has been shown to increase the velocity of reperfusion when administered in combination with streptokinase.

E. Monoclonal Antiplatelet Glycoprotein IIb/IIIA Antibody

The inhibition of the platelet GP IIb/IIIa receptor by murine monoclonal antibodies (7E3) inhibits ex vivo platelet aggregation by 90% and has been shown to prevent platelet thrombus formation and accelerate thrombolysis in vivo. In a pilot study, 7E3 was well tolerated in combination with rt-PA, aspirin, and heparin. TIMI 2/3 patency was 91% (31/43) after a median of 118 hours. When 7E3 was given in the highest dose and started early after thrombolysis (3 hours), there seemed to be a trend toward fewer ischemic events.

F. Platelet GPIIb/IIIa Competitive Antagonists

Integrelin, a cyclic peptide, is a potent antagonist specific for platelet GPIIb/IIIa. In experimental models it was able to enhance fibrinolysis and prevent reocclusion. It has not yet been tested in patients with acute myocardial infarction.

IV. THROMBIN-DIRECTED AGENTS

A. Heparin

At present, the most widely used agent for conjunctive anticoagulation is heparin, a complex glycosaminoglycan that compromises fractions of molecular weights between 3,000 and 30,000. Anticoagulant effects result from the binding of heparin to specific sites on antithrombin III. Its effectiveness is limited by the relative inaccessibility of fibrin-bound thrombin to heparin–antithrombin III complexes.

Experimental studies have demonstrated a facilitative interaction between heparin and rt-PA for increasing fibrinolytic activity. However, in a randomized trial, early administration of a bolus of 10,000 U heparin did not improve 90-minute patency, when compared to rt-PA alone (79% versus 79%). In contrast, in the HART study, 7–24-hour coronary patency was significantly better with intravenous heparin (82%) than with oral aspirin (52%). The rate of reocclusions up to day 7, recurrent ischemic events, and bleeding complications were similar in both groups.

In a trial with 84 patients, coronary artery patency 3 days after rt-PA fibrinolysis was higher with heparin (71%) than without heparin (43%); it should be noted that neither group received aspirin. The European Cooperative Study Group (ECSG) showed, in a double-blind randomized trial, that intravenous heparin enhanced angiographic patency 48 to 120 hours after rt-PA treatment when compared to placebo (83.4% versus 74.7%). Consistent with these results are the findings of the LIMITS trial, in which pretreatment with a bolus of heparin improved patency of the infarct-related artery 6 to 12 hours after thrombolysis with saruplase (80.8% in the heparin group versus 60.4% in the placebo group).

Administration of heparin seems to be most important during the first 24 hours after thrombolysis with rt-PA. Prolonged infusions for more than 24 hours showed no beneficial effect on 7- to 10-day patency rates, reinfarction rate, and recurrent angina in comparison to an oral antiplatelet treatment. In a small randomized trial in low-risk patients with successful reperfusion in acute myocardial infarction, no difference in reocclusions or recurrent ischemic events after 7 days was observed when intravenous heparin for ≤24 hours was compared to a prolonged infusion of ≥72 hours. However, small sample sizes may have limited power for detection of small differences with more prolonged heparin.

A crucial point is the level of prolongation of aPTT achieved by heparin. In patients with adequate aPTT prolongation (greater than two times control), a significantly higher coronary artery patency was seen in both the HART trial and the ECSG-6 trial (Figure 3).

The findings of GISSI-2 and ISIS-3 must be interpreted in light of these results. The heparin regimen used in both trials (12.500 U subcutaneously b.i.d., starting 12 and 4 hours after thrombolysis, respectively) does not adequately prolong aPTT

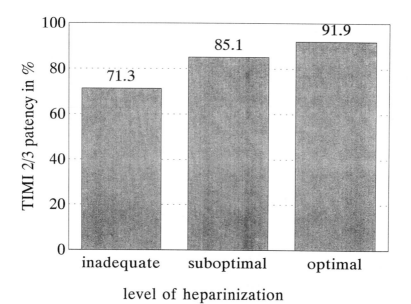

Figure 3   Correlation between level of heparinization and patency of the infarct-related artery 18–120 hours after treatment with rt-PA—pooled data from the HART study and the ECSG-6 trial. Inadequate anticoagulation was defined as at least one aPTT < 130% of baseline, suboptimal as lowest aPTT between 130 and 200% of baseline, and optimal as all aPTTs over 200% of baseline. APTTs were determined between 3 and 36 hours after thrombolysis. (Data from Arnout et al., 1992; Hsia et al., 1992.)

during the crucial interval for the prevention of early reocclusion. This may explain why there was no difference in mortality and reinfarction between rt-PA alone and rt-PA plus subcutaneous heparin in both trials. Based on our present knowledge, the use of intravenous heparin for at least 24 hours is highly recommended with fibrin-specific agents to achieve adequate anticoagulation.

Still controversial is the use of heparin in addition to the first-generation drugs streptokinase and urokinase. These drugs produce a systemic lytic state. The high levels of fibrinogen degradation products exert anticoagulation and antiplatelet effects and diminish the likelihood of reocclusion.

Despite these facts, the addition of 12,500 U subcutaneous heparin b.i.d. to streptokinase led to a significantly lower in-hospital mortality in the SCATI trial (4.5% versus 8.8%). Reperfusion time was reduced in comparison to placebo when intravenous heparin was given as a conjunct to streptokinase and aspirin in the OSIRIS trial.

In a retrospective analysis of the ISIS-2 trial, of all patients randomized to aspirin and streptokinase, mortality after 5 weeks was highest (9.6%) in the group receiving no heparin, lower (7.6%) in those receiving subcutaneous heparin, and lowest (6.4%) in those patients receiving intravenous heparin. Interestingly, the beneficial effect of heparin was limited to patients receiving aspirin in addition to streptokinase. In contrast, in ISIS-3—in which heparin was given in a randomized fashion—there was no difference between streptokinase and streptokinase plus heparin. Thus, at present, anticoagulation with heparin does not seem to be mandatory, although it may be desirable, after streptokinase.

B. Low-Molecular-Weight Heparin

In experimental models of thrombosis, low-molecular-weight heparin (LMWH) was able to sustain coronary artery patency after rt-PA thrombolysis, but there was still residual thrombus and platelet as well as fibrin deposition. In patients, LMWH was more effective than heparin in the therapy of deep-vein thrombosis. To date, LMWH efficacy has not been evaluated in patients with acute myocardial infarction.

C. Hirudin and Analogs

The naturally occurring hirudin is a 65-amino-acid anticoagulant derived from the leech, *Hirudo medicinalis*, but it has recently become available in larger quantities produced by recombinant DNA techniques. Hirudin reacts specifically with thrombin to form an inactive enzyme-inhibitor complex and, unlike heparin, does not require antithrombin III for inhibitory activity. In contrast to heparin, hirudin does inactivate clot-bound thrombin as well. In experimental animals, hirudin was effective in facilitating thrombolysis and preventing

reocclusion. Because of its pathway of renal elimination, hirudin carries the potential risk of accumulation in patients with
impaired renal function.

In the TIMI-5 trial, a randomized, open-label, dose-
ranging study, recombinant desulfatohirudin (CGP-39393) was
compared to heparin. Patients with acute myocardial infarction
received front-loaded rt-PA, aspirin, and either heparin as a
5000 U bolus + 1000 U/hour infusion, adjusted every 12 hours
to maintain an APTT of 65–90 seconds, or hirudin as a bolus
followed by a constant infusion at one of four different dose
levels. TIMI-3 patency at 90 minutes in all hirudin groups was
66% (102 of 155) compared with 56% (45 of 80) after heparin. At
18–36 hours, TIMI-3 flow was present in 113 of 131 (86%) of all
hirudin patients compared to 48 of 67 (72%) of heparin-treated
patients ($p = 0.01$); TIMI 2/3 patency was seen in 98% of
hirudin-treated patients compared to 86% of heparin-treated
patients ($p = 0.002$). Reocclusions occurred in 2% of the hirudin patients and in 7% of the heparin patients. The in-hospital
incidence of death or reinfarction was lower after hirudin (2%
and 6%) as compared to heparin (6% and 10%). Spontaneous
hemorrhage occurred in 3% of both groups.

Another recombinant hirudin (HBW 023) was used in a pilot trial with front-loaded rt-PA (100 mg/90 minutes) in 40 patients. After a bolus of 0.07 mg/kg, patients received an
infusion of 0.05 mg/kg per hour over 48 hours. TIMI-3 patency
after 60 minutes, 90 minutes, and 36–48 hours was 64.1, 71.1,
and 80.0%, respectively. Reocclusion occurred in eight patients; four of them had had a PTCA after 90 minutes. During
hirudin treatment there was no spontaneous hemorrhage. The
only in-hospital death was due to late retroperitoneal bleeding.
Subsequently a dose-escalation study was started, which was
completed recently. Preliminary results showed a significant
reduction of reocclusion by hirudin in higher doses. This effect
might be due at least in part to the stable and effective prolongation of aPTT and ACT during hirudin treatment.

Hirulog, a 20-amino-acid hirudin analog, was compared
to heparin as a conjunct to streptokinase in 42 patients by

Ridon et al. In this small series, TIMI-3 patency after 90 minutes was significantly better after hirulog (61%) than after heparin (29%).

According to these results, direct thrombin inhibition by hirudin or analogs seems to enhance thrombolysis and, maybe more importantly, maintain coronary patency more effectively than heparin.

D. Argatroban

Argatroban, a synthetic competitive thrombin inhibitor, was significantly more effective than heparin in preventing experimental platelet-rich arterial occlusion. In a small nonrandomized trial, argatroban was more effective in preventing reocclusion within 1 month (0% = 0 of 22 patients) compared to heparin (15% = 11 of 74 patients). Larger randomized studies are necessary to confirm these results.

V. IMPLICATIONS FOR CLINICAL PRACTICE

The significant benefit of thrombolytic treatment in patients with acute myocardial infarction has been shown unequivocally. Conjunctive treatment with antiplatelet agents has been proven to be of significant additional benefit, no matter which thrombolytic drug is used. Thrombin inhibition with heparin has been shown to be useful at least in some settings. When given as a conjunct to streptokinase, intravenous heparin slightly increases the risks of bleeding without much of an advantage in mortality over subcutaneous heparin. For second-generation fibrinolytics such as rt-PA, thrombin inhibition during the first days after thrombolysis seems mandatory to preserve patency of the infarct-related artery.

PERTINENT REFERENCES

Andreotti F, Kluft C, Ujang M S, et al.: Enhanced thrombin suppression by high-dose aspirin during coronary angioplasty. *Circulation* 1992;86(Suppl I):I-249.

Arnout J, Simoons M, de Bono D, et al.: Correlation between level of heparinization and patency of the infarct-related coronary artery after treatment of acute myocardial infarction with alteplase. *J Am Coll Cardiol* 1992;20:513–519.

Baer F W, Meyer J, Uebis R, et al.: The value of Taprostene on patency and reocclusion in myocardial infarction. Results of the "START" study. *Eur Heart J* 1991;12(abstract suppl):30.

Balsano F, Rizzon P, Violi F, et al.: Antiplatelet treatment with ticlopidine in unstable angina. A controlled multicenter clinical trial. *Circulation* 1990; 82:17–26.

Bleich S D, Nichols T C, Schumacher R R, et al.: Effect of heparin on coronary arterial patency after thrombolysis with tissue plasminogen activator in acute myocardial infarction. *Am J Cardiol* 1990;66:1412–1417.

Cannon C P, McCabe C H, Henry T D, et al.: Hirudin reduces reocclusion compared to heparin following thrombolysis in acute myocardial infarction: results of the TIMI 5 trial. *J Am Coll Cardiol* 1993;21:136A.

Cercek B, Lew A S, Hod H, Yano J, Reddy N K N, Ganz W: Enhancement of thrombolysis with tissue-type plasminogen activator by pretreatment with heparin. *Circulation* 1986;74:583–587.

Col J, Decoster O, Hanique G, et al.: Infusion of heparin conjunct to streptokinase accelerates reperfusion of acute myocardial infarction: results of a double blind randomized study (OSIRIS). *Circulation* 1992;86(suppl I):I-259.

Coller B S: Platelets and thrombolytic therapy: *N Engl J Med* 1990;322:33–42.

Dabaghi S F, Kamat S, Hendricks O, et al.: Low dose aspirin inhibits in vitro platelet aggregation within minutes after ingestion. *Circulation* 1992;86 (suppl I):I-261.

De Bono D P, Simoons M L, Tijssen J, et al.: Effect of early intravenous heparin on coronary patency, infarct size, and bleeding complications after alteplase thrombolysis: results of a randomized double blind European Cooperative Study Group trial. *Br Heart J* 1992;67:122–128.

Diaz R, Paolasso E, Piegas L S, et al.: The Ridogrel versus aspirin patency trial (RAPT). Circulation 1992;86(suppl I):I-642.

GISSI: GISSI-2: A factorial randomized trial of alteplase versus streptokinase and heparin versus no heparin among 12,490 patients with acute myocardial infarction. *Lancet* 1990;336:65–71.

Gold H K, et al.: Rapid and sustained coronary artery recanalization with combined bolus injection of recombinant tissue type plasminogen activator and monoclonal antiplatelet GPIIb/IIIa antibody in a canine preparation. *Circulation* 1988;77:670–677.

Granger B G, Ohman E M, Bates E: Pooled analysis of angiographic patency rates from thrombolytic therapy trials. *Circulation* 1992;86(suppl I):I-269.

Haskel E J, Prager N A, Sobel B E, Abendschein D R: Relative efficacy of antithrombin compared with antiplatelet agents in accelerating coronary thrombolysis and preventing early reocclusion. *Circulation* 1991; 83:1048–1056.

Hirsh J: Drug therapy: heparin. *N Engl J Med* 1991;324:1565–1574.

Hsia J, Hamilton W P, Kleiman N, et al.: A comparison between heparin and low-dose aspirin as conjunctive therapy with tissue plasminogen activator for acute myocardial infarction. *N Engl J Med* 1990;323:1433–1437.

Hsia J, Kleiman N, Aguirre F, et al.: Heparin-induced prolongation of partial thromboplastin time after thrombolysis: relation to coronary artery patency. *J Am Coll Cardiol* 1992;20:31–35.

Hull R D, Raskob G E, Pineo G F, et al.: Subcutaneous low-molecular-weight heparin compared with continuous intravenous heparin in the treatment of proximal-vein thrombosis. *N Engl J Med* 1992;326:975–982.

ISIS-2 Collaborative Group: Randomised trial of intravenous streptokinase, oral aspirin, both, or neither among 17187 cases of suspected acute myocardial infarction: ISIS-2. *Lancet* 1988;ii:349–360.

ISIS-3 Study Group: ISIS-3: a randomized comparison of streptokinase vs tissue plasminogen activator vs anistreplase and of aspirin plus heparin vs aspirin alone among 41,299 cases of suspected acute myocardial infarction. *Lancet* 1992;339:753–770.

Jang I K, Gold H K, Ziskind A A, et al.: Prevention of platelet-rich arterial thrombosis by selective thrombin inhibition. *Circulation* 1990;81:219–225.

Kander N H, Holland K J, Pitt B, Topol E J: A randomized pilot trial of brief versus prolonged heparin after successful reperfusion in acute myocardial infarction. *Am J Cardiol* 1990;65:139–142.

Kleiman N S, Ohman E M, Ellis G E, et al.: Infarct vessel patency is enhanced by profound platelet inhibition of fibrinogen receptor blockade with 7E3 in patients receiving thrombolysis for acute myocardial infarction. *Circulation* 1992;86(suppl I):I-260.

Lidón R M, Théroux P, Bonan R, et al.: Hirulog as adjunctive therapy to streptokinase in acute myocardial infarction. *J Am Coll Cardiol* 1993; 21:419A.

Lincoff A M, Topol E J: The illusion of reperfusion. *JAMA*. In press.

Neuhaus K L, von Essen R, Tebbe U, et al.: Improved thrombolysis in acute myocardial infarction with front loaded administration of alteplase: results of the rt-PA-APSAC patency study (TAPS). *J Am Coll Cardiol* 1992; 19:885–891.

Neuhaus K L, von Essen R, Tebbe U, Vogt A, Jessel A, Zeymer U: Hirudin and thrombolysis with front-loaded alteplase in acute myocardial infarction: results of a pilot study. *J Am Coll Cardiol* 1992;21:418A.

Nicolino F A, Nichols W W, Saldeen T G P, et al.: Adjunctive therapy with low molecular weight heparin with recombinant tissue-type plasminogen activator causes sustained reflow in canine coronary thrombosis. *Am Heart J* 1992;124:280–288.

Ohman E M, Califf R M, Topol E J, et al.: Consequences of reocclusion after successful reperfusion therapy in acute myocardial infarction. *Circulation* 1990;82:781–791.

Owen J, Friedman K D, Grossman B A, Wilkins C, Berke A D, Powers E R: Thrombolytic therapy with tissue plasminogen activator or streptokinase induces transient thrombin activity. *Blood* 1988;72:616–620.

Ratnatunga C P, Edmonson S F, Rees G M, Kovacs I B: High-dose aspirin inhibits shear-induced platelet reaction involving thrombin generation. *Circulation* 1992;85:1077–1082.

Sharma B, Wyeth R P, Gimenez H J, Franciosa J A: Intracoronary prostaglandin E1 plus streptokinase in acute myocardial infarction. *Am J Cardiol* 1986;58:1161–1166.

Sobel B E, Hirsh J: Principles and practice of coronary thrombolysis and conjunctive treatment. *Am J Cardiol* 1991;68:382–388.

Song A, Scarborough R M, Phillips D R, et al.: Intregelin enhances fibrinolysis and prevents acute arterial reocclusion following thrombolysis in a canine anodal current model with high grade stenosis. *Circulation* 1992; 86(suppl I):I-410.

Stein B, Fuster V, Israel D H, et al.: Platelet inhibitor agents in cardiovascular disease: an update. *J Am Coll Cardiol* 1989;14:813–836.

Tabata H, Mizuno K, Miyamoto A, et al.: The effect of a new thrombin inhibitor (Argatroban) in the prevention of reocclusion after reperfusion therapy in patients with acute myocardial infarction. *Circulation* 1992;86 (suppl I):I-260.

Tebbe U, Wasberg I, Windeler J, for the LIMITS Study Group: Einfluss von Heparin auf die thrombolytische Wirkung von Saruplase. *Z Kardiol* 1991; 80(suppl 3):32.

The ISAM Study Group: A prospective trial of intravenous streptokinase in acute myocardial infarction (I.S.A.M.). *N Engl J Med* 1986;314:1465–1471.

The SCATI Group: Randomised controlled trial of subcutaneous calcium-heparin in acute myocardial infarction. *Lancet* 1989;ii:182–186.

Thompson P L, Aylward P E, Federman J, et al.: A randomized comparison of intravenous heparin with oral aspirin and dipyridamol 24 hours after recombinant tissue-type plasminogen activator for acute myocardial infarction. *Circulation* 1991;83:1534–1542.

Topol E J, Ellis S G, Califf R M, et al.: Combined tissue-type plasminogen activator therapy and prostacyclin therapy for acute myocardial infarction. *J Am Coll Cardiol* 1989;14:877–884.

Topol E J, George B S, Kereiakes D J, et al.: A randomized controlled trial of intravenous tissue plasminogen activator and early intravenous heparin in acute myocardial infarction. *Circulation* 1989;79:281–286.

Van der Wieken L R, van den Brand M, Larman G J, et al.: Ridogrel as adjunct to thrombolysis in acute myocardial infarction. *Circulation* 1992; 86(suppl I):I-47.

Verstraete M, Tranchesi B: Ridogrel: superior to aspirin in MI? Clinical trial results. 8th International Workshop: Thrombolysis and Interventional Therapy in Acute Myocardial Infarction, New Orleans, LA, Nov 15, 1992.

Vogt A, Tebbe U, von Essen R, Feuerer W, Niederer W, Alber G, Appel K F, Zeymer U, Neuhaus K L: 90-minute patency and optimal perfusion of infarct related coronary arteries. *Circulation* 1992; 86(suppl I):I-268.

Vogt A, von Essen R, Tebbe U, Feuerer W, Appel K F, Neuhaus K L: Impact of early perfusion status of the infarct-related artery on short-term mortality after thrombolysis for acute myocardial infarction: retrospective analysis of four German multicenter studies. *J Am Coll Cardiol*. In Press.

White C W, Chaitman B, Lassar T A, et al.: Antiplatelet agents are effective in reducing the immediate complications of PTCA: results from the ticlopidine multicenter trial. *Circulation* 1987;76(suppl IV):IV-400.

Zeymer U, Jessel A, Neuhaus K L: Hirudin as adjunctive therapy in patients with thrombolysis for acute myocardial infarction produced stable prolongation of ACT and aPTT. *Eur Heart J* 1993(abstract suppl). In press.

15

Myocardial Reperfusion Injury
Concepts, Mechanisms, and Therapeutic Strategies

Jean-Louis J. Vanoverschelde and Steven R. Bergmann
Washington University School of Medicine
St. Louis, Missouri

I. INTRODUCTION

Although reduction of myocardial work, relief of pain, and prevention of malignant arrhythmias have been the mainstay of treatment of myocardial infarction, the advent of reperfusion therapy has provided a practical approach for actual salvage of ischemic myocardium. The dramatic reduction in morbidity and mortality from acute ischemia observed in clinical trials of reperfusion therapy has led to embracement of the use of thrombolytic therapy as the treatment of choice. Nonetheless, the benefits of reperfusion therapy can be compromised by the presence of severe residual stenosis, which can limit flow, and also by coronary reocclusion. In addition, reperfusion appears to trigger specific biochemical, functional, and ultrastructural changes, which may limit maximal myocardial salvage (Table 1). For example, after reperfusion, contractile function of myocardium destined to ultimately recover often remains depressed for a period of time. These sequelae and results of studies showing that they can be modified by treat-

Table 1   Mechanisms Potentially Preventing Maximal Salvage of Myocardium by Reperfusion and Amendable to Adjunctive Pharmacological Manipulation

Metabolic
  Inhibition of glycolysis
  Accumulation of fatty acid intermediates
  Supply/Demand balance
Vascular
  Residual stenosis
  Endothelial damage
  Extravascular compression
  Microcirculatory plugging
  Vasoconstriction and loss of vasorelaxation
  Intravascular generation of oxygen-centered free radicals
Direct
  Increased calcium influx and diminished myofibrillar calcium
    sensitivity
  Oxygen-centered free radicals

ments given at the time of reperfusion have led to the speculation that reperfusion per se could precipitate a series of specific events that mitigate the full benefits of recanalization therapy.

The major controversy regarding the nature of this "reperfusion injury" is whether it simply represents an acceleration of damage that would have occurred anyway, or whether there is a specific, additional component caused by reperfusion itself. This is a complex question since although reperfusion injury may represent a specific entity, it occurs only if the myocardium has been injured or "primed" by an antecedent ischemic episode. Until recently, the existence of a specific injury precipitated by reperfusion has largely remained speculative and definite evidence supporting the phenomenon has been lacking.

A. Relation of Reperfusion Injury to the Magnitude and Duration of the Antecedent Ischemic Episode

The magnitude and duration of ischemia markedly influences the severity and extent of damage observed upon reperfusion. Very short periods of ischemia result in rapid and complete restoration of contractile performance during reperfusion (Fig. 1). There is no infarction, and myocardial ultrastructure appears normal. More prolonged periods of ischemia, up to 15–20 minutes, do not usually result in tissue necrosis or enzyme release but are associated with calcium overload during early reperfusion and prolonged, albeit reversible, dysfunction, which has been termed "myocardial stunning." Further increases in the duration of ischemia results in appearance of

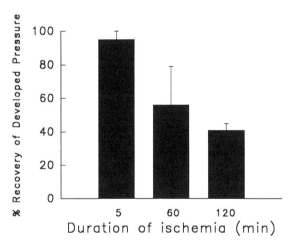

Figure 1   Histogram showing the recovery of left ventricular developed pressure early during reperfusion as a function of the duration of ischemia in isolated perfused rabbit hearts subjected to low-flow ischemia followed by 45 minutes of reperfusion. The data demonstrate the temporal dependence of myocardial stunning and the effectiveness of early reperfusion in attenuating contractile dysfunction.

cell damage during ischemia, the ultrastructural characteristics of which include cellular swelling, membrane rupture, and cell contracture with reperfusion. It is associated with a marked gain in cellular calcium, worsening of contracture, exaggerated enzyme release, and failure to replenish high energy phosphate. Both experimental and clinical studies have demonstrated that reperfusion can decrease the extent of myocardial infarction. However, the efficacy of reperfusion therapy is related to the duration of antecedent ischemia. Thus, in the experimental setting, late reperfusion, although effective in reestablishing macrovascular flow, does not limit ultimate infarct size (Fig. 2). Extending this to the human setting is more complex since factors such as territory effected, levels of collateral flow, duration of ischemia, and the magnitude and mode of recanalization are more variable.

The absolute magnitude of the flow deficit that occurs during ischemia and the size of the territory involved as well as the mode and abruptness of reperfusion and the level of residual stenosis all influence ultimate injury. It appears that there may be a threshold of myocardial flow above which it is difficult to demonstrate that irreversible injury will occur. Likewise, the larger the territory involved in an ischemic episode, the more devastating the deficit will be. Interestingly, it is patients with large territories at risk that benefit most from reperfusion therapy. Although it has been shown experimentally that ultimate infarct size can be reduced by decreasing oxygen requirements during ischemia, results of this approach in patients were ineffectual, and only with prompt, early reperfusion can the ultimate size of the jeopardized region be diminished.

Using positron emission tomography (PET) we demonstrated that the extent of restoration of uptake of 1-^{11}C-palmitate (a fatty acid used by aerobic myocardium for energy production) was markedly dependent on, and inversely proportional to, the duration of ischemia prior to reperfusion (Fig. 2). Reperfusion documented angiographically 6–12 hours after the onset of ischemia failed to restore intermediate me-

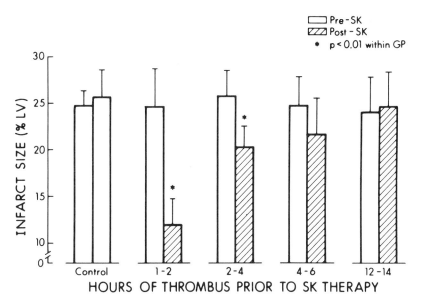

Figure 2   Graph showing temporal dependence of salvage of myocardium by reperfusion. Infarct size was estimated tomographically
in terms of diminished accumulation of 1-^{11}C-palmitate as a percentage of the left ventricle (LV) in jeopardized tissue in dogs with coronary thrombolysis induced with streptokinase (SK) at selected
intervals after induction of coronary thrombosis. The histogram dem-
onstrates the marked temporal dependence of salvage induced by
reperfusion. Dogs in the control group had persistent occlusion. The
results indicate that maximum salvage occurs when reperfusion is established early after coronary occlusion. (From Bergmann et al. 1982.)

tabolism. This result is consistent with the time course of beneficial effects delineated in clinical trials. Although arbitrary
numbers do not apply universally, and late reperfusion may
exert benefits in terms of improved ventricular remodeling or
decreased arrhythmias and salvage in patients with high collateral flow, it appears that the temporal window of induction
of salutary effects in terms of diminished infarct size comprise
only a few hours after the onset of ischemia. This temporal de-

pendence of salutary effects probably accounts for the lack of objective benefits observed in many clinical studies.

B. Metabolism as the Major Determinant of Reperfusion-Mediated Events

Several lines of evidence suggest that the severity of ischemic and reperfusion injury is closely related to myocardial energy metabolism, particularly levels of aerobic and anaerobic glycolysis and overall levels of oxidative metabolism. The heart is an aerobic organ, which requires high levels of energy production to sustain cellular homeostasis as well as contractile activity. Although the heart can oxidatively metabolize a number of substrates, under physiological conditions it has a preference for nonesterified fatty acids. However, with the onset of ischemia or hypoxia, β-oxidation of fatty acids is rapidly impaired, and myocardial glycolysis increases. Although it is generally accepted that rates of glycolysis cannot generate enough high-energy phosphate to maintain contractile function, they may be sufficient to maintain cellular viability. However, with severe degrees of ischemia or its prolonged duration, glycolysis becomes impaired due to buildup of protons and other inhibitory regulators, and energy production, even at a minimal level, fails.

In isolated hearts, one can prevent the development of both ischemic contracture and contractile failure during reperfusion by increasing the rate of anaerobic glycolysis during ischemia. We recently demonstrated that, in isolated perfused rabbit hearts subjected to one hour of low-flow ischemia followed by reperfusion, maintenance of high rates of anaerobic glycolysis during ischemia by diverse mechanisms (increasing endogenous or exogenous glucose supply, directly stimulating glycolytic enzymes, or stimulation of adenosine receptors), prevented the onset of ischemic contracture, preserved adenine nucleotide content, lessened ischemic membrane damage, and allowed faster and more complete recovery of contractile function during reperfusion. Although lactate production (indicative of anaerobic metabolism) has typically been interpreted as an adverse sign of myocardial ischemia, in our studies, maintenance of anaerobic glycolysis (i.e., continued production of lactate throughout the ischemic episode) had a profound salutary effect on preventing ischemic contracture (Fig. 3) and on enhancing contractile recovery during reflow.

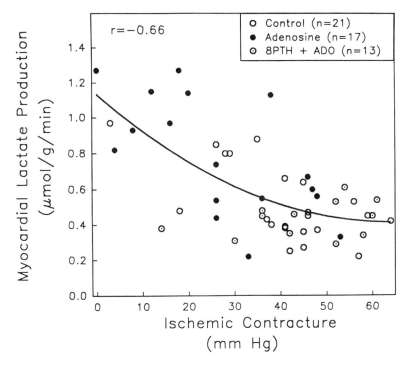

Figure 3   Relationship between levels of ischemic contracture in isolated perfused hearts and myocardial lactate production at the end of the ischemic period. Thus, hearts that were not able to maintain anaerobic glycolysis underwent ischemia contracture and were subsequently unable to recover function with reperfusion. Data was obtained from 21 hearts without intervention, 17 receiving 1 μM adenosine, in 13 in which adenosine receptors were blocked with 8 phenyltheophylline (8PTH). (From Janier et al., 1993.)

Similarly, while contractile function only recovered to 56% of baseline in control hearts, it returned to 90% or more of baseline in hearts with enhanced glycolysis during ischemia. Similar observations were made by Owen et al. and by Eberli et al.

Since ischemic contracture can increase mechanical tension on sarcolemmal membranes and result in vascular compression that may compromise full restoration of nutritive flow at the time of reperfusion (the no-reflow phenomenon, see below) and either directly or indirectly determine the extent of recovery of contractile function following reperfusion, it is postulated that its prevention constitutes a primary mechanism by which enhanced glycolytic flux protects the ischemic myocardium and improves the recovery of function during reperfusion. Alternatively, anaerobic adenosine triphosphate (ATP) production could favorably influence membrane function and cellular calcium homeostasis during ischemia. There is evidence that glycolysis is the preferential source of high-energy phosphates supporting membrane function and preventing irreversible damage during ischemia. The basis for this compartmentalization of ATP production may be related to localization of key glycolytic enzymes at specific sites in the cell that maintain adenine nucleotides locally at concentrations not necessarily reflected by total tissue levels of ATP. Glycolysis has been shown to be the major source of ATP supporting the Na^+/ K^+ ATPase, an enzyme critical to maintenance of cell volume and electrolyte homeostasis. Additionally, studies in isolated membrane vesicles from smooth muscle cells have shown that membrane calcium transport was preferentially supported by glycolysis and thereby prevented the deleterious actions of calcium at reflow.

In addition to rates of glycolysis, levels of overall oxidative metabolism may be key in the maintenance of myocardial viability in patients. In patients with left ventricular dysfunction due to coronary artery disease, maintenance of levels of oxidative metabolism (assessed with ^{11}C-acetate and PET) within the normal range predicted myocardium that would recover after revascularization. Similar results were observed in patients with evolving myocardial infarction treated with thrombolytic therapy. Thus, recovery of function was observed only when levels of oxidative metabolism were maintained. In an experimental study, we recently demonstrated that reperfusion after short periods of ischemia was associated with more rapid and complete recovery of oxidative metabolism (and function) compared to reperfusion after more prolonged periods of ischemia. In concert, these observations suggest that energy depletion and, specifically, insufficient energy production (both aerobic and anaerobic) to maintain cellular homeostasis is the main contributor to myocardial ischemic and reperfusion damage, and reinforce the hypothesis that reperfusion-mediated events are precipitated by injury occurring during the antecedent ischemic interval. Prevention of these ischemia-specific events preclude reperfusion-induced injury.

II. SPECIFIC ASPECTS OF REPERFUSION INJURY

Even after brief periods of ischemia, reperfused myocardium exhibits prolonged depression of contractile performance, which may extend for hours or days despite adequate restoration of blood flow and in the absence of tissue necrosis. This condition has been termed "myocardial stunning" and has been the focus of several investigations since its original description by Heyndrickx et al. Early studies documented that postischemic dysfunction was associated with depletion of tissue ATP, which slowly replenished at rates that paralleled the return of normal contractile function. However, recent studies have shown that stunning appears to be independent of tissue high-energy phosphate content. Thus, low tissue ATP does not preclude contractile recovery, nor does high tissue ATP content predict functional recovery. More recently, attention has focused on calcium homeostasis and myofibrillar sensitivity to calcium as the cause of myocardial stunning (see below).

It has been shown that pharmacological manipulations administered at the time of reperfusion can decrease the ultimate extent of infarction and stunning to a greater extent than achievable with reperfusion alone. Thus, although it is unclear whether reperfusion injury represents an entity into itself, independent of modulating injury induced by ischemia, it is clear that specific biochemical and physiological events only occur with reperfusion. Since clinically, any adjunctive therapy that could enhance the salutary effects of reperfusion is likely to be administered concurrently with thrombolytic therapy, it is these reperfusion-specific events that are target of pharmacological manipulation.

A. Role of Calcium in Myocardial Stunning and Reperfusion Injury

The effects of reperfusion on myocardial calcium content have been scrutinized over the past two decades. The prototype experiments were performed by Jennings et al. Upon reperfusion, tissue calcium content increases much more than if coronary occlusion is maintained. This is associated with the appearance of contraction band necrosis and intramitochondrial dense bodies, likely corresponding to deposition of calcium phosphate. Jennings and Ganote showed that these phenomena were strikingly similar to those of the calcium paradox, an experimental condition in which calcium is first removed from the extracellular space and then reintroduced. This manipulation results in severe cellular damage with massive membrane disruption, enzyme release and contracture. Although a true calcium paradox cannot occur in vivo since extracellular calcium never drops below 50 µM (the threshold required for the calcium paradox to occur), a modified form of the calcium paradox, perhaps linked to the reintroduction of oxygen as well, could be a plausible explanation for reperfusion injury.

Several lines of evidence support the hypothesis that transient calcium overload during early reperfusion is critical in the pathogenesis of myocardial stunning. Marban and coworkers showed that when isolated ferret hearts are exposed to elevated extracellular calcium during reperfusion, stunning inevitably ensues, whereas reperfusion with low calcium in the perfusion medium improves postischemic recovery. The same group also showed that a transient increase in cellular calcium in the absence of ischemia mimics stunning functionally, metabolically, and histologically. Additional evidence for the role of calcium overload in the genesis of myocardial stunning is provided by the results of experiments in which transmembrane calcium transport was specifically manipulated at the time of reperfusion. Administration of ryanodine, an agent that inhibits calcium release from the sarcoplasmic reticulum, has been shown to protect isolated rat hearts from stunning.

Although the cause of impaired calcium homeostasis during early reperfusion is still debated, there is evidence that the rise in cytosolic calcium during ischemia is related to myocardial energy depletion, either global or compartmentalized. Jeremy et al. showed that myocardial energy regulation, and particularly ATP production via anaerobic glycolysis, was the most important factor governing calcium homeostasis during early reperfusion. Increasing glucose oxidation during reperfusion also improves the recovery of postischemic myocardium.

The mechanics by which reperfusion-mediate calcium overload provokes stunning is currently under intense investigation. The most recent explanation relates stunning to decreased sensitivity of the myofibrils to calcium. The observation that calcium transients are increased in stunned myocardium, while function is severely depressed, supports this hypothesis. One possible mechanism could be that, during the initial period of overload, calcium triggers a series of deleterious biochemical events, such as activation of calcium-dependent proteases or protein kinases, which subsequently modify the properties of the contractile proteins and leads to a different state of calcium sensitivity. The reduction in the maximal calcium-activated force observed in stunned hearts, as well as the time course of recovery of stunned myocardium, which corresponds to the natural turnover rate of the contractile proteins in vivo, would support this hypothesis.

B. Oxygen-Centered Free Radicals as an Etiology for Reperfusion Injury

The reintroduction of oxygen after a period of deprivation provokes a syndrome, known as the oxygen paradox, that closely resembles the calcium paradox with very similar morphological features. Like the calcium paradox, it results in massive cell disruption, appearance of contracture, and release of macromolecules from damaged cells. In addition, the fundamentals of the oxygen paradox appear to be identical to those of the calcium paradox, i.e., a rapid and excessive uptake of calcium upon reoxygenation, which may be linked to the generation of oxygen-centered free radicals.

There is experimental evidence that oxygen-centered free radicals are generated upon reperfusion of ischemic or hypoxic myocardium. These reactive moieties are produced most rapidly in the first few minutes after reperfusion, but their production may continue for more prolonged intervals. Hypothetically, oxygen-centered free radicals can induce tissue damage by causing lipid peroxidation of membranes which would be expected to alter membrane integrity, thereby permitting altered ion fluxes and organelle dysfunction. However, the locus or loci of free radical generation is controversial. Because of their high reactivity and thus short life, it is not anticipated that these species can travel for any distance from their site of production in order to induce damage. Although it has been shown that direct production of free radical species such as hydrogen peroxide have a negative inotropic effect on myocardium, it is felt that most oxygen-centered free radicals are produced in the vasculature (as opposed to the interstices of the myocyte), and it is possible that these moieties influence vascular function (and perhaps contribute to the no-reflow phenomenon) rather than have a direct effect on myocyte function. In addition, it is unclear whether oxygen-centered free radicals are causative in inducing myocardial injury during reperfusion. Experimental studies have been variable, and scavenging of oxygen-centered free radicals has not been uniformly salutary.

In patients, it has been shown that lipid peroxidation (one potential biochemical marker of free-radical induced damage) can occur after transient coronary artery occlusion induced by balloon angioplasty or after thrombolytic therapy. Most clinical studies have assayed malondialdehyde in coronary venous blood and have shown a relatively transient rise of this lipid peroxidation metabolite during angioplasty. In patients studied 2 hours after streptokinase administration for treatment of acute myocardial infarction, thiobarbituric acid-reactive material (an indirect and nonspecific assay for malondialdehyde) was increased in patients with angiographically documented reperfusion but not in those with unsuccessful lysis. Whether the appearance of lipid-peroxidation products is specific for oxygen-centered free-radical–induced damage and, if so, whether it is causative of reperfusion injury or merely an epiphenomenon remains unsettled.

Release of oxygen-centered free radicals has been proposed as a triggering event for altering calcium homeostasis. The potential role of oxygen-centered free radicals in the pathogenesis of stunned myocardium is supported by results of several studies in which free-radical–scavenging agents attenuated the severity of stunning. However, the results of other studies has not been concordant.

In isolated perfused hearts, Corretti et al. showed that exogenous administration of free radicals induced glycolytic inhibition. It is therefore tempting to hypothesize that myocardial stunning might result from damage to the anaerobic energy–producing machinery, perhaps mediated by free radicals, leading secondarily to impaired calcium homeostasis and consequently calcium overload.

In summary, although there is good evidence that oxygen-centered free radicals are generated during reperfusion, and that they can be deleterious to myocardium, the extent to which free radicals are involved in limiting salvage due to reperfusion is currently unresolved. The variable results observed in experimental studies suggest that scavengers of free radicals will have limited efficacy in enhancing the benefits of reperfusion.

C. The No-Reflow Phenomenon

The no-reflow phenomenon refers to vascular damage that occurs upon recanalization, which prevents restoration of flow to reperfused tissue. This phenomenon was first described in the heart by Krug et al. and expanded upon by Kloner and coworkers. Impairment in blood flow can be due to a number of factors, such as microvascular damage; extravascular compression due to hemorrhage, edema, or contracture; obstruction of the microcirculation by thrombi and cellular blood cell elements, particularly neutrophils and platelets; and release of vasoactive agents or loss of vasorelaxing agents by the endothelium. In dogs, after 90 minutes of coronary occlusion followed by reperfusion, portions of the previously ischemic area failed to stain with Thioflavine-S, a fluorescent dye used as a perfusion marker. In the poorly perfused areas, severe capillary damage was present and coagulation necrosis was observed. These findings lent considerable support to the hypothesis that the no-reflow phenomenon was the consequence of severe damage to the microvasculature during ischemia and that it was largely established at the time of reperfusion. Recent studies have suggested, however, that part of the vascular damage could develop during reperfusion, either secondary to myocyte damage or as a result of direct vascular injury.

Granulocytes have been shown to rapidly invade the previously ischemic area after reperfusion. Accumulation and plugging of leukocytes in the microvasculature have been proposed as alternative mechanisms for the occurrence of the no-reflow phenomenon. Ambrosio and coworkers have shown that the severity and the extent of the no-reflow zone was larger after 30 minutes of reperfusion than immediately upon restoration of flow. The zone of diminished flow was, however,

always included within the area of cell necrosis, which suggests that the no-reflow phenomenon is more a consequence
than a cause of cell damage in the previously ischemia zone.
One possible explanation for its progression during early
reperfusion is the occurrence of progressive contracture. Humphrey et al. showed that ischemic contracture could alter the
normal transmural distribution of nutritive perfusion, with less
flow distributed to the subendocardium, and that this phenomenon is perpetuated during reperfusion so that large regions of the endocardium do not reperfuse upon restoration
of macrovascular flow. The additional contribution of leukocyte plugging might further contribute to this phenomenon,
potentially amenable to pharmacological manipulation. Administration of adenosine or perfluorocarbons, two agents that
decrease leukocyte activation, and maneuvers that reduce neutrophil number or function have been shown to reduce the severity of the no-reflow phenomenon. These interventions also
resulted in decreased infarct size, suggesting that the progression of the no-reflow zone might partially contribute to the extent of final injury.

In addition to the relatively early no-reflow response observed in experimental preparations, a delayed diminution of
flow in the reperfused zone has also been described. In a canine preparation in which myocardial perfusion was followed
sequentially, early, complete restoration of flow was followed
24–48 hours later by a decrease in perfusion, which then improved over 4 weeks. Whether this delayed reflow reflects altered autoregulation of flow due to diminished myocardial
demand, contracture of myocytes and extravascular compression effects, or other mechanisms, is not clear.

Clinical evidence of the no-reflow phenomenon in patients has been more controversial, likely because of the techniques utilized to assess nutritive flow. Using positron
emission tomography and the freely diffusible tracer, oxygen-
15 labeled water, Henes et al. demonstrated that 24 hours after
treatment with tissue-type plasminogen activator, absolute

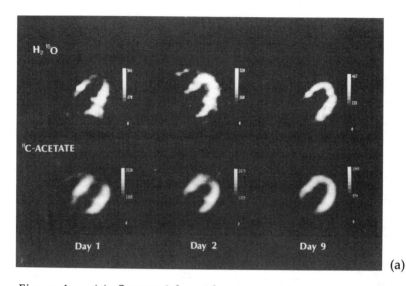

(a)

Figure 4   (a) Sequential, midventricular transaxial tomograms showing restoration of myocardial perfusion (top row of images) assessed with oxygen-15–labeled water and positron emission tomography and the recovery of oxidative metabolism (assessed with 1-^{11}C-acetate, bottom row) in a patient treated with thrombolytic therapy for evolving myocardial infarction. Lateral free wall is to the right, anterior myocardium uppermost, myocardial septum to the left, and the mitral valve plane bottommost. (b) Restoration of perfusion in the reperfused zone (solid bars) was prompt and equivalent to flow in remote myocardium (open bars) as assessed using a mathematical model that provides quantitative assessment of perfusion. Oxidative metabolism recovered more slowly but was required for ultimate recovery of function. (From Henes et al., 1990.)

myocardial blood flow (measured in ml/g/min) in the reperfused territory was restored to normal levels and was maintained at this level until the time of hospital discharge (Fig. 4). In contrast, Schofer et al. demonstrated reduced uptake of intracoronarily administered thallium-201– and technetium-99m–labeled albumin microspheres in patients after thrombolytic therapy. Further characterization of myocardial perfusion after recanalization therapy will be necessary to determine whether

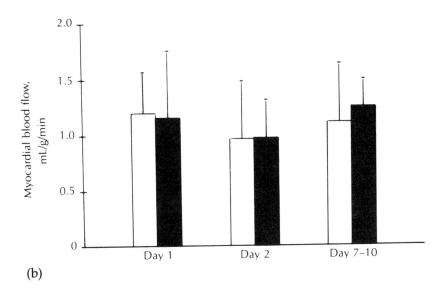

(b)

the no-reflow phenomena exists in humans and its relationship to the duration and magnitude of antecedent ischemia, and the mode and success of recanalization.

III. PHARMACOLOGICAL MANIPULATION OF REPERFUSION INJURY

A. Increasing Energy Production

Prompt reperfusion, with or without specific pharmacological adjunctives, is the most effective way to salvage ischemic myocardium (Figs. 1 and 2). In addition, prevention or minimization of the metabolic consequences of ischemia and manipulation of reperfusion-specific events can maximize the beneficial effects of reperfusion.

Several approaches have been proposed to improve myocardial metabolism during ischemia. Among these, stimulation of glycolytic energy production has received much attention over the past decade. Despite initial reports suggesting that accumulation of glycolytic byproducts were harmful during severe ischemia, we and others have shown that the severity of membrane damage during ischemia and functional recovery during reperfusion critically depended on the rate of anaerobic glycolysis during ischemia. In our studies, whatever the means used to increase glucose flux during low-flow ischemia—increased exogenous provision of glycolytic substrate, increased preischemic glycogen, direct activation of glycolytic enzymes—resulted in protection of ischemic myocardium. Although most of the data presently available were obtained in isolated hearts, preliminary reports indicate that similar results can be expected in vivo and that the same mechanisms of protection are effective in humans as well. Gradinac et al. recently showed that increasing glucose and insulin supply to postischemic myocardium in patients after aortocoronary bypass surgery was beneficial. The incidence of postoperative ventricular dysfunction (including the time of weaning from counterpulsation and the need for inotropic support) was significantly reduced in treated patients.

Exogenous administration of adenosine or adenosine analogs may also benefit the ischemic myocardium. Recent studies from our laboratory provided evidence that the myocardial protection afforded by exogenous adenosine resulted from the stimulation of anaerobic glycolysis. In isolated perfused rabbit hearts, adenosine reduced the amplitude and severity of ischemic contracture, decreased enzyme release, and improved functional recovery during reperfusion. These beneficial effects were associated with preservation of total ATP content and with a significant increase in the amount of energy produced during ischemia via anaerobic metabolism. Alternative effects of adenosine include direct repletion of high-energy phosphates, scavenging of oxygen-centered free radicals, reducing neutrophil activation, coronary vasodilation, and effects on inotropy. Forman and colleagues have demonstrated that adenosine administered after the onset of reperfusion prevents the no-reflow phenomenon and reduces myocardial injury.

An alternative approach to enhancing myocardial metabolism during ischemia and with reperfusion involves agents that shift myocardial metabolism from fatty acid to glucose. Thus, agents that diminish the buildup of long-chain fatty acid intermediates (specifically acyl-CoA and acyl-carnitine), diminish fatty acid–mediated effects on contractile function, and de-inhibit the effects of fatty acids on glucose metabolism would be anticipated to be beneficial. Indeed, such agents have been shown to improve myocardial function during reperfusion.

B. Reduction of Myocardial Demands

Although preservation of intermediary metabolism is one way to protect myocardium and enhance the effects of reperfusion, decreasing energy needs would also be expected to improve the heart's supply/demand balance and may enhance the effects of reperfusion.

Drugs that reduce energy demands, including calcium-channel antagonists, β-adrenergic blocking agents, or angiotensin converting enzyme (ACE) inhibitors, would be expected to reduce ischemic as well as reperfusion injury. The effects of the latter agents are likely to be nonspecific with actions mediated by reduction of metabolic needs by decreasing work although direct protective mechanisms have been suggested. The role of calcium-channel antagonists is considered below. In addition to reducing metabolic needs during ischemia and thereby favoring influencing the supply/demand balance, some experimental studies have demonstrated that administration of β-blockers at the time of reperfusion results in decreased infarct size and reduced myocardial stunning. However, results of a recently reported study where the β-blocker metoprolol was administered at the time of thrombolytic therapy demonstrated diminished recurrent ischemia but no other major salutary effects. Similarly, administration of the afterload-reducing ACE inhibitor captopril was associated with favorable hemodynamics although overall global ventricular function was not markedly improved. The limited effectiveness of these adjunctive agents may reflect the relatively late administration of thrombolytic therapy relative to the benefits that can be achieved by adjunctive maneuvers.

C. Use of Calcium-Channel Antagonists

Definite evidence that administration of calcium-channel antagonists lessens reperfusion injury has remained controversial. Although a number of experimental studies have demonstrated that calcium-channel antagonists diminish ultimate infarct size and improve myocardial stunning even when administered solely during the reperfusion period, results have not been consistent. In studies from our laboratory, the administration of diltiazem had an additive salutary effect on reperfusion. When diltiazem was administered to intact dogs starting 90 minutes after ischemia concurrently with the administration of intravenous streptokinase, infarct size estimated both by the accumulation of radiolabeled palmitate and PET as well as with direct analysis of myocardial creatine kinase depletion was reduced by nearly half over that achieved by reperfusion alone (Fig. 5). Territories at risk were not different between the groups, nor were systemic hemodynamics or myocardial blood flow during ischemia or after reperfusion. Thus, the effectiveness of diltiazem in this study was attributable to direct myocardial protective effects. In a subsequent study in isolated perfused rabbit hearts, we demonstrated that diltiazem can reduce lipid peroxidation in reperfused myocardium, suggesting that the mechanism of efficacy in vivo may be related to direct effects on the production or action of oxygen-centered free radicals or, alternatively, on the rates of potentially deleterious calcium-mediated proteases in decreasing myocardial damage.

Despite these promising experimental studies, clinical data using calcium-channel antagonists in conjunction with thrombolytic therapy is limited. In one report, administration of nifedipine late in the course of reperfusion exacerbated injury. In that study, nifedipine, administered sublingually in the emergency room and readministered intracoronarily later, failed to improve the results of intracoronary streptoki-

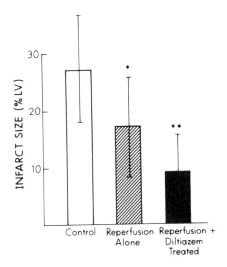

Figure 5   Efficacy of diltiazem in reducing infarct size in intact dogs. In this study, streptokinase was administered concomitantly with diltiazem 90 minutes after coronary artery occlusion. Diltiazem reduced infarct size by nearly 50% over the salvage achievable with reperfusion alone. The effects of diltiazem were attributable to direct myocardial protection since systemic hemodynamics and myocardial perfusion were not different in the groups subjected to reperfusion. The control group did not receive reperfusion therapy. (From Knabb et al., 1986.)

nase and, in fact, tended to increase reinfarction rates and mortality. The apparent negative effects of nifedipine were mostly attributable to a decrease in systematic blood pressure (and hence, coronary perfusion) with a compensatory tachycardia that may have increased energy needs. The results also suggest that the potentially beneficial effects of calcium entry blockade at the cellular level may be overcome in vivo by the systematic action of these drugs. Whether newer classes of calcium antagonists with less vascular effects will prove more useful in decreasing reperfusion injury in the clinical setting remains to be determined.

D. Scavengers of Oxygen-Centered Free Radicals

The administration of oxygen-centered free radical scavengers has been shown to attenuate infarct size and myocardial stunning in some studies, but their efficacy is controversial. Of 13 animal studies recently reviewed by Opie, seven failed to demonstrate any reduction of infarct size. Among the three studies in which scavengers were administered at the time of reperfusion, only one had positive results. The reasons for the disparate results of these studies is unclear but may include variable contributions of the different free radical species to injury, differences in the timing of administration, in the concentrations used or in the tissue penetration of the different scavengers. More recently, attention has focused on the role of activated neutrophils in generation of oxygen-centered free radicals (see below).

Results of clinical trials of scavengers of free radicals have been limited. In a preliminary study, there was no difference in mortality or global function in patients receiving recombinant superoxide dismutase compared with those not receiving this agent. Thus, it appears premature to recommend their routine utilization as adjunctive agents in humans.

E. Prevention of the No-Reflow Phenomenon

Although some studies have suggested that the no-reflow phenomena exists in humans after reperfusion, results obtained with positron emission tomography have not demonstrated any decrement in myocardial perfusion after thrombolytic therapy (Fig. 4). The differences reported may reflect the mode or agents used to induce recanalization, the adequacy of maintained patency, or differences in the completeness and rapidity of reperfusion. In the 2nd International Study of Infarct Survival (ISIS-2) Trial, aspirin, as an adjunctive agent given with streptokinase, reduced mortality to a greater extent than reperfusion therapy alone, presumably related to its efficacy in maintaining vessel patency, although alternative mechanisms of aspirin cannot be excluded. The results of studies using adjunctive agents that influence the coagulation/fibrinolytic system are covered elsewhere in this monograph.

Interventions that decrease the no-reflow phenomenon have been shown to be beneficial in experimental animals. These include pharmacological maneuvers that decrease neutrophil and/or platelet activation or adhesion with the use of perfluorocarbons or with specific antiplatelet or antineutrophil antibodies or depletion of these cellular elements with filtering. In experimental studies, these maneuvers have been shown to enhance reperfusion flow, decrease ultimate injury, and protect the myocardium from stunning. Other maneuvers that may aid reflow are prevention of contracture, hemorrhage, and monocyte swelling—all which would decrease the extent of extravascular compression; normalization of endothelial function and regulation of vasoconstrictor/vasodilatory mechanisms; and prevention of endothelial damage. The relevance of any of these maneuvers, however, will first require better characterization of whether the no-reflow phenomenon exists in human subjects.

Forman et al. recently demonstrated that patients receiving intracoronary perfluorocarbon following emergent coronary angioplasty for acute myocardial infarction had better regional function and diminished infarct size (delineated with thallium-201) than patients treated with angioplasty alone. Although the mechanism of this improvement is unclear, the potent antineutrophil properties of perfluorocarbon may have resulted in improved perfusion to the reperfused territory by diminishing neutrophil activation and accumulation, or perhaps by eliminating the generation oxygen-centered free radicals from activated neutrophils. However, the Forman study for the first time demonstrated that jeopardized myocardium can be favorably influenced clinically by therapies given in the reperfusion period.

IV. CONCLUSIONS AND THERAPEUTIC IMPLICATIONS

It is not at all clear that "reperfusion injury" represents an entity unto itself as opposed to a modulation of the events that occur during ischemia. Nonetheless, both experimental and clinical studies have demonstrated that these events can be beneficially modified by adjunctive therapy. However, the benefit that can be achieved by adjunctive agents given at the time of reperfusion is likely to be modest, reflecting the more prolonged period of ischemia that patients endure compared to protocols in most experimental studies, which involve briefer periods and more prompt, complete reperfusion compared to that typical in the clinical setting. Most patients receiving thrombolytic therapy have residual high-grade stenosis, which may impair full recanalization, impair subendocardial flow, and limit salvage.

Reperfusion therapy has revolutionized the treatment of myocardial infarction. Prompt reperfusion with maintenance of sustained patency is paramount for myocardial salvage. Effects of adjunctive therapy are likely to be modest, are dependent on the primary restoration of flow, and cannot be viewed as a substitute for full recanalization. Clearly, prevention or minimization of ischemic damage precludes reperfusion-mediated damage.

From a therapeutic point of view the following appears reasonable to minimize infarction and increase functional recovery following reperfusion:

1. Minimize the duration of ischemia, i.e., reperfuse early. However, it should be recognized that thrombolysis is only an initial step. Since residual stenosis is common after recanalization and high-grade residual stenosis is a progenitor of reocclusion, maintenance of patency is critical.
2. Optimize the metabolic status of the myocardium before and during reperfusion. This includes decreasing the metabolic needs of the ischemic myocardium (calcium-channel antagonists, β-blockers, and/or ACE

inhibitors) and increasing metabolic capacity. Stimulation of glycolysis, perhaps with drugs that selectively stimulate adenosine A_1 receptors or enhance glycolysis specifically in low pH or oxygen environments, may constitute an elegant approach to achieve this goal.

3. Although specific agents that modulate calcium flux or scavengers of oxygen-centered free radicals may be efficacious, their routine use clinically for their specific ability to reduce reperfusion-mediated events appears premature.

ACKNOWLEDGEMENTS

The authors thank Becky Leonard for secretarial assistance. Work from the author's laboratory was funded in part by grants HL-17646 and HL-468 95 from the National Institutes of Health and the American Heart Association, Missouri Affiliate.

PERTINENT REFERENCES

Ambrosio G, Weisman H F, Mannisi J A, Becker L C: Progressive impairment of regional myocardial perfusion after initial restoration of postischemic blood flow. *Circulation* 1989;80:1846–1861.

Apstein C S, Gravino F N, Haudenschild C C: Determinants of a protective effect of glucose and insulin on the ischemic myocardium: effects on contractile function, diastolic compliance, metabolism, and ultrastructure during ischemia and reperfusion. *Circ Res* 1983;52:515–526.

Babbitt D G, Vormani R, Forman M B: Intracoronary adenosine administered after reperfusion limits vascular injury after prolonged ischemia in the canine model. *Circulation* 1989;80:1388–1399.

Bajaj A K, Cobb M A, Virmani R, Gay J C, Light R T, Forman M B: Limitation of myocardial reperfusion injury by intravenous perfluorochemicals. Role of neutrophil activation. *Circulation* 1989;79:645–656.

Becker L C, Ambrosio G: Myocardial consequences of reperfusion. *Prog Cardiovasc Dis* 1987;30:23–44.

Bergmann S R, Lerch R A, Fox K A A, Ludbrook P A, Welch M J, Ter-Pogossian M M, Sobel B E: Temporal dependence of beneficial effects of coronary thrombolysis characterized by positron emission tomography. *Am J Med* 1982;73:573–581.

Bolli R: Mechanism of myocardial "stunning." *Circulation* 1990;82:723–738.

Bolli R: Myocardial 'stunning' in man. *Circulation* 1992;86:1671–1691.

Braunwald E, Kloner R A: The stunned myocardium: prolonged, post-ischemic ventircular dysfunction. *Circulation* 1982;66:1146–1149.

Christian T F, Schwartz R S, Gibbons R J: Determinants of infarct size in reperfusion therapy for acute myocardial infarction. *Circulation* 1992; 86:81–90.

Corretti M C, Koretsune Y, Chacko V P, Zweier J L, Marban E: Glycolytic inhibition and calcium overload as consequences of exogenously-generated free radicals in rabbit hearts. *J Clin Invest* 1991;88:1014–1025.

Davies S W, Ranjadayalan K, Wickens D G, Dormardy T L, Timmis A D: Lipid peroxidation associated with successful thrombolysis. *Lancet* 1990;335:741–743.

Downey J M: Free radicals and their involvement during long-term myocardial ischemia and reperfusion. *Annu Rev Physiol* 1990;52:487–504.

du Toit E F, Opie L H: Modulation of severity of reperfusion stunning in the isolated rat heart by agents altering calcium flux at onset of reperfusion. *Circ Res* 1992;70:960–967.

Eberli F R, Weinberg E O, Grice W N, Horiwitz G L, Apstein C S: Protective effect of increased glycolytic substrate against systolic and diastolic dysfunction and increased coronary resistance from prolonged global underperfusion and reperfusion in isolated rabbit hearts perfused with erythrocyte suspensions. *Circ Res* 1991;68:466–481.

Ely S W, Berne R M: Protective effects of adenosine in myocardial ischemia. *Circulation* 1992;85:893–904.

Engler R L, Dahlgren M D, Morris D, Peterson M S, Schmid-Schonbein G W: Role of leukocytes in the response to acute myocardial ischemia and reflow in dogs. *Am J Physiol* 1986;251:H314–323.

Erbel R, Pop T, Meinertz T, Olshausen K V, Treese N, Henrichs K J, Schuster C J, Rupprecht H J, Schlurmann W, Meyer J: Combination of calcium channel blocker and thrombolytic therapy in acute myocardial infarction. *Am Heart J* 1988;115:529–538.

Forman M B, Perry J M, Wilson B H, Verani M S, Kaplan P R, Shawl F A, Friesinger G C: Demonstration of myocardial reperfusion injury in humans: results of a pilot study utilizing acute coronary angioplasty with perfluorochemical in anterior myocardial infarction. *J Am Coll Cardiol* 1991;18:911–918.

Forman M B, Virmani R, Puett D W: Mechanisms and therapy of myocardial reperfusion injury. *Circulation* 1990;81(suppl IV):69–78.

Fox K A A, Saffitz J E, Corr P B: Pathophysiology of myocardial reperfusion. *Cardiol Clin* 1987;5:31–48.

Garcia-Dorado D, Théroux P, Duran J M, Solares J, Alonso J, Sanz E, Munoz R, Elizaga J, Botas J, Fernandez-Avilés F, Soriano J, Esteban E: Selective inhibition of the contractile apparatus: a new approach to modification of infarct size, infarct composition, and infarct geometry during coronary artery occlusion and reperfusion. *Circulation* 1992;85:1160–1174.

Gradinac S, Coleman G M, Taegtmeyer H, Sweeney M S, Frazier O H: Improved cardiac function with Glucose-Insulin-Potassium after aortocoronary bypass grafting. *Ann Thorac Surg* 1989;48:484–489.

Gropler R J, Geltman E M, Sampathkumaran K, Perez J E, Conversano A, Sobel B E, Bergmann S R: Delineation of viable myocardium by positron tomographic assessment of oxidative metabolism. *J Am Coll Cardiol* (in press).

Gropler R J, Geltman E M, Sampathkumaran K, Perez J E, Moerlein S M, Sobel B E, Bergmann S R, Siegel B A: Functional recovery after coronary revascularization for chronic coronary artery disease is dependent on peroxidation. *Circ Res* 1990;66:1449–1452.

Gropler R J, Siegel B A, Sampathkumaran K, Perez J E, Sobel B E, Bergmann S R, Geltman E M: Dependence of recovery of contractile function on maintenance of oxidative metabolism after myocardial infarction. *J Am Coll Cardiol* 1992;19:989–997.

Hammerman H, Kloner R A, Briggs L L: Enhancement of salvage of reperfused myocardium by early beta-adrenergic blockade (timolol). *J Am Coll Cardiol* 1984;3:1438–1443.

Henes C G, Bergman S R, Perez J E, Sobel B E, Geltman E M: The time course of restoration of nutritive perfusion, myocardial oxygen consumption, and regional function after coronary thrombolysis. *Coronary Artery Disease* 1990;1:687–696.

Heyndrickx G R, Millard R W, McRitchie R J, Maroko P R, Vatner S F: Regional myocardial functional and electrophysiological alterations after brief coronary occlusions in conscious dogs. *J Clin Invest* 1975;56:978–985.

Humphrey S M, Gavin J B, Herdson P B: The relationship of ischemic contracture to vascular reperfusion in the isolated heart. *J Mol Cell Cardiol* 1980;12:1397–1406.

ISIS-2 (Second International Study of Infarct Survival) Collaborative Group: Randomized trial of intravenous streptokinase, oral aspirin, both or neither among 17,187 cases of suspected acute myocardial infarction. *Lancet* 1988;11:349–360.

Janier M F, Vanoverschelde J -L, Bergmann S R: Adenosine protects ischemic and reperfused myocardium by receptor-mediated mechanisms. *Am J Physiol:Heart Circ Physiol* 1993;264:H163–H170.

Jennings R B, Ganote C: Mitochondrial structure and function in acute myocardial ischemic injury. *Circ Res* 1976;38(suppl I):80–91.

Jennings R B, Sommers H M, Smyth G A, Flack H H, Linn H: Myocardial necrosis induced by temporary occlusion of a coronary artery in the dog. *Arch Pathol* 1960;70:68–78.

Jeremy R W, Koretsune Y, Marban E, Becker L C: Relation between glycolysis and calcium homeostasis in postischemic myocardium. *Circ Res* 1992;70:1180–1190.

Kitakaze M, Weisman H F, Marban E: Contractile dysfunction and ATP depletion after transient calcium overload in perfused ferret hearts. *Circulation* 1988;77:685–695.

Kloner R A: Does reperfusion injury exist in humans? *J Am Coll Cardiol* 1993;21:537–545.

Kloner R A, Ganote C E, Jennings R B: The 'no-reflow' phenomenon after temporary coronary occlusion in the dog. *J Clin Invest* 1974;54:1496–1508.

Kloner R A, Przyklenk K, Whittaker P: Deleterious effects of oxygen radicals in ischemia/reperfusion. Resolved and unresolved issues. *Circulation* 1989;80:1115–1127.

Knabb R M, Bergmann S R, Fox K A A, Sobel B E: The temporal pattern of recovery of myocardial perfusion and metabolism delineated by positron emission tomography after coronary thrombolysis. *J Nucl Med* 1987;28:1563–1570.

Knabb R M, Rosamond T L, Fox K A A, Sobel B E, Bergmann S R: Enhancement of salvage of reperfused ischemic myocardium by diltiazem. *J Am Coll Cardiol* 1986;8:861–871.

Kobyashi K, Neely J R: Control of maximum rates of glycolysis in rat cardiac muscle. *Circ Res* 1979;44:166–175.

Koller P T, Bergmann S R: Reduction of lipid peroxidation in reperfused isolated rabbit hearts by diltiazem. *Circ Res* 1989;65:838–846.

Krug A, deRochemont W M, Korb G: Blood supply of the myocardium after temporary coronary occlusion. *Circ Res* 1966;19:57–62.

Kusuoka H, Koretsune Y, Chacko V P, Weisfelt M L, Marban E: Excitation-contraction coupling in postischemic myocardium: Does failure of activator Ca2+ transients underlie "stunning?" *Circ Res* 1990;66:1268–1276.

Kusuoka H, Porterfield J K, Weisman H F, Weisfeldt M L, Marban E: Pathophysiology and pathogenesis of stunned myocardium: depressed Ca^{++}

activation of contraction as a consequence of reperfusion-induced cellular calcium overload in ferret hearts. *J Clin Invest* 1987;79:950–961.

Liedtke A J, DeMaison L, Nellis S H: Effects of L-propionylcarnitine on mechanical recovery during reflow in intact hearts. *Am J Physiol:Heart Circ Physiol* 1988;255:H169–H176.

Lopaschuk G D, McNeil G F, McVeigh J J: Glucose oxidation is stimulated in reperfused ischemic hearts with the carnitine palmitoyltransferase 1 inhibitor, Etomoxir. *Mol Cell Biochem* 1989;88:175–179.

Mak I T, Weglicki W B: Comparative antioxidant activities of propranolol, nifedipine, verapamil, and diltiazem against sarcolemmal membrane lipid peroxidation. *Circ Res* 1990;66:1449–1452.

Mauser M, Hoffmeister H M, Nienaber C, Schaper W: Influence of ribose, adenosine, and "AICAR" on the rate of myocardial adenosine triphosphate synthesis during reperfusion after coronary artery occlusion in the dog. *Circ Res* 1985;56:220–230.

McVeigh J J, Lopaschuk G D: Dichloroacetate stimulation of glucose oxidation improves recovery of ischemic rat hearts. *Am J Physiol* 1990; 259:H1079–H1085.

Murdock R H, Chu A, Grubb M, Cobb F R: Effects of reestablishing blood flow on extent of myocardial infarction in conscious dogs. *Am J Physiol: Heart Circ Physiol* 1985;249:H783–H791.

Myears D W, Nohara R, Abendschein D R, Saffitz J E, Sobel B E, Bergmann S R: Compromise of beneficial effects of reperfusion on myocardium supplied by vessels with critical residual stenosis. *J Am Coll Cardiol* 1988;11:1078–1086.

Nabel E G, Topol E J, Galeana A, Ellis S G, Bates E R, Werns S W, Walton J A, Muller D W, Schwaiger M, Pitt B: A randomized placebo-controlled trial of combined early intravenous captopril and recombinant tissue-type plasminogen activator therapy in acute myocardial infarction. *J Am Coll Cardiol* 1991;17:467–473.

Opie L H: Hypothesis: glycolytic rates control cell viability in ischemia. *J Appl Cardiol* 1988;3:407–414.

Opie L H: Reperfusion injury and its pharmacologic modification. *Circulation* 1989;80:1049–1062.

Owen, P, Dennis S, Opie L H: Glucose flux rate regulates onset of ischemic contracture in globally underperfused rat hearts. *Circ Res* 1990;66: 344–354.

Paul R J, Hardin C D, Raeymaekers L, Wuytack F, Casteels R: Preferential support of Ca^{++} uptake in smooth muscle plasma membrane vesicles by an endogenous glycolytic cascade. *FASEB J* 1989;3:2298–2301.

Pitarys C J, Virmani R, Vildibill H D, Jackson E K, Forman M B: Reduction of myocardial reperfusion injury by intravenous adenosine administered during the early reperfusion period. *Circulation* 1991;83:237–247.

Przyklenk K, Vivaldi M T, Schoen F J, Arnold J M O, Kloner R A: Salvage of ischaemic myocardium by reperfusion: importance of collateral blood flow and myocardial oxygen demand during occlusion. *Cardiovasc Res* 1986;20:403–414.

Roberts R: Thrombolysis and its sequelae. Calcium antagonists as potential adjunctive therapy. *Circulation* 1989;80(suppl IV):93–101.

Roberts R, Rogers W J, Mueller H S, Lambrew C T, Diver D J, Smith H C, Willerson J T, Knatterud G L, Forman S, Passamani E, Zaret B L, Wachers F J T, Braunwald E: Immediate versus deferred β-blockade following thrombolytic therapy in patients with acute myocardial infarction. Results of the thrombolysis in myocardial infarction (TIMI) II-B study. *Circulation* 1991;83:422–437.

Schofer J, Montz R, Mathey D G: Scintigraphic evidence of the "no reflow" phenomenon in human beings after coronary thrombolysis. *J Am Coll Cardiol* 1985;5:593–598.

Simoons M L: Thrombolytic therapy in acute myocardial infarction. *Ann Rev Med* 1989;40:181–200.

Taegtmeyer H, Roberts A F C, Raine A E G: Energy metabolism in reperfused hearts muscle: metabolic correlate to return of function. *J Am Coll Cardiol* 1985;6:864–870.

Tiefenbrunn A J, Sobel B E: The impact of coronary thrombolysis on myocardial infarction. *Fibrinolysis* 1989;3:1–15.

Vanoverschelde J -L, Janier M, Bakke J E, Marshall D R, Bergmann S R: Increasing glycolytic flux during ischemia limits tissue damage and enhances functional recovery with reperfusion (abstr). *J Am Coll Cardiol* 1992;19(suppl A):335A.

Weinheimer C J, Brown M A, Nohara R, Perez J E, Bergmann S R: Functional recovery after reperfusion is predicated on recovery of myocardial oxidative metabolism. *Am Heart J* 1993;125:939–949.

Weiss J, Hiltbrand B: Functional compartmentation of glycolytic versus oxidative metabolism in isolated rabbit heart. *J Clin Invest* 1985;75:436–447.

Weiss J N, Lamp S T: Cardiac ATP-sensitive K^+ channels: evidence for preferential regulation by glycolysis. *J Gen Physiol* 1989;94:911–935.

Werns S, Brinker J, Gruber J, Rothbaum D, Heuser R, George B, Burwell L, Kereiakes D, Mancini G B J, Flaherty J: A randomized, double-blind trial of recombinant human superoxide dismutase (SOD) in patients undergoing PTCA for acute MI (abstr). *Circulation* 1989;80(suppl II):II–113.

West P N, Connors J P, Clark R E, Weldon C S, Ramsey D L, Roberts R, Sobel B R, Williamson J R: Compromised microvascular integrity in ischemic myocardium. *Lab Invest* 1978;38:677–684.

Yamazaki S, Fujibayashi Y, Rajagopalan R E, Meerbaum S, Corday E: Effects of staged versus sudden reperfusion after acute coronary occlusion in the dog. *J Am Coll Cardiol* 1986;7:564–572.

EPILOGUE

Controversy and Clarification
Preliminary Results of the GUSTO Trial

Burton E. Sobel
Washington University School of Medicine and Barnes Hospital
St. Louis, Missouri

Désiré Collen
University of Leuven
Leuven, Belgium

The "perspective" in the title of this monograph is, simply stated, the following: Coronary thrombolysis exerts its benefits on the heart and on the patient by recanalizing coronary arteries; benefit is dependent on the rapidity and persistence of recanalization and the brevity of ischemia preceding reperfusion; and fibrinolysis is not monotherapy but rather an intervention requiring conjunctive anticoagulation to attenuate the concomitant thrombosis that can retard recanalization, precipitate early thrombotic reocclusion, or both.

Efforts in this field have focused on development of clot-selective fibrinolytic agents to avoid nonspecific proteolysis associated with induction of a systemic lytic state and the plasminemia typical with intravenous use of non-clot-selective agents. Results of early studies indicated that clot-selective agents were remarkably effective in initiating early recanalization. Subsequently, two phenomena, both associated with limitation of plasminemia, have been implicated as contributors to their increased efficacy—namely, the relative paucities of procoagulant effects induced with clot-selective agents and of "plasminogen steal" encountered with plasminemia.

When the clot-selective agent tissue-type plasminogen activator, t-PA (initially melanoma-cell t-PA and subsequently human t-PA produced by recombinant DNA technology), was first administered to laboratory animals with induced coronary thrombosis, prompt coronary thrombolysis occurred without concomitant induction of a systemic lytic state. When patients with coronary occlusion were first treated with t-PA (initially melanoma-cell t-PA and subsequently t-PA produced by recombinant DNA technology), similar salutary effects were evident.

Despite accumulating evidence over the next 5 years supporting the concept that 1) coronary thrombolysis exerted its beneficial effects by promptly resupplying jeopardized ischemic myocardium with blood and oxygen, thereby avoiding irreversible injury, and 2) clot-selective agents initiated recanalization more often and more promptly than non-clot-selective drugs, results of two mega-trials (GISSI/International and ISIS-3) failed to reflect thrombolytic drug-dependent differences in clinical outcome.

Recently—and after this book was virtually finished—results of the GUSTO trial were presented in Washington, D.C., at the annual meeting of the American Federation for Clinical Research. They appear to resolve disparities between results of carefully controlled, mechanistic investigations that had demonstrated advantages of clot-selective agents and the necessity of conjunctive therapy in contrast to the negative results in the GISSI/International (GISSI-2 and its international extension) and ISIS-3 trials. The GUSTO trial studied four randomized groups of approximately 10,000 patients each (treatment with streptokinase plus subcutaneous heparin, streptokinase plus intravenous heparin, accelerated t-PA plus intravenous heparin, and a combination of streptokinase and t-PA plus intravenous heparin). An angiographic substudy was performed to define relationships between early patency and clinical out-

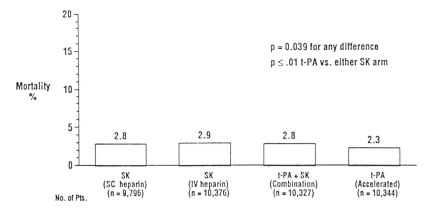

Figure 1   GUSTO Trial: 24-hour mortality.

come. Results of GUSTO were internally consistent and compatible with results of antecedent mechanistic laboratory and clinical studies. They were highly statistically significant. Salient observations included the following:

1. Twenty-four-hour mortality was lower with accelerated t-PA and intravenous heparin than with streptokinase with either intravenous or subcutaneous heparin and lower than mortality with streptokinase plus t-PA in combination with intravenous heparin (Figure 1).

2. Thirty-day mortality was lower with accelerated t-PA and intravenous heparin than with streptokinase with intravenous or subcutaneous heparin and lower than that seen with streptokinase plus t-PA in combination with intravenous heparin (Table 1).

3. Net clinical benefit (survival without disabling stroke) was greater with accelerated t-PA and intravenous heparin than with streptokinase with subcutaneous heparin or streptokinase with intravenous heparin and greater than that seen with streptokinase plus t-PA in combination with intravenous heparin (Table 2).

Table 1   GUSTO Trial: 30-Day Mortality

	SK (s.q.)	SK (i.v.)	t-PA	t-PA + SK	Total
No. of patients	9,796	10,376	10,344	10,327	40,843
No. of deaths	708	763	652	723	2,846
Mortality rate	7.2%	7.4%	6.3%	7.0%	7.0%

Table 2   GUSTO Trial: Net Clinical Benefit

Treatment	n	30-day mortality (%)	Disabling stroke (%)
t-PA	10,344	6.3	0.6
t-PA + SK	10,328	7.0	0.6
SK (s.q.)	9,796	7.2	0.5
SK (i.v.)	10,377	7.4	0.5

4. The accelerated t-PA and intravenous heparin strategy was superior to the streptokinase with intravenous or subcutaneous heparin and to the streptokinase plus t-PA in combination with intravenous heparin strategies with respect to the incidence of diverse cardiac complications (Table 3).

5. The relative mortality reduction with accelerated t-PA and intravenous heparin compared with streptokinase was 14% for the trial as a whole and even greater in patients randomized within 2 hours of the onset of symptoms (Table 4).

6. Mortality reduction favored accelerated t-PA with intravenous heparin regardless of patient age (Figure 2).

7. Survival was dependent on the induction of patency (TIMI flow grade 2 or 3) within 90 minutes of onset of treatment with all the regimens tested (Figure 3).

8. Induction of patency within 90 minutes of the onset of treatment was much more frequent with accelerated t-PA with intravenous heparin compared with strep-

Table 3　GUSTO Trial: Complications and Arrhythmias

	SK (s.c.)	SK (i.v.)	t-PA	t-PA + SK
n	8669	9260	9235	9193
Worst Killip class (%)				
II	24.7	25.2	23.9[a]	25.2
III	4.8	4.4	4.1[a]	4.2
IV	5.0	4.9	4.3[a]	4.8
Fever, chills, allergic reaction (%)	5.7	5.8	1.6[a]	5.4
Anaphylaxis (%)	0.7	0.6	0.2[a]	0.6
Sustained hypotension (%)	13.3	12.5	10.1[a]	12.4
2° or 3° AV block (%)	9.5	8.7	7.3[a]	8.4
Sustained VT (%)	6.8	6.5	5.6[a]	6.1
VF (%)	7.1	6.9	6.3[a]	6.9
Asystole (%)	6.0	6.4	5.3[a]	6.4
Atrial fib./flutter (%)	9.9	9.8	8.6[a]	9.1
Acute MR (%)	1.6	1.6	1.3[a]	1.4

[a]Significant versus SK alone.

Age	Percent of Patients	Mortality Rates SK	Mortality Rates t-PA
< 55	32%	2.0%	1.8%
55–64	29%	4.7%	3.6%
65–74	27%	10.4%	8.3%
75+	12%	20.4%	19.2%

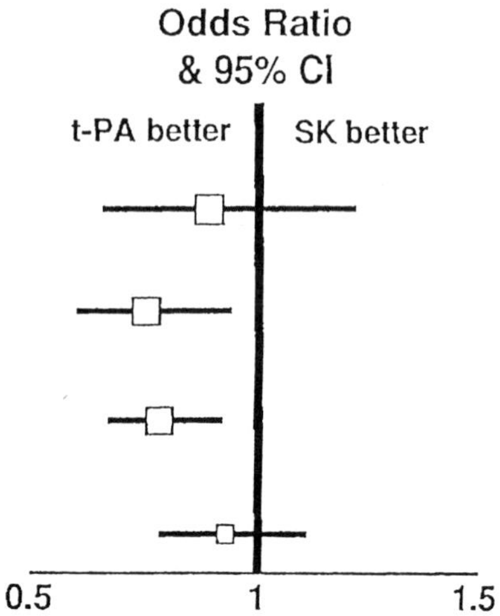

Figure 2   GUSTO Trial: 30-day mortality subdivided by age.

tokinase with intravenous or subcutaneous heparin (Table 5).

Taken together, the results of the GUSTO trial underscore the validity of the hypotheses explored in this monograph. They demonstrate that:

1. Clinical benefit induced by coronary thrombolysis is dependent on the rapidity and frequency of sustained recanalization.
2. Effective fibrinolysis requires prompt and vigorous conjunctive anticoagulation.
3. The increased rapidity and frequency of early recanalization induced by clot-selective fibrinolytic agents is accompanied by clinical benefit compared with results with non-clot-selective drugs.

An even broader lesson can be learned from GUSTO and the controversy that preceded it. It concerns the nature and impact of large-scale clinical trials. As we have noted previously,

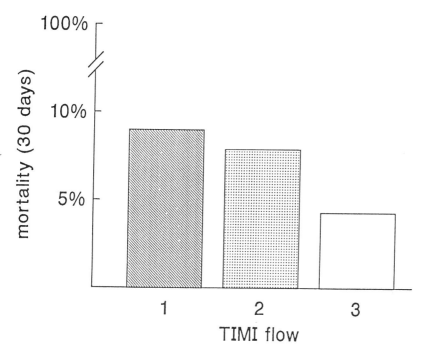

Figure 3   GUSTO Trial: Angiographic study.

large numbers of patients do not ensure the validity of conclusions in a mega-trial if the design is flawed. A hypothetical example would be the failure of a massive study of penicillin in
the treatment of streptococcal pneumonia to demonstrate mortality reduction if such a study were performed several decades
ago when penicillin was in very short supply mandating a
dose of only 1000 units per day. No matter how large the study
population, a favorable impact of penicillin on mortality would
not be evident. An analogous failure would occur if a repeat
study were performed decades later when the supply of penicillin was virtually unlimited and the cost profoundly diminished. If such a study were performed with a dose of 100
million units of penicillin per day, no matter how large the
study population, an overall reduction of mortality might be

Table 4   GUSTO Trial: 30-Day Mortality by Time to
Randomization

	SK (s.c.)	SK (i.v.)	t-PA	t-PA + SK	Total
0–2 hours[a]					
No. of patients	5,210	5,434	5,350	5,449	21,443
No. of deaths	327	366	286	340	1,319
Mortality rate	6.3%	6.7%	5.4%	6.2%	6.2%
2–4 hours[a]					
No. of patients	3,362	3,638	3,728	3,620	14,348
No. of deaths	263	270	247	271	1,051
Mortality rate	7.8%	7.4%	6.6%	7.5%	7.3%
4–6 hours[a]					
No. of patients	1,133	1,209	1,176	1,160	4,678
No. of deaths	107	119	110	104	440
Mortality rate	9.4%	9.8%	9.4%	9.0%	9.4%

[a]Time from onset of symptoms until randomization.

offset by the excess mortality attributable to overdosing and
consequent superinfections, anaphylaxis, seizures, and aspiration, among other deleterious phenomena.

The risk of reaching erroneous conclusions in mega-trials
is greatest when the design fails to take into account principles
that have been delineated in cause–consequence, mechanistic
studies, often involving only small numbers of patients. Such
studies are generally predicated on progress in fundamental
research in biochemistry, molecular and cell biology, physiology, and pharmacology elucidated in studies of laboratory
animals.

In the case of coronary thrombolysis, it had been well established in mechanistic studies that acute myocardial infarction was a dynamic process that can be modified by early
reperfusion, that the outcome after infarction is dependent
largely on the extent of irreversible myocardial injury sustained, that clot-selective fibrinolytic agents open more infarct-
related arteries in the first 60 to 90 minutes than nonselective

Table 5   GUSTO Trial: Angiographic Substudy—Infarct Artery Patency at 90 Minutes

	SK (s.c. heparin)		SK (i.v. heparin)		t-PA (Accelerated)		t-PA + SK (Combination)
No. of patients	295		282		291		297
TIMI 2 flow	26.1%		28.4%		27.2%		35.7%
TIMI 3 flow	29.5%		32.6%		53.6%		37.4%
Patent (TIMI 2 or 3)	55.6%	n.s.	61.0%	0.001	80.8%	0.001	73.1%

Table 6   30–35-Day Mortality in GISSI/International, ISIS-3, and GUSTO

	SK	t-PA	RR (95% CI)
GISSI/International	958 (10,067)	993 (10,028)	0.96 (0.87–1.05)
ISIS-3	1,455 (13,780)	1,418 (13,746)	1.03 (0.95–1.11)
Combined			1.00 (0.94–1.06)
GUSTO	1,471 (20,172)	652 (10,344)	1.17 (1.06–1.28)

Homogeneity test: GISSI/International vs. ISIS-3: $p = 0.26$; GISSI/International vs. ISIS-3 vs. GUSTO: $p = 0.012$.   RR = relative risk.

agents do, and that fibrinolytic agents induce unavoidable procoagulant effects mediated by plasminemia when given intravenously in therapeutically effective doses. It had also been
established that concomitant thrombosis can delay recanalization induced by fibrinolytic agents and increase the incidence
of early, thrombotic reocclusion precipitated also by persistence of thrombogenic atheroma and platelet activation secondary to high shear forces in narrowed vascular segments,
and, finally, that optimal thrombolysis requires prompt and
vigorous anticoagulation (currently accomplished clinically
with heparin administered by bolus and subsequent infusion)
and other conjunctive measures such as administration of antiplatelet agents.

   Carefully controlled but small clinical trials comparing
clot-selective and nonselective fibrinolytic agents given with
conjunctive anticoagulation yielded results consistent with
these principles. A formal meta-analysis of results of such
studies demonstrated a more favorable outcome and lower
mortality with clot-selective than with nonselective drugs.
Other studies demonstrated the dependence of optimal benefit
of fibrinolysis with clot-selective fibrinolytic agents on conjunctive anticoagulation with intravenous heparin. Thus, it
should not be surprising that the two mega-trials (GISSI/
International and ISIS-3) that did not incorporate protocol-
mandated intravenous heparin failed to demonstrate thrombolytic drug-dependent differences in outcome.

   It is not appropriate to combine results of GISSI/Interna-
tional and ISIS-3 with those of the GUSTO trial. The 30- to 35-
day mortalities in the GISSI/International, ISIS-3, and GUSTO
trails are shown in Table 6. The relative risk of dying after
streptokinase versus t-PA was 0.96 (95% CI: 0.87–1.05) and
1.03 (95% CI: 0.95–1.11) in the GISSI/International and ISIS-3
studies, respectively. Homogeneity testing yields a p value of
0.26, permitting meta-analysis of the data, which yields a relative risk of 1.00 (95% CI: 0.94–1.06). In the GUSTO study,
however, the relative risk of dying after streptokinase versus
t-PA was 1.17 (95% CI: 1.06–1.28). Homogeneity testing of the

three studies yields a p value of 0.012, precluding meta-analysis of the data combining results from the three studies. Furthermore, because the confidence intervals on the relative risk of dying in GUSTO do not overlap either unity or the confidence intervals in the combined GISSI/International and ISIS-3 trials, the results are consistent with a disparate and significantly greater effect of accelerated t-PA and intravenous heparin on reduction of mortality in GUSTO compared with that seen with the standard t-PA and delayed subcutaneous heparin regimens used in GISSI/International and ISIS-3.

The GUSTO results are consistent with principles established in mechanistic research. They are compelling not only because of their statistical significance but also because of their internal consistency across numerous subsets and their acquisition under conditions in which differences would not be obscured by omission of intravenous heparin. They underscore the concept that the design of large-scale clinical trials undertaken to reduce fundamental advances in biomedical research to practice must be consistent with principles established in cause–consequence research.

PERTINENT REFERENCES

Bergmann S R, Fox K A A, Ter-Pogossian M M, Sobel B E, Collen D: Clot-selective coronary thrombolysis with tissue-type plasminogen activator. *Science* 1983;220:1187–1183.

Chesebro J H, Knatterud G, Roberts R, Borer J, Cohen L S, Dalen J, Dodge H T, Francis C K, Hillis D, Ludbrook P, Markis J E, Muller H, Passamani E R, Powers E R, Rao A K, Robertson T, Ross A, Ryan T J, Sobel B E, Willerson J, Williams D O, Zaret B L, Braunwald E: Thrombolysis in Myocardial Infarction (TIMI) Trial, Phase I: A comparison between intravenous tissue plasminogen activator and intravenous streptokinase. Clinical findings through hospital discharge. *Circulation* 1987;76:142–154.

Collen D: Thrombolysis: is there a future for thrombolytic therapy in acute myocardial infarction? *Curr Opin Cardiol* 1991;6:552–558.

Eisenberg P R, Sherman L, Rich M, Schwartz D, Schechtman K, Geltman E M, Sobel B E, Jaffe A S: Importance of continued activation of thrombin reflected by fibrinopeptide A to the efficacy of thrombolysis. *J Am Coll Cardiol* 1986;7:1255–1262.

The GUSTO Investigators: A global randomized trial of aggressive vs. standard thrombolytic strategies in 41,021 patients with acute myocardial infarction. *N Engl J Med* 1993;329(10): in press.

The GUSTO Angiographic Investigators: The angiographic sub-study in GUSTO (global utilization of streptokinase and tissue plasminogen activator for occluded coronary arteries). Presented at the Clinical Meetings of the American Federation for Clinical Research, Washington, DC, April 1993.

Sobel B E: Thrombolysis in the treatment of acute myocardial infarction. In: Fuster V, Verstraete M, eds. Thrombosis in Cardiovascular Disorders. Philadelphia: W B Saunders, 1992:289–326.

Sobel B E, Collen D: Questions unresolved by the third International Study of Infarct Survival. *Am J Cardiol* 1992;70:385–389.

Sobel B E, Collen D: ISIS-3 and GISSI-2: Critique of the meta-analysis. *Am J Cardiol* 1993;71:1128–1129.

The TIMI Study Group: Comparison of invasive and conservative strategies after treatment with intravenous tissue plasminogen activator in acute myocardial infarction: Results of the Thrombolysis in Myocardial Infarction (TIMI) Phase II Trial. *N Engl J Med* 1989;320:618–627.

Torr S R, Nachowiak D A, Fujii S, Sobel B E: "Plasminogen steal" and clot lysis. *J Am Coll Cardiol* 1992;19:1085–1090.

Van de Werf F, Bergmann S R, Fox K A A, de Geest H, Hoyng C F, Sobel B E, Collen D: Coronary thrombolysis with intravenously administered human tissue-type plasminogen activator produced by recombinant DNA technology. *Circulation* 1984;69:605–610.

Van de Werf F, Ludbrook P A, Bergmann S R, Tiefenbrunn A J, Fox K A A, de Geest H, Verstraete M, Collen D, Sobel B E: Coronary thrombolysis with tissue-type plasminogen activator in patients with evolving myocardial infarction. *N Engl J Med* 1984;310:609–613.

Index

[Atherosclerotic plaque]
  stabilization, 46–47
  thrombosis inhibition and,
    47–48
  treatment implications, 46–50
  trigger reduction, 47
  volume, as risk factor, 44, 45
  vulnerability, 36–38
ATIII-independent factor Xa inhib-
    itors, 158, 161–162 (see also
    specific inhibitors)
ATIII-independent inhibitors, 159–
    160 (see also specific inhibitors)
  advantages, 159
  animal studies, 160–161
  types, 159
ATIII-independent thrombin in-
    hibitors, 158
ATP (adenosine triphosphate),
    278, 279
Attributable risk, 198
Auckland, New Zealand Group, 57
Australian National Heart Founda-
    tion Study, 246
Autocatalysis, thrombin-induced,
    inhibitor of, 145

Bernard-Soulier syndrome, 110
Beta blockers
  conjunctive, 222, 224
  reduction of myocardial
    demand, 289
  for trigger reduction, 47
Bleeding complications
  of alteplase with heparin,
    235, 237
  cerebral, 16, 28–29, 156
  of GPIIb-IIIa antagonists,
    113–114
  of heparin, 156
  of low-molecular-weight hepa-
    rin, 159
  platelet adhesion inhibition
    and, 112

[Bleeding complications]
  streptokinase and, 15
  of t-PA, 28–29
Blood flow, cyclic variations,
    thrombus formation and,
    41, 43
Boroarginine tripeptide
    (DuP 714), 128
Bradycardia, streptokinase and, 14

Calcium
  homeostasis, oxygen-centered
    free radicals and, 283
  in myocardial stunning,
    280–282
  overload
    myocardial ischemia
      and, 273
    in myocardial stunning, 281
  paradox, 280, 282
  in reperfusion injury, 280–282
Calcium-channel antagonists
  reduction of myocardial
    demand, 289
  for reperfusion injury, 290–291
  for trigger reduction, 47
Catch-up phenomenon, 70
Cerebral bleeding
  alteplase and, 28–29
  heparin and, 156
  streptokinase and, 16, 28–29
Cerebrovascular accidents, anis-
    treplase treatment and, 18
CGP-39393 (recombinant deasulfa-
    tohirudin), 264 (see also
    TIMI-5 trial)
Chlormethylketones, 145 (see also
    PPACK)
Circadian-triggering concept, of
    atherosclerotic plaque rup-
    ture, 36–37
Clamp injury and thrombin injec-
    tion method, for thrombosis
    induction, 132

Low-molecular-weight heparin
    (LMWH)
  anticoagulant effect, 158
  bioavailability, 158–159
  bleeding complications, 159
  clearance, 147
  conjunctive, 263
  predictable anticoagulant re-
      sponse, 157–158
Lytic therapy (see Thrombolytic
    therapy)

Malondialdehyde, 283
Mega-trials (see Clinical trials,
    large-scale)
Meta-analysis, of mortality,
    214–216
Metoprolol, 224
MITI trial
  interpretation, ambiguous,
      70, 72
  mortality, 202, 211, 213
Monoclonal antibodies
  Fab fragments, 163
  against factor VIIa, 139
  against tissue factor, 139
Monoclonal antibody 7E3, 113, 260
Mortality
  absolute vs. relative, 213–214
  aspirin and, 48, 77, 155–156
  of aspirin with heparin, 77
  as clinical trial endpoint, 193
  clot-selective agents and, 6, 210
  of conjunctive heparin, 263
  coronary thrombolysis and,
      202–207
  as end point
    mega-trial results and,
        209–212
    obfuscating factors, 198–200
    statistical power and, 200–201
  fibrinolytic agents and, 213
  flow grades and, 185–186
  in GUSTO trial, 305–306, 308

[Mortality]
  heparin and, 155–156
  high, in mega-trials, 209–212
  hypothetical rate, 214
  in-hospital studies, 207–209
  meta-analysis, 214–216
  non-fibrin-selective agents, 210
  non-fibrin-selective agents
      and, 213
  streptokinase with subcutane-
      ous heparin and, 263
  studies, weaknesses of, 193–194
Myocardial infarction
  aspirin and, 153
  clot-selective fibrinolytic agents
      for, 6
  conceptualization of, 3
  coronary thrombosis and, 53–54
  fibrinolytic agents for, 3
  left ventricular function and,
      168–170
  survival, 167–170
  thrombosis as cause of, 4
Myocardial ischemia
  contracture, 278
  glycolysis in, 276
  lactate production and, 276–277
  magnitude and duration,
      273–276
  salvage and, 3, 7
  ultrastructural character-
      istics, 274
Myocardial reperfusion injury (see
    Reperfusion injury)
Myocardial stunning
  calcium in, 280–282
  causes, 279
  decreasing, 279–280
  mechanism, 273
  protection from, 281
Myocardium
  demand reduction, 289–290
  energy metabolism
    increasing, during ischemia,
        287–289
    optimizing, 294–295

About the Editors

Burton E. Sobel is the Tobias and Hortense Lewin Distinguished Professor in Cardiovascular Disease at the Washington University School of Medicine in St. Louis, Missouri, where he has taught since 1973. He serves as Head, Cardiovascular Division and Center for Cardiovascular Research, at the Washington University School of Medicine and Cardiologist-in-Chief, Barnes Hospital in St. Louis, and he is Adjunct Professor of Chemistry at Washington University. The author or coauthor of over 630 articles and book chapters, he has lectured at universities and conferences throughout the world. He has served as Editor of the journals *Circulation, Coronary Artery Disease,* and *Current Opinion in Cardiology,* and as an Associate Editor and editorial board member of, among many others, the *Journal of Clinical Investigation, Annals of Internal Medicine, Circulation Research,* and *American Journal of Physiology: Heart and Circulatory Physiology.* He is a Fellow of The Royal Society of Medicine in the U.K., the American College of Cardiology (which he served as Governor), and the American College of Physicians, and he is a member of numerous societies, including the American Society for Clinical Investigation, the American Physiological Society, the Society for Experimental Biology and Medicine, and the Association of Professors of Cardiology (President-elect). Dr. Sobel received the A.B. degree (1958) from Cornell University, Ithaca, New York, and the M.D. degree (1962) magna cum laude from Harvard Medical School, Boston, Massachusetts.

Désiré Collen is Professor in the Faculty of Medicine at the University of Leuven in Belgium, where he serves in addition as Associate Head of Clinic at the University Hospitals. He is also Professor of Biochemistry and Medicine at the University of Vermont's College of Medicine and Visiting Professor at Harvard Medical School, Boston, Massachusetts. His research focuses on the molecular biology and pathophysiology of hemostasis and thrombosis as well as the development of new thrombolytic and antithrombotic agents. A member of the Royal Academy of Medicine of Belgium, he has been awarded numerous honors for his work, including the Servier Prize for Research in Fibrinolysis (1978), the A. Faes Prize (1981), the Francqui Prize (1984), and the Louis Jeantet Prize for Medicine (1986). Since 1974 a higher associate in the Faculty of Medicine, Dr. Collen received the M.D. (1968), M.S. (1969; medical sciences), and Ph.D. (1974; chemistry) degrees from the University of Leuven, Belgium.